USMLE Step 1 Review

1st Edition

1200
Questions & Answers

Alfred Olusegun Fayemi, MSc(Path), MD

Associate Clinical Professor of Pathology
Mount Sinai School of Medicine
City University of New York
New York, New York
Director of Pathology and Laboratories
Franciscan Health System of New Jersey
St. Mary Hospital, Hoboken, New Jersey
St. Francis Hospital, Jersey City, New Jersey

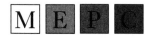

APPLETON & LANGE
Stamford, Connecticut

Notice: The authors and the publisher of this volume have taken care to make certain that the doses of drugs and schedules of treatment are correct and compatible with the standards generally accepted at the time of publication. Nevertheless, as new information becomes available, changes in treatment and in the use of drugs become necessary. The reader is advised to carefully consult the instruction and information material included in the package insert of each drug or therapeutic agent before administration. This advice is especially important when using new and infrequently used drugs. The publisher disclaims any liability, loss, injury, or damage incurred as a consequence, directly or indirectly, of the use and application of any of the contents of this volume.

Prentice Hall International (UK) Limited, *London*
Prentice Hall of Australia Pty. Limited, *Sydney*
Prentice Hall Canada, Inc., *Toronto*
Prentice Hall Hispanoamericana, S.A., *Mexico*
Prentice Hall of India Private Limited, *New Delhi*
Prentice Hall of Japan, Inc., *Tokyo*
Simon and Schuster Asia Pte. Ltd., *Singapore*
Editora Prentice Hall do Brasil Ltda., *Rio de Janeiro*
Prentice Hall, *Englewood Cliffs, New Jersey*

ISSN: 1082-8567   ISBN 0-8385-6269-8

9 780838 562697   90000

Aquisitions Editor: Marinita Timban
Production Editor: Sondra Greenfield
Production Service: Rainbow Graphics, Inc.
Cover Designer: Mary Skudlarek

PRINTED IN THE UNITED STATES OF AMERICA

CONTENTS

CONTRIBUTORS

Alfred Olusegun Fayemi, MSc(Path), MD
Associate Clinical Professor of Pathology
Mount Sinai School of Medicine
City University of New York
New York, New York
Director of Pathology and Laboratories
Franciscan Health System of New Jersey
St. Mary Hospital, Hoboken, New Jersey
St. Francis Hospital, Jersey City, New Jersey

David M. Glick, PhD
Department of Biological Chemistry
The Hebrew University of Jerusalem
Jerusalem, Israel
Adjunct Associate Professor
Department of Biochemistry
The Medical College of Wisconsin
Milwaukee, Wisconsin

Charles W. Kim, MSPH, PhD
Professor
Department of Microbiology and
Department of Medicine
Division of Infectious Diseases
School of Medicine
Health Sciences Center
State University of New York at Stony Brook
Stony Brook, New York

Joseph J. Krzanowski, Jr., PhD
Professor and Vice Chair
Department of Pharmacology and Therapeutics
University of South Florida
College of Medicine
Tampa, Florida

David G. Penney, BS, MS, PhD
Professor of Physiology and Occupational and Environmental Health
Department of Physiology
Wayne State University School of Medicine
Cardiology Research Coordinator
St. John's Hospital
Detroit, Michigan

Steven Steury, MD
Associate Professor
Department of Psychiatry and Mental Health Sciences
Medical College of Wisconsin
Milwaukee, Wisconsin

Jack L. Wilson, PhD
Professor of Anatomy and Neurobiology
College of Medicine
The University of Tennessee at Memphis
The Health Science Center
Memphis, Tennessee

PREFACE

USMLE Step 1 Review offers a comprehensive review of the basic medical sciences in a question-and-answer format. The material herein has been specifically written for medical students preparing for the United States Medical Licensing Examination (USMLE) Step 1.

This book contains 1200 multiple-choice questions with referenced explanatory answers devoted to Anatomy, Biochemistry, Microbiology, Pathology, Pharmacology, Behavioral Sciences, and Physiology. The topics covered reflect the USMLE content outline of The Federation of State Medical Boards of the U.S., Inc. and the National Board of Medical Examiners. The questions have been modeled after those used on the Step 1 examination and are arranged by type within each subject section to provide practice in dealing with the test format. Answers, with explanatory responses and references, are conveniently placed at the end of the section containing the corresponding questions. The reference list for each section appears after the answers.

Using this book, you may identify areas of relative strength and weakness in your command of the constituent disciplines. Specific references to widely used textbooks allow you to return to authoritative sources for further study. The explanatory statements accompanying each answer are intended to put the responses in broadened perspective, and to add to your fund of knowledge. In composite, the material in this book emphasizes problem solving and application of underlying principles in addition to factual recall.

The publisher would like to extend a special thank you to all of the authors whose work appears in this volume.

1

Anatomy
Jack L. Wilson

DIRECTIONS (Questions 1 through 126): Each of the questions or incomplete statements below is followed by five suggested answers or completions. Select the ONE that is best in each case.

---

1. The posterior boundary of the intervertebral foramina is formed by the
   - **A.** intervertebral disk
   - **B.** body of the vertebra
   - **C.** zygopophyseal joint
   - **D.** pedicle
   - **E.** posterior longitudinal ligament

2. Each of the following are correct statements regarding the vertebral column EXCEPT
   - **A.** there are 31 vertebrae
   - **B.** the vertebra are separated by fibrocartilaginous intervertebral disks
   - **C.** the vertebrae are larger and more massively constructed toward the lower end of the column
   - **D.** there are seven cervical vertebrae
   - **E.** the column consists of four curvatures

3. All of the following nerves approach the surface in the posterior triangle of the neck at about the middle of the posterior border of the sternocleidomastoid muscle EXCEPT
   A. the lesser occipital
   B. the great auricular
   C. the transverse cervical
   D. the supraclavicular
   E. the auriculotemporal

4. Each of the following muscles are responsible for rotational movements of the scapular EXCEPT the
   A. latissimus dorsi
   B. rhomboideus major
   C. trapezius
   D. levator scapulae
   E. rhomboideus minor

5. Each of the following open into the pterygopalatine fossa EXCEPT for the
   A. foramen rotundum
   B. pterygoid canal
   C. pharyngeal canal
   D. sphenopalatine foramen
   E. infraorbital foramen

6. Loss of action of the muscle inserting on the crest of the lesser tubercle of the humerus would result from damage of which nerve?
   A. musculocutaneous
   B. radial
   C. axillary
   D. lower subscapular
   E. ulnar

7. General sensation from the posterior one-third of the tongue is mediated by the
   A. lingual nerve
   B. glossopharyngeal nerve
   C. vagus nerve
   D. hypoglossal nerve
   E. chorda tympani nerve

8. The inferior mesenteric artery supplies all of the following organs EXCEPT the
   A. rectum
   B. ascending colon
   C. transverse colon
   D. descending colon
   E. sigmoid colon

9. In the anatomical position, the distal end of the radius articulates primarily with which of the following bones at the wrist joint?
   A. triquetrum
   B. pisiform
   C. hamate
   D. capitate
   E. scaphoid

10. The humerus is flexed at the shoulder joint by all of the following muscles EXCEPT the
    A. pectoralis minor
    B. coracobrachialis
    C. anterior fibers of the deltoid
    D. pectoralis major
    E. biceps brachii

11. Which of the following muscles inserts into the lesser trochanter of the femur?
    A. gluteus medius
    B. gluteus minimus
    C. obturator externus
    D. gemellus
    E. iliopsoas

12. The elbow joint is an example of a
    A. sliding joint
    B. pivot joint
    C. hinge joint
    D. ball-and-socket joint
    E. saddle joint

13. Which of the following movements of the mandible would be affected by injury to the nerve supplying the lateral pterygoid muscle?
    A. depression
    B. lateral rotation
    C. elevation
    D. retrusion
    E. no movements

14. Damage to the ulnar nerve at the medial epicondyle of the elbow would result in
    A. loss of abduction of the thumb
    B. loss of flexion of the distal interphalangeal joint of the fourth finger
    C. loss of extension of metacarpophalangeal joints of the fourth and fifth fingers
    D. loss of general sensation from the skin overlying the thenar eminence
    E. loss of function of the first two lumbricales

15. All of the following structures are located within the carotid sheath EXCEPT the
    A. common carotid artery
    B. cervical sympathetic trunk
    C. vagus nerve
    D. internal carotid artery
    E. internal jugular vein

16. Each of the following statements concerning the femoral triangle is correct EXCEPT the
    A. femoral artery is lateral to the femoral vein
    B. inguinal ligament forms its base
    C. iliopsoas muscle forms part of its floor
    D. adductor longus muscle forms its lateral boundary
    E. great saphenous vein terminates in the triangle

17. Which of the following structures passes through the aortic hiatus of the diaphragm?
    A. vagus nerve
    B. esophagus

C. inferior vena cava
D. sympathetic trunk
E. azygos vein

18. The space between the buccopharyngeal fascia anteriorly and the prevertebral fascia posteriorly is known as the
   A. suprasternal space
   B. lateral pharyngeal space
   C. axillary space
   D. retropharyngeal space
   E. masticator space

19. The common carotid artery divides into its external and internal branches at the level of the upper border of the
   A. hyoid bone
   B. cricoid cartilage
   C. thyroid cartilage
   D. first cervical vertebra
   E. jugular notch

20. The inferior thyroid artery is a branch of which of the following arteries?
   A. external carotid
   B. dorsal scapular
   C. thyrocervical
   D. internal thoracic
   E. common carotid

21. All of the following arteries arise in the carotid triangle EXCEPT the
   A. maxillary
   B. superior thyroid
   C. lingual
   D. facial
   E. ascending pharyngeal

22. The formation of primordial cells (oogonia) in the human ovary ceases
    A. at menopause
    B. at puberty
    C. shortly after birth
    D. at the end of puberty
    E. between 40 and 50 years of age

23. Nerve impulses responsible for contraction of the detrusor muscle during emptying of the bladder are carried in the
    A. sacral splanchnic nerves
    B. lumbar splanchnic nerves
    C. pelvic splanchnic nerves
    D. thoracic splanchnic nerves
    E. white rami communicantes

24. All of the following pass through the inguinal canal EXCEPT for the
    A. spermatic cord
    B. ilioinguinal nerve
    C. testicular vessels
    D. cremaster muscle
    E. hypogastric artery

25. Taste from the epiglottis and palate is mediated by the
    A. facial nerve
    B. trigeminal nerve
    C. glossopharyngeal nerve
    D. vagus nerve
    E. hypoglossal nerve

26. The vagus nerve leaves the skull through which of the following foramina?
    A. foramen rotundum
    B. jugular foramen
    C. foramen ovale
    D. foramen spinosum
    E. foramen lacerum

27. Inability to elevate the tip of the shoulder would indicate damage to which of the following muscles?
- **A.** rhomboideus major
- **B.** latissimus dorsi
- **C.** trapezius
- **D.** teres major
- **E.** supraspinatus

28. The anterior belly of the digastric muscle is innervated by which of the following nerves?
- **A.** facial nerve
- **B.** trigeminal nerve
- **C.** vagus nerve
- **D.** abducens nerve
- **E.** first cervical nerve

29. Which of the following muscles are abductors of the vocal fold?
- **A.** transverse arytenoid
- **B.** posterior cricoarytenoid
- **C.** thyroarytenoid
- **D.** cricothyroid
- **E.** oblique arytenoid

30. The portal vein directly receives each of the following tributaries EXCEPT the
- **A.** superior mesenteric
- **B.** splenic
- **C.** left gastric
- **D.** paraumbilical
- **E.** inferior mesenteric

31. It is possible to recognize primary chorionic villi by the end of the
- **A.** first week
- **B.** second week
- **C.** third week
- **D.** fourth week
- **E.** fifth week

32. Each of the following is part of the limbic system EXCEPT the
    A. amygdaloid nucleus
    B. hypothalamus
    C. claustrum
    D. parahippocampal gyrus
    E. dentate gyrus

33. The meeting and union of the mature human sex cells at fertilization normally occur in the
    A. cervix
    B. upper third of the uterine tube
    C. fundus of the uterus
    D. body of the uterus
    E. vagina

34. In the formation of a sperm, part of the Golgi apparatus gives rise to the
    A. acrosome
    B. cytoplasmic sheath
    C. axial filament
    D. neck
    E. flagellum

35. The hypoblast cell layer develops from the
    A. inner cell mass
    B. trophoblast
    C. cytotrophoblast
    D. syncytiotrophoblast
    E. blastocyst cavity

36. General sensations from the head region are transmitted to the brain stem by each of the following cranial nerves EXCEPT the
    A. trigeminal
    B. oculomotor
    C. facial
    D. glossopharyngeal
    E. vagus

37. The major body cavities develop within the
    A. intermediate mesoderm
    B. primitive streak

C. paraaxial mesoderm
D. lateral mesoderm
E. extraembryonic coelom

38. The costocoracoid membrane in the axilla is pierced by the
    A. axillary vein
    B. medial pectoral nerve
    C. lateral pectoral nerve
    D. axillary artery
    E. brachial vein

39. The deltoid muscle is innervated by the
    A. medial pectoral nerve
    B. long thoracic nerve
    C. axillary nerve
    D. subscapular nerve
    E. suprascapular nerve

40. Each of the following muscles plays a role in plantar flexion of the foot EXCEPT the
    A. gastrocnemius
    B. soleus
    C. plantaris
    D. tibialis posterior
    E. popliteus

41. The inferior mesenteric artery directly supplies each of the following EXCEPT the
    A. upper third of the rectum
    B. proximal transverse colon
    C. descending colon
    D. sigmoid colon
    E. middle third of the rectum

42. The diencephalon is bounded laterally by the
    A. internal capsule
    B. lamina terminalis
    C. optic tract
    D. tela choroidea
    E. third ventricle

43. The striate arterial branches of the middle cerebral artery supply the
    A. tectum of the midbrain
    B. putamen
    C. pulvinar
    D. uncus
    E. preoptic region of the thalamus

44. The middle mediastinum contains which of the following structures?
    A. thymus
    B. heart
    C. esophagus
    D. azygos veins
    E. arch of the aorta

45. The bilaminar embryonic disc consists of which of the following two components?
    A. trophoblast and cytotrophoblast
    B. trophoblast and syncytiotrophoblast
    C. hypoblast and epiblast
    D. amnion and exocoelomic (Heuser's) membrane
    E. extraembryonic mesoderm and cytotrophoblast

46. Intramembranous bone development can be seen in the growth of which one of the following bones?
    A. ulnar
    B. femur
    C. humerus
    D. frontal
    E. tibia

47. The endometrium of the human uterus is lined by which of the following types of epithelium?
    A. simple cuboidal
    B. stratified squamous
    C. transitional
    D. simple columnar
    E. simple squamous

48. The apex of the heart is located in which of the following left intercostal spaces?
   A. third
   B. fourth
   C. fifth
   D. sixth
   E. seventh

49. Compared to companion arteries, veins show all of the following EXCEPT
   A. same general structure
   B. smaller caliber
   C. lower blood pressure within them
   D. less muscle
   E. less elastic tissue

50. All of the following anastomoses play an important role in collateral circulation after ligation of the external iliac artery EXCEPT the
   A. iliolumbar with iliac circumflex
   B. lateral femoral circumflex with superior gluteal
   C. obturator with medial femoral circumflex
   D. superior gluteal with external pudendal
   E. external pudendal with internal pudendal

51. The thoracic duct
   A. begins at the cisterna chyli on the posterior abdominal wall at the second lumbar vertebra
   B. courses through the esophageal hiatus of the diaphragm
   C. ascends the posterior thoracic wall lateral to the aorta
   D. receives lymphatic flow from the right and left halves of the thoracic wall and neck
   E. drains into the right brachiocephalic vein

52. Aggregated lymph nodules are found mainly in the
   A. duodenum
   B. jejunum
   C. ileum
   D. stomach
   E. cecum

53. A histologic characteristic which helps to distinguish the prostate gland is the presence of
   A. interstitial cells
   B. cilia
   C. corpora amylacea
   D. simple squamous epithelium
   E. spermatozoa

54. If the surgical neck of the humerus was crushed in an accident, which of the following nerves would likely be damaged?
   A. radial
   B. axillary
   C. lateral cord of brachial plexus
   D. ulnar
   E. median

55. A hypofunction of which of the following endocrine glands can lead to cretinism in the adult?
   A. posterior pituitary
   B. thyroid
   C. adrenal cortex
   D. anterior pituitary
   E. parathyroid

56. The muscles of facial expression are characterized by each of the following EXCEPT
   A. they generally originate from bone and insert into the skin
   B. they are functionally important in closing the eyes and mouth and in chewing
   C. they develop from the second branchial arch
   D. the cell bodies of the nerve fibers innervating these muscles are located in the geniculate ganglion of the seventh cranial nerve
   E. they are not all physically located on the face

57. Phagocytic cells lining the sinusoids of the liver are called
   A. Kupffer cells
   B. chief cells
   C. guard cells
   D. mast cells
   E. crest cells

58. Which of the following veins drains directly into the inferior vena cava?
- **A.** splenic
- **B.** hepatic
- **C.** inferior mesenteric
- **D.** renal
- **E.** superior rectal

59. The basophilia seen in the cytoplasm of conventionally stained cells has been shown under the electron microscope to be due to the
- **A.** mitochondria
- **B.** Golgi apparatus
- **C.** nucleus
- **D.** lysosomes
- **E.** ribosomes

60. The muscularis mucosae of which segment of the digestive tract contains smooth and striated muscles?
- **A.** pharnyx
- **B.** stomach
- **C.** esophagus
- **D.** small intestine
- **E.** large intestine

61. The prochordal plate
- **A.** is formed at the caudal end of the hypoblast
- **B.** contributes to the formation of the notochord
- **C.** gives rises to the extraembryonic mesoderm
- **D.** develops into the chorionic villi
- **E.** indicates the future location of the mouth and forms the oropharyngeal membrane

62. The mesencephalon receives its blood supply primarily from the
- **A.** internal carotid artery
- **B.** middle cerebral artery
- **C.** pontine arteries
- **D.** posterior cerebral artery
- **E.** basilar artery

63. The superior boundary of the triangle of auscultation is formed by the
   A. rhomboid major muscle
   B. trapezius muscle
   C. latissimus dorsi muscle
   D. rhomboid minor muscle
   E. teres minor muscle

64. Pseudostratified columnar ciliated epithelium is characteristic of the
   A. esophagus
   B. large excretory ducts of the salivary glands
   C. male urethra
   D. ureter
   E. primary bronchus

65. The notochordal process develops from the
   A. primitive node
   B. caudal end of the primitive streak
   C. prochordal plate
   D. intraembryonic mesoderm
   E. embryonic endoderm

66. Damage to which of the following structures in the pelvis would affect muscular functions of the thigh?
   A. internal pudendal artery
   B. inferior hypogastric nerve plexus
   C. obturator nerve
   D. pelvic splanchnic nerves
   E. uterine artery

67. The parasympathetic nervous system has central connections with the brain through all of the following cranial nerves EXCEPT
   A. III
   B. VII
   C. X
   D. V
   E. IX

68. The ductus venosus connects the left portal vein to the
  A. superior vena cava
  B. inferior vena cava
  C. placenta
  D. femoral vein
  E. umbilical vein

69. Which of the following regions is NOT drained directly by the afferent vessels of the submandibular lymph nodes?
  A. chin
  B. anterior aspect of tongue
  C. soft palate
  D. corners of the lips
  E. gums

70. The cell organelle which contains a number of hydrolytic enzymes is the
  A. lysosome
  B. Golgi apparatus
  C. mitochondrion
  D. centriole
  E. ribosome

71. Following ovulation, the collapsed and shriveled vesicular follicle forms the
  A. corona radiata
  B. stigma
  C. oogonium
  D. corpus luteum
  E. corpus albicans

72. The largest concentration of centers controlling visceral functions is located in the
  A. septal area
  B. amygdaloid formation
  C. hippocampal formation
  D. hypothalamus
  E. motor cortex

73. Cerebrospinal fluid reaches the subarachnoid cavity directly by way of the
  - **A.** arachnoid granulations
  - **B.** choroid plexus
  - **C.** fourth ventricle
  - **D.** cerebral aqueduct
  - **E.** third ventricle

74. Loss of eversion and dorsiflexion of the foot would result from damage to which of the following nerves?
  - **A.** tibial
  - **B.** common (fibular) peroneal
  - **C.** femoral
  - **D.** superficial (fibular) peroneal
  - **E.** obturator

75. All of the following structures are enclosed within the cervical visceral fasciae EXCEPT the
  - **A.** trachea
  - **B.** thyroid gland
  - **C.** spinal cord
  - **D.** pharynx
  - **E.** larynx

76. The buccopharyngeal fascia provides an external investment for all of the following muscles EXCEPT the
  - **A.** platysma
  - **B.** buccinator
  - **C.** superior pharyngeal constrictor
  - **D.** middle pharyngeal constrictor
  - **E.** inferior pharyngeal constrictor

77. At birth, the spinal cord extends only to vertebral level
  - **A.** T-3
  - **B.** T-4
  - **C.** T-6
  - **D.** L-3
  - **E.** L-6

78. During maturation of the egg, three rudimentary ova are produced, known as
  A. gametocytes
  B. zygotes
  C. oogonia
  D. polocytes
  E. ootids

79. The arterial bypass in the fetus that allows blood to go directly from the right to the left atrium is the
  A. ductus venosus
  B. foramen ovale
  C. ductus arteriosum
  D. umbilical vein
  E. fossa ovalis

80. Cerebrospinal fluid is returned directly to the venous system by means of the
  A. cerebral veins
  B. arachnoid granulations
  C. choroid plexus
  D. cerebral aqueduct
  E. apertures in the third ventricle

81. The uterus and vagina are formed by the fusion of the
  A. mesonephric tubules
  B. mesonephric ducts
  C. urogenital sinuses
  D. paramesonephric ducts
  E. metanephros

82. One of the principal components of the Nissl substance of nerve tissue is
  A. lipid
  B. glycoprotein
  C. glycogen
  D. ribonucleoprotein
  E. enzymes

83. Meningitis can result from an infected thrombus in the nose because progression can pass to the
    A. superior sagittal sinus
    B. cavernous sinus
    C. great cerebral vein (Galen)
    D. inferior sagittal sinus
    E. transverse sinus

84. The great saphenous vein is characterized by all of the following EXCEPT that it
    A. is the longest vein in the body
    B. ends in the femoral vein
    C. runs along the medial side of the thigh
    D. begins posterior to the lateral malleolus
    E. ascends anterior to the medial malleolus

85. Tributaries of the portal vein include all of the following EXCEPT the
    A. superior mesenteric
    B. paraumbilical
    C. uterine
    D. pyloric
    E. lienal (splenic)

86. The mitochondria play an important role in
    A. cell division
    B. phagocytosis
    C. forming hydrolytic enzymes
    D. energy requirements of the cell
    E. protein synthesis

87. The coronary sinus opens into the
    A. right atrium
    B. left atrium
    C. left ventricle
    D. conus arteriosus
    E. inferior vena cava

88. Each of the following structures is found in an osteon of adult bone EXCEPT the
    A. circumferential lamella
    B. Haversian canal
    C. concentric lamella
    D. lacuna
    E. canaliculi

89. The innermost layer of the neopallial cortex or isocortex is the
    A. internal pyramidal layer
    B. internal granular layer
    C. external pyramidal layer
    D. external granular layer
    E. multiform or plexiform layer

90. A lesion of the otic ganglion would be expressed clinically by a loss of
    A. function of the sublingual gland
    B. taste on the posterior one-third of the tongue
    C. sensory innervation to the parotid gland
    D. secretion of the parotid gland
    E. function of the stylopharyngeus muscle

91. All of the following nerves are cutaneous branches of the maxillary division of the trigeminal EXCEPT the
    A. auriculotemporal nerve
    B. zygomaticofacial nerve
    C. inferior palpebral nerve
    D. superior labial nerve
    E. external nasal nerve

92. The ligamentum teres represents an obliterated
    A. ductus venosus
    B. ductus arteriosus
    C. internal iliac artery
    D. umbilical vein
    E. porta hepatis

93. All of the following pass through the carpal tunnel at the wrist formed by the flexor retinaculum and the carpal bones EXCEPT the
    A. flexor pollicis longus
    B. flexor digitorum superficialis
    C. median nerve
    D. ulnar nerve
    E. flexor digitorum profundus

94. The principal cutaneous nerves of the face are derived from which of the following nerves?
    A. facial
    B. cervical
    C. hypoglossal
    D. trigeminal
    E. glossopharyngeal

95. The opening into the inferior meatus of the nose is from the
    A. maxillary sinus
    B. frontal sinus
    C. ethmoid sinus
    D. sphenoid sinus
    E. nasolacrimal duct

96. The emissary vein, which is found in the foramen ovale, is a means of communication between the pterygoid plexus and the
    A. sigmoid sinus
    B. sphenoparietal sinus
    C. cavernous sinus
    D. superior petrosal sinus
    E. inferior petrosal sinus

97. Types of neuroglia include each of the following EXCEPT
    A. astrocytes
    B. microglia
    C. plasmocytes
    D. ependymal cells
    E. oligodendrocytes

98. All of the following are characteristic of the tetralogy of Fallot EXCEPT
   A. overriding of the aorta
   B. ventricular septal defect
   C. pulmonary stenosis
   D. hypertrophy of the right ventricular wall
   E. hypoplasia of the aorta

99. The ventral lateral nucleus of the thalamus is an important synaptic site for fibers from the
   A. cerebellum and basal ganglia
   B. medial lemniscus
   C. superior colliculus
   D. amygdala and hypothalamus
   E. thalamus

100. The laminae of adjacent vertebrae are united by the
   A. supraspinous ligament
   B. annulus fibrosus
   C. fibroelastic cartilage
   D. dentate ligament
   E. ligamentum flavum

101. The primordium of the ureter, calices, and collecting tubules of the kidney is the
   A. mesonephric duct
   B. metanephric mesoderm
   C. mesonephric tubules
   D. pronephros
   E. metanephric diverticulum

102. The sarcomere of skeletal muscle is defined as the segment between two successive
   A. I bands
   B. H bands
   C. Z lines
   D. M bands
   E. A bands

103. Each of the following is a direct branch of the axillary artery EX-CEPT the
  A. thoracodorsal artery
  B. subscapular artery
  C. highest thoracic artery
  D. posterior humeral circumflex artery
  E. thoracoacromial artery

104. The chief characteristic common to all lymphatic organs is the presence of
  A. trabeculae
  B. sinusoids
  C. cortical nodules
  D. medullary cords
  E. lymphocytes

105. The medial wall of the axilla is formed by the
  A. pectoralis major muscle
  B. subscapularis muscle
  C. serratus anterior muscle
  D. humerus
  E. teres major muscle

106. A complete cut through the facial nerve just distal to the greater petrosal nerve would result in each of the following EXCEPT
  A. dry mouth
  B. decreased taste function at the tip of the tongue
  C. dry eye
  D. weakness in muscles of the cheek
  E. closing of the eye

107. Cleavage splits the fertilized egg into smaller cells called
  A. gastromeres
  B. blastomeres
  C. gametes
  D. zygotes
  E. oocytes

108. Each of the following nerves is located in the wall or lumen of the cavernous sinus EXCEPT the
   A. optic
   B. trochlear
   C. oculomotor
   D. mandibular
   E. abducens

109. Anterior division fibers that are located in the inferior trunk of the brachial plexus contribute to which of the following nerves?
   A. radial and axillary
   B. ulnar and median
   C. median and radial
   D. musculocutaneous and ulnar
   E. axillary and median

110. Which of the following nerves provide parasympathetic fibers through the otic ganglion to the parotid gland?
   A. facial
   B. glossopharyngeal
   C. vagus
   D. trigeminal
   E. oculomotor

111. The proximal segment of the right and left sixth aortic arch gives rise to the
   A. pulmonary artery
   B. internal carotid arteries
   C. common carotid arteries
   D. aortic arch
   E. ascending aorta

112. The middle meningeal artery enters the cranium through the
   A. foramen spinosum
   B. foramen rotundum
   C. foramen magnum
   D. foramen ovale
   E. foramen lacerum

113. Which of the following organs is supplied by the celiac artery?
   A. spleen
   B. ascending colon
   C. jejunum
   D. rectum
   E. appendix

114. Elastic cartilage is found in the
   A. intervertebral discs
   B. trachea
   C. auditory tube
   D. sternal ends of the ribs
   E. articular cartilage

115. Nonkeratinized stratified squamous epithelium is found in each of the following EXCEPT the
   A. epidermis
   B. mouth
   C. upper pharynx
   D. esophagus
   E. vagina

116. Synapses may be classified on the basis of each of the following EXCEPT
   A. position
   B. membrane specialization
   C. organelle content
   D. synaptic vesicle content
   E. shape of end bulb

117 Corticobulbar axons terminate on all of the following motor nuclei EXCEPT
   A. nucleus ambiguus
   B. Edinger–Westphal nucleus
   C. hypoglossal motor nucleus (XII)
   D. motor nucleus of V (masticator nucleus)
   E. facial motor nucleus (VII)

118 Which of the following muscles is derived from the third branchial arch?
A. styloglossus
B. palatopharyngeus
C. stylopharyngeus
D. superior pharnygeal constrictor
E. levator veli palatini

119. When the mandible is elevated from a wide-open position, the articular disk moves
A. medially
B. posteriorly
C. anteriorly
D. laterally
E. inferiorly

120. All of the muscles of the pharynx are innervated by the vagal fibers of the pharyngeal plexus EXCEPT the
A. middle constrictor
B. superior constrictor
C. stylopharyngeus
D. palatopharyngeus
E. salpingopharyngeus

121. All of the following structures are found within the parotid gland EXCEPT the
A. maxillary artery
B. facial nerve
C. internal carotid artery
D. retromandibular vein
E. auticulotemporal nerve

122 The calcarine branch of the posterior cerebral artery is important because it supplies the
A. primary visual cortex
B. motor areas
C. premotor areas
D. auditory projection areas
E. somesthetic areas

123. Which one of the following nerves provides innervation for the infrahyoid muscle?
   A. ansa cervicalis
   B. vagus
   C. ansa subclavia
   D. facial
   E. glossopharyngeal

124. Each of the following functions could be affected by a cavernous sinus infection EXCEPT
   A. somatic sensation from the cornea
   B. abduction of the eye
   C. closure of the eyelids
   D. action of the muscle that functions through a pulley
   E. reduced ability to constrict the pupil

125. The anterior and middle scalene muscles that border the scalene triangle in the neck are useful surgical landmarks for each of the following EXCEPT
   A. trunks of brachial plexus
   B. subclavian artery
   C. phrenic nerve
   D. suprascapular artery
   E. second cervical spinal nerve

126. The submandibular duct is crossed twice by which of the following nerves?
   A. hypoglossal
   B. facial
   C. lingual
   D. vagus
   E. glossopharyngeal

DIRECTIONS (Questions 127 through 158): Each group of questions below consists of lettered headings followed by a list of numbered words, phrases, or statements. For each numbered word, phrase, or statement, select the ONE lettered heading that is most closely associated with it. Each lettered heading may be selected once, more than once, or not at all.

Questions 127 through 133

- **A.** liver
- **B.** tongue
- **C.** ureter
- **D.** thymus
- **E.** stomach
- **F.** trachea
- **G.** colon
- **H.** submandibular gland

127. Serous demilune

128. Hyaline cartilage

129. Tenia coli

130. Kupffer cells

131. Glands of von Ebner

132. Parietal cells

133. Transitional epithelium

Questions 134 through 138

    A. anterior spinocerebellar tract
    B. pyramidal tract
    C. reticulospinal tract
    D. rubrospinal tract
    E. vestibulospinal tract
    F. cuneocerebellar tract

134. Derived from the cells of the accessory cuneate nucleus; fibers terminate in the ipsilateral cerebellar cortex

135. The largest and most important descending fiber system in the human neuraxis

136. Fibers descend in the anterior and anterolateral portions of the spinal cord; may function in voluntary movement, muscle tone, and respiration

137. Situated along the lateral periphery of the spinal cord; anterior to the posterior spinocerebellar tract

138. Relays impulses from specific portions of the cerebellum; associated with the eighth cranial nerve

Questions 139 through 143

    A. lenticular nucleus
    B. fornix
    C. claustrum
    D. red nucleus
    E. caudate nucleus
    F. ventral posterior nucleus

139. A thin plate of gray matter lying in the medullary substance of the hemisphere between the lenticular nucleus and the cortex of the insula

140. An elongated, arched, gray mass related throughout its extent to the ventricular surface of the lateral ventricle

141. Divided into the putamen and globus pallidus

142. A band of white fibers constituting the main efferent fiber system of the hippocampal formation

143. The largest primary somatic relay nucleus of the thalamus

Questions 144 through 148

    A. obturator nerve
    B. femoral nerve
    C. pudendal nerve
    D. sciatic nerve
    E. saphenous nerve
    F. superior gluteal nerve

144. Leaves the pelvis through the greater sciatic foramen to enter the gluteal region

145. Accompanies the femoral artery through the femoral triangle and adductor canal

146. Forms the greatest part of the sacral plexus

147. Supplies three abductors and medial rotators of the hip

148. Enters the thigh behind the inguinal ligament; cannot enter the femoral sheath because it is extrafascial

Questions 149 through 153

    A. related to the radial bursa
    B. abduction of the hand at the wrist
    C. supination of forearm
    D. abduction of digits 2 through 4
    E. flexion of distal phalanx of digits 2 through 5

149. Flexor carpi radialis muscle

150. Biceps brachii muscle

151. Dorsal interossei muscle

152. Flexor pollicis longus muscle

153. Flexor digitorum profundus

Questions 154 through 158

    A. receives a blood supply from the superior mesenteric artery
    B. receives a blood supply from the inferior mesenteric artery
    C. receives a blood supply from the celiac artery

154. Duodenum

155. Ascending colon

156. Spleen

157. Rectum

158. Traverse colon

DIRECTIONS (Questions 159 through 175): Each of the questions or incomplete statements below is followed by five suggested answers or completions. Select the ONE that is best in each case.

---

159. On examination of a motorcyclist who suffered a head injury, you suspect oculomotor nerve involvement because of paralysis of each of the following eye muscles EXCEPT the
    A. superior rectus
    B. medial rectus
    C. levator palpebrae superioris
    D. inferior oblique
    E. superior oblique

160. In describing the trochlear nerve, it can be said to
    A. supply the superior oblique muscle
    B. innervate a muscle that abducts the eye
    C. run through the lumen of the cavernous sinus

D. be sensory from the sclera

E. course in the floor of the orbit

161. The maxillary division of the trigeminal nerve supplies sensory fibers from each of the following EXCEPT the
   A. lower eyelid
   B. upper lip
   C. temporomandibular joint
   D. upper incisors
   E. skin of the cheek

162. The facial nerve supplies motor fibers to which of the following muscles?
   A. stapedius
   B. mylohyoid
   C. anterior belly of the digastric
   D. geniohyoid
   E. lateral pterygoid

163. Branches of the external carotid artery include each of the following EXCEPT the
   A. ascending pharyngeal
   B. thyrocervical trunk
   C. lingual
   D. maxillary
   E. superior thyroid

164. Derived from the posterior cord of the brachial plexus is the
   A. upper subscapular nerve
   B. pectoral nerve
   C. ulnar nerve
   D. median nerve
   E. musculocutaneous nerve

165. The tibial nerve supplies muscles of the posterior leg and thigh that includes each of the following muscles EXCEPT the
   A. soleus
   B. gastrocnemius
   C. popliteus
   D. abductor hallucis
   E. semitendinosus

166. The outflow of the parasympathetic division of the autonomic nervous system includes fibers in each of the following EXCEPT the
    A. oculomotor
    B. trigeminal
    C. glossopharyngeal
    D. vagus
    E. pelvic splanchnics

167. The retina of the adult eye is derived from the
    A. lens placode
    B. surface ectoderm
    C. optic cup
    D. mesoderm
    E. lens vesicle

168. Contents of the middle ear include the
    A. lateral semicircular canal
    B. utricle
    C. scala vestibuli
    D. promontory
    E. cochlea

169. Each of the following openings communicate with the pterygopalatine fossa EXCEPT the
    A. foramen rotundum
    B. pterygoid canal
    C. interior orbital fissure
    D. sphenopalative foramen
    E. ovale

170. Each of the following muscles would be involved in elevation of the mandible EXCEPT the
    A. temporalis, anterior fibers
    B. masseter, superficial fibers
    C. medial pterygoid
    D. lateral pterygoid
    E. masseter, deep fibers

171. Ectoderm will give rise to all of the following EXCEPT
  A. smooth muscle
  B. lens
  C. brain
  D. pituitary gland
  E. peripheral nerves

172. Derivatives of endoderm include
  A. kidney
  B. cartilage
  C. heart
  D. suprarenal cortex
  E. pancreas

173. Chondrocytes are nourished by
  A. dissolved nutrients passing through cartilage matrix
  B. a system of canaliculi between lacunae
  C. the vascular network within the territorial matrix
  D. glycogen and lipid stores
  E. calcified matrix channels

174. Which of the following muscles is derived from the second branchial arch?
  A. posterior belly of the digastric
  B. geniohyoid
  C. temporalis
  D. styloglossus
  E. stylopharyngeus

175. The urinary bladder is lined with
  A. stratified squamous epithelium
  B. transitional epithelium
  C. pseudostratified squamous epithelium
  D. simple squamous epithelium
  E. cuboidal epithelium

DIRECTIONS (Questions 176 through 275): Each group of questions below consists of lettered headings followed by a diagram with numbered components. For each numbered component, select the ONE lettered heading that is most closely associated with it. Each lettered heading may be selected once, more than once, or not at all.

Questions 176 through 188

Figure 1.1 depicts a schematic horizontal section of the inguinal canal. Identify the structures indicated by the guidelines.

A. transversus abdominis muscle
B. obliterated umbilical artery
C. internal oblique muscle
D. extraperitoneal fat
E. transversalis fascia
F. dartos muscle
G. external oblique muscle
H. superficial fascia
I. skin
J. inferior epigastric artery
K. urachus
L. external spermatic fascia
M. cremaster muscle

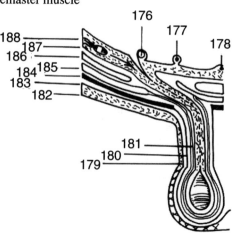

Figure 1.1. (Reproduced, with permission, from Dershwitz M, *National Boards Examination Review for Part 1*, 3rd ed. East Norwalk, Ct: Appleton & Lange; 1987.)

Questions 189 through 205

In Figure 1.2, identify the contents and landmarks associated with the diaphragm and pericardial sac.

A. sternal reflection of right pleura
B. internal thoracic vessels
C. right phrenic nerve
D. external oblique muscle
E. left phrenic nerve
F. fat pat
G. costomediastinal recess
H. sternal reflection of left pleura
I. transversus thoracis muscle
J. latissimus dorsi muscle
K. serratus posterior inferior
L. costal pleura
M. costodiaphragmatic recess
N. diaphragmatic pleura
O. costotransverse ligament
P. azygos vein, thoracic duct
Q. anterior mediastinum

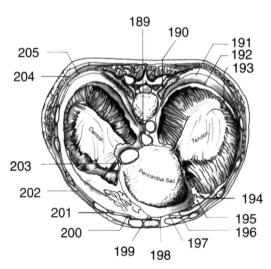

Figure 1.2. (Reproduced, with permission, from Dershwitz M, *National Boards Examination Review for Part 1*, 3rd ed. East Norwalk, Ct: Appleton & Lange; 1987.)

Questions 206 through 213

In Figure 1.3, identify the interior of the right atrium as indicated by the guidelines.

- **A.** tricuspid orifice
- **B.** crista terminalis
- **C.** valve of coronary sinus
- **D.** valve of inferior vena cava
- **E.** fossa ovalis
- **F.** pectinate muscle
- **G.** superior vena cava
- **H.** limbus fossa ovalis

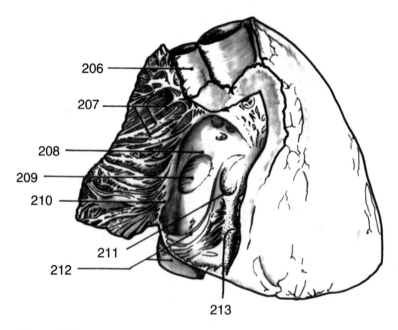

Figure 1.3. (Reproduced, with permission, from Dershwitz M, *National Boards Examination Review for Part 1*, 3rd ed. East Norwalk, Ct: Appleton & Lange; 1987.)

Questions 214 through 227

Figure 1.4 depicts the extrahepatic bile passages and the pancreatic ducts. Identify the structures indicated by the guidelines.

- **A.** body of gallbladder
- **B.** neck of gallbladder
- **C.** mucous membrane of gallbladder
- **D.** cystic duct
- **E.** common hepatic duct
- **F.** ducts from left lobe
- **G.** ducts from the caudate lobe
- **H.** accessory pancreatic duct
- **I.** common bile duct
- **J.** second portion of duodenum
- **K.** right and left hepatic ducts
- **L.** ducts from the quadrate lobe
- **M.** ducts from the bed of gallbladder
- **N.** main pancreatic duct

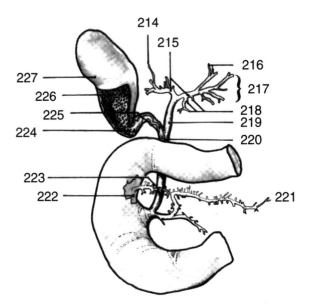

Figure 1.4. (Reproduced, with permission, from Dershwitz M, *National Boards Examination Review for Part 1*, 3rd ed. East Norwalk, Ct: Appleton & Lange; 1987.)

Questions 228 through 239

Figure 1.5 depicts the diaphragm viewed from below. Identify the structures indicated by the guidelines.

    A. vena caval foramen
    B. arch for psoas major muscle
    C. anterolateral hiatus
    D. right crus
    E. anteromedial hiatus
    F. lateral lumbocostal arch
    G. esophageal hiatus
    H. costal margin of diaphragm
    I. medial lumbocostal arch
    J. left crus
    K. aortic hiatus
    L. lumbocostal triangle

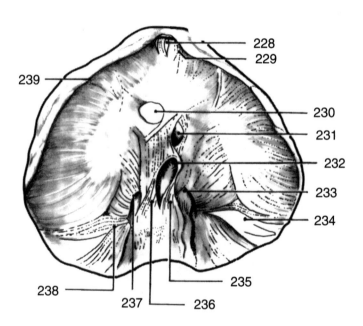

Figure 1.5. (Reproduced, with permission, from Dershwitz M, *National Boards Examination Review for Part 1,* 3rd ed. East Norwalk, Ct: Appleton & Lange; 1987.)

Questions 240 through 259

Figure 1.6 depicts the femoral triangle. Identify the structures indicated by the guidelines.

A. lateral cutaneous nerve
B. perforating artery
C. obturator nerve
D. pectineus and pectineal fascia
E. superficial circumflex iliac artery
F. deep circumflex iliac artery
G. iliac muscle and fascia
H. deep femoral artery
I. adductor longus
J. femoral nerve, artery, vein

K. sartorius muscle
L. iliotibial tract
M. gracilis muscle
N. great saphenous vein
O. femoral ring
P. lacunar ligament
Q. pubic tubercle
R. inguinal ligament
S. rectus femoris muscle
T. intermediate and medial cutaneous nerves

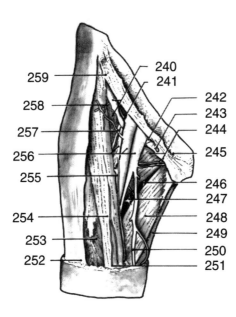

Figure 1.6. (Reproduced, with permission, from Dershwitz M, *National Boards Examination Review for Part 1,* 3rd ed. East Norwalk, Ct: Appleton & Lange; 1987.)

Questions 260 through 275

Figure 1.7 depicts a lateral view of the skull. Identify the structures indicated by the guidelines.

A. glabella
B. mastoid process
C. nasion
D. base of mandible
E. nasal bone
F. bregma
G. tympanic portion of temporal bone
H. pterion
I. external occipital protuberance
J. styloid process
K. ramus of mandible
L. mental protuberance
M. anterior nasal spine
N. anterior nasal aperture
O. lacrimal bone
P. external auditory meatus

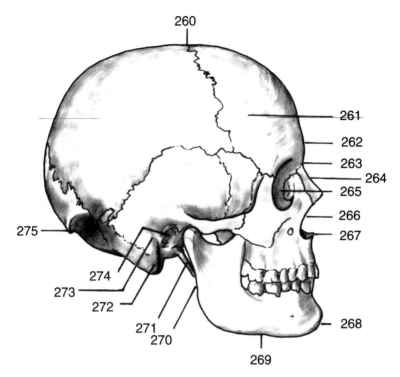

Figure 1.7. (Reproduced, with permission, from Dershwitz M, *National Boards Examination Review for Part 1,* 3rd ed. East Norwalk, Ct: Appleton & Lange; 1987.)

Anatomy

Answers and Comments

1. **(C)** The capsule of the zygopophyseal joint attaches to the articular processes of the adjacent vertebrae and forms the posterior boundary of the foramen. The joint is immediately posterior to the exit of the spinal nerve, which is often involved in disease processes involving the joint. The other structures are anterior, superior, and inferior to the intervertebral foramen. (**Ref. 1,** p. 347)

2. **(A)** The vertebral column consists of 33 vertebrae superimposed on one another in a series that provides a flexible supporting column for the trunk and head. The intervertebral disks and ligaments provide critical strength to the column. (**Ref. 1,** pp. 339–347)

3. **(E)** The cutaneous branches of the cervical plexus (lesser occipital, great auricular, transverse cervical, and supraclavicular nerves) approach the surface in the posterior triangle of the neck about the middle of the posterior border of the sternocleidomastoid muscle. The auriculotemporal nerve is sensory from the scalp and temporal region. (**Ref. 1,** p. 220)

4. **(A)** Scapular rotation is essential for the wide range of motion available at the shoulder joint. All of the muscles listed provide either superior or inferior rotation of the scapula except for the

latissimus dorsi. This muscle does not have any functional attachments to the girdle and attaches directly to the humerus, thus bypassing the scapular. (**Ref. 1**, p. 91)

5. **(E)** The infraorbital foramen transmits the infraorbital nerve and vessels onto the face. It has no connection with the pterygopalatine fossa. The other openings transmit branches of the maxillary nerve from the fossa. (**Ref. 1**, pp. 243, 265)

6. **(D)** The teres major muscle inserts on the crest of the lesser tubercle and functions as an extensor, medial rotator, and adductor at the shoulder joint. It is innervated by the lower subscapular nerve, which is a branch of the posterior card of the brachial plexus. (**Ref. 1**, p. 96)

7. **(B)** The glossopharyngeal nerve mediates general sensation and taste from the posterior one-third of the tongue. It reaches the tongue by coursing between the superior and middle pharyngeal muscles. (**Ref. 1**, p. 239)

8. **(B)** The ascending colon is supplied by the superior mesenteric artery via the ileocolic and right colic branches. The inferior mesenteric arteries supply the hindgut derivatives. (**Ref. 1**, p. 479)

9. **(E)** Within the capsule of the wrist (radiocarpal) joint, the radius articulates with the scaphoid bone, the most lateral bone in the proximal row of carpal bones. The lunate and triquetrum bones articulate more medially with the articular disk. (**Ref. 1**, p. 179)

10. **(A)** The pectoralis minor inserts on the coracoid process and draws the scapula anteriorly and inferiorly. It also aids in inspiration by lifting the ribs. The muscle contributes to the anterior wall of the axilla. (**Ref. 1**, p. 113)

11. **(E)** The gluteus medius and minimus insert into the greater trochanter, the obturator externus into the trochanteric fossa, the gemellus above and anterior to the trochanteric fossa, and the iliopsoas into the lesser trochanter (**Ref. 1**, pp. 589–590)

12. **(C)** The elbow joint is classified as a hinge or ginglymus joint wherein the distal end of the humerus articulates with the proximal end of the bones of the forearm. (**Ref. 1**, p. 174)

13. **(A)** The lateral pterygoid muscle is extremely important in movements involving protrusion, depression, and lateral excursion of the mandible. The muscle pulls the mandibular condyle anteriorly out of the mandibular fossa. (**Ref. 1**, p. 261)

14. **(B)** The ulnar nerve innervates the flexor carpi ulnaris muscle and the medial two parts of the flexor digitorum profundus muscle. The profundus muscle is responsible for flexing the distal phalanx of the fourth and fifth digits. (**Ref. 1**, p. 141)

15. **(B)** The carotid sheath is a tubular investment of the internal and common carotid arteries, the internal jugular vein, and the vagus nerve. The cervical sympathetic trunk lies behind the sheath but is not included within it. (**Ref. 1**, p. 239)

16. **(D)** The femoral triangle occupies the superior aspect of the anterior thigh. It conducts the femoral vessels and nerve. The adductor longus muscle forms the medial boundary of the femoral triangle. (**Ref. 1**, p. 585)

17. **(E)** The azygos vein passes through the aortic hiatus of the diaphragm and ascends the posterior mediastinum of the thoracic cavity. The other structures listed pass through other openings. (**Ref. 1**, p. 411)

18. **(D)** The retropharyngeal space is located between the buccopharyngeal fascia anteriorly and the prevertebral fascia posteriorly. The space descends inferiorly to reach the mediastinum of the thorax. (**Ref. 1**, p. 195)

19. **(C)** The common carotid artery divides into its external and internal branches at the level of the upper border of the thyroid cartilage. The external carotid exits the carotid sheath. (**Ref. 1**, p. 202)

20. (C) The inferior thyroid artery is the largest branch of the thyrocervical trunk of the subclavian artery. The artery courses medially and deep to the carotid sheath to reach the inferior pole of the thyroid gland. (**Ref. 1,** p. 222)

21. (A) The superior thyroid, lingual, facial, and ascending pharyngeal arteries arise from the external carotid in the carotid triangle. The maxillary artery is one of the two terminal branches of the external carotid artery. (**Ref. 1,** p. 203)

22. (C) The formation of human oogonia ceases shortly after birth and the resulting cells are called primary oocytes. These cells develop into a primary follicle that is surrounded by the zona pellucida. (**Ref. 3,** p. 18)

23. (C) The contraction of the detrusor muscle of the bladder is a function of parasympathetic nerves carried in the pelvic splanchnic nerves. These splanchnic nerves branch from the second, third, and fourth sacral ventral rami in the floor of the pelvis. (**Ref. 1,** p. 540)

24. (E) The hypogastric or internal iliac artery commences at the bifurcation of the common iliac adjacent to the lumbosacral articulation and supplies pelvic viscera and parietal branches. It is not found in the inguinal canal. (**Ref. 1,** p. 553)

25. (D) The vagus nerve mediates taste from the epiglottis and base of the tongue via the internal branch of the superior laryngeal nerve. (**Ref. 1,** p. 276)

26. (B) The vagus nerve leaves the skull through the jugular foramen and enters the carotid sheath where it descends the neck. The vagus nerve has communication with other nerves of the neck. (**Ref. 1,** p. 205)

27. (D) The upper fibers of the trapezius muscle connect the posterior skull and cervical vertebrae with the lateral one-third of the clavicle. These fibers elevate the shoulder and prevent it from sagging. The trapezius muscle is innervated by the accessory nerve. (**Ref. 1,** p. 90)

28. (B) The anterior belly of the digastric muscle is innervated by the mandibular division of the trigeminal nerve. The inferior alveolar nerve gives rise to the mylohyoid nerve that innervates the mylohyoid muscle. (**Ref. 1,** p. 213)

29. (B) The posterior cricoarytenoid muscles are the abductors of the vocal folds. These muscles arise from the lamina of the cricoid cartilage and insert on the muscular process of the arytenoid cartilage. (**Ref. 1,** p. 232)

30. (E) The portal vein receives directly the superior mesenteric, splenic, left gastric, right gastric, posterior superior pancreaticoduodenal, and paraumbilical veins. The inferior mesenteric vein is usually a tributary of the splenic vein. (**Ref. 1,** p. 488)

31. (B) A distinctive feature of the second week of human development is the appearance of primary chorionic villi. A rapid growth and differentiation of the chorion occurs from the ninth day until the fourth week. (**Ref. 3,** p. 65)

32. (C) The limbic system consists of the amygdaloid nucleus, subcallosal gyrus, cingulate gyrus, parahippocampal gyrus, and dentate gyrus. Also included are the hypothalamus and epithalamus. The claustrum is a layer of gray matter found between the lenticular nucleus and the insula. Its function is not known, and it is not a part of the limbic system. (**Ref. 4,** p. 384)

33. (B) It is generally believed that fertilization, the meeting and union of the human germ cells, occurs in the upper third of the uterine tube. The process lasts about 24 hours for the sperm to penetrate into the secondary oocyte. (**Ref. 3,** p. 30)

34. (A) The sperm head arises from the nucleus of each spermatid. Part of the Golgi apparatus within the nucleus becomes the acrosome and constitutes a head cap covering the apical half of the head. (**Ref. 3,** p. 29)

35. (A) At about seven days following fertilization, the hypoblast cells appear on the surface of the inner cell mass. The blastocyst is partially implanted in the endometrium at this time. (**Ref. 3,** p. 36)

36. (B) Sensations are conveyed to the brain stem by the sensory components of the vagus, glossopharyngeal, facial, and trigeminal nerves. The oculomotor nerve carries impulses to muscles of the orbit. (**Ref. 1,** p. 295)

37. (D) During the third week, the process of gastrulation establishes three germ layers. Spaces begin to form in the lateral mesoderm and then coalesce to initiate the beginnings of the body cavities. (**Ref. 3,** p. 63)

38. (C) The costocoracoid membrane is pierced by the lateral pectoral nerve, thoracoacromial artery, and the cephalic vein. (**Ref. 1,** p. 113)

39. (C) The deltoid is the thick, strong muscle that contributes to the prominence of the shoulder. It is innervated by the axillary nerve derived from the fifth and sixth cervical nerves off the brachial plexus. (**Ref. 1,** p. 94)

40. (E) All of the muscles listed play a role in the plantar flexion of the foot except the popliteus, which acts at the knee joint (flexion). The other muscles are located in the posterior compartment of the leg. (**Ref. 1,** p. 615)

41. (B) The inferior mesenteric artery arises from the aorta at the level of the third lumbar vertebra. Its branches supply all regions listed except for the proximal transverse colon, which is supplied by the superior mesenteric artery. (**Ref. 1,** p. 486)

42. (A) The diencephalon is bounded laterally by the posterior limb of the internal capsule. The optic tract bounds the ventral surface of the diencephalon. (**Ref. 4,** p. 448)

43. (B) The anterolateral (striate) arteries arise from the middle cerebral artery. They supply the caudate nucleus, putamen, and internal capsule. These branches also supply the globus pallidus. (**Ref. 4,** p. 443)

44. (B) The middle mediastinum includes the pericardial sac and its contents. Anteriorly is the sternum and posteriorly is the esophagus. The heart and great vessels are the primary contents of the middle mediastinum. (**Ref. 1,** p. 370)

45. (C) At the beginning of the second week, the embryoblast undergoes changes that result in the formation of the bilaminar disc composed of the hypoblast adjacent to the blastocyst cavity and the epiblast adjacent to the amniotic cavity. (**Ref. 3,** p. 40)

46. (D) The flat bones of the skull develop only by intramembranous bone formation. Examples of these flat bones are the frontal, parietal, and temporal. This type of bone formation takes place in mesenchymal tissue. (**Ref. 2,** p. 150)

47. (D) The endometrium of the human uterus is characteristically lined by simple columnar epithelium which consists of patches of ciliated cells among which are nonciliated cells. (**Ref. 2,** p. 451)

48. (C) The outline of the heart when projected anteriorly is defined by its relation to its base, the right end of the diaphragmatic surface, and its apex. The apex of the heart is located about 8 cm from the midline in the left fifth interspace. (**Ref. 1,** p. 378)

49. (B) The structure of veins is similar to their companion arteries. However, the blood pressure within them is lower; they have less muscle, their caliber is larger, and they have much less elastic tissue. (**Ref. 2,** pp. 222–227)

50. (D) An anastomosis between the superior gluteal and external pudendal arteries does not occur in the collateral circulation after ligation of the external iliac artery. (**Ref. 1,** p. 653)

51. (A) The thoracic duct originates at the cisterna chyli on the posterior abdominal wall at the L2 vertebra and then courses through the aortic hiatus of the diaphragm. It then ascends the posterior thoracic wall between the aorta and azygos and courses to the left into the root of the neck to drain into the junction of the left subclavian and internal jugular vein. (**Ref. 1,** p. 412)

52. (C) A characteristic feature of the ileum is the aggregated lymph nodules which are located on the side of the gut opposite the mesentery. They extend through the lamina propria to the submucosa. (**Ref. 2,** p. 297)

53. (C) The presence of corpora amylacea in the alveoli of much of the prostate gland helps to distinguish this organ. In histologic sections they appear as concentric layers and are composed of protein and carbohydrates. **(Ref. 2,** pp. 437–438)

54. (B) The axillary nerve is one of the terminal branches of the posterior cord of the brachial plexus. It courses through the quadrangular space around the surgical neck of the humerus where it could be damaged in this type of break. **(Ref. 1,** p. 121)

55. (B) A hypothyroidism which begins in infancy and continues in the adult can lead to cretinism and mental retardation. It may be secondary to pituitary gland failure. **(Ref. 2,** p. 420)

56. (D) The muscles of facial expression are important muscles involving movments of the eyes and mouth. They form from the second branchial arch and are innervated by nerve fibers of the seventh cranial nerve, which have their cell bodies located in the brain. **(Ref. 1,** p. 244)

57. (A) Phagocytic cells lining the sinusoids of the liver are named Kupffer cells. They belong to the reticuloendothelial system. They are found on the luminal surface of the endothelial cells. **(Ref. 2,** p. 321)

58. (D) The inferior vena cava is formed by the junction of the common iliac veins. It receives the lumbar veins, the right testicular vein, the renal veins, the right suprarenal vein, the right inferior phrenic vein, and the hepatic veins. **(Ref. 1,** p. 509)

60. (C) The esophagus has the widest muscularis mucosae of any segment of the digestive tract. There is a mixture of smooth and skeletal muscle in the middle and proximal ends. **(Ref. 2,** p. 289)

61. (E) The prochordal plate is a thickened area at the cranial aspect of the hypoblast cells. The plate indicates the location of the future mouth and the cranial end of the embryo. It forms the oropharyngeal membrane. **(Ref. 3,** p. 43)

62. **(E)** The primary blood supply to the mesencephalon is from the basilar artery with contribution from the internal carotid. (**Ref. 4,** p. 454)

63. **(B)** The superior boundary of the triangle of auscultation is formed by the trapezius muscle. The other boundaries are the latissimus and rhomboideus major muscles. This triangle provides a space for an auscultation. (**Ref. 1,** p. 92)

64. **(E)** Pseudostratified columnar ciliated epithelium is characteristic of the respiratory system from the nasal passages to the bronchial passages of the lungs. (**Ref. 2,** p. 76)

65. **(A)** The notochordal process develops in the third week as a crainal cellular growth from the primitive node. The notochord grows cranially until it abuts the prochordal plate. Cells migrate laterally from the process as it develops. (**Ref. 3,** p. 57)

66. **(C)** The obturator nerve courses on the lateral pelvic wall at the ovarian fossa and then passes through the obturator foramen to the thigh. Damage to this nerve would impair the medial adductor muscles of the thigh. (**Ref. 1,** pp. 516, 581)

67. **(D)** The cranial nerves containing preganglionic general visceral efferent components of the parasympathetic system are the oculomotor, facial, glossopharnygeal, and vagus or III, VII, IX, and X, respectively. (**Ref. 1,** pp. 332–333)

68. **(B)** In the fetal circulation, the ductus venosus joins the left portal vein to the inferior vena cava, allowing pure blood to reach the heart directly through this main channel. (**Ref. 3,** pp. 341–344)

69. **(C)** The submandibular nodes do not drain the soft palate. The soft palate drains into the superior deep cervical nodes. These nodes are numerous and extend along the carotid sheath. (**Ref. 1,** p. 210)

70. **(A)** The lysosomes, one of the more recently discovered organelles, have been shown to contain a number of hydrolytic enzymes which act as an internal digestive system. (**Ref. 2,** pp. 39–43)

71. **(D)**   Upon ovulation, the Graafian follicle collapses and folds upon itself. It is now a new structure called the corpus luteum. It is located in the cortex of the ovary and secretes estrogen and progesterone. (**Ref. 2,** p. 448)

72. **(D)**   The hypothalamus has connections with the limbic system, pituitary gland, and brain stem and controls many of the visceral functions including feeding, drinking, temperature, sexual activity, and gut motility. (**Ref. 4,** p. 303)

73. **(C)**   The cerebrospinal fluid is produced by the choroid plexus of the lateral, third, and fourth ventricles and reaches the subarachnoid cavity by means of foramina in the roof of the fourth ventricle. (**Ref. 4,** p. 9)

74. **(B)**   The common peroneal nerve derives from the sciatic nerve in the lower third of the posterior compartment of the thigh. The nerve courses laterally across the head of the fibula where it divides into the superficial peroneal (eversion) and deep peroneal (dorsiflexion) nerves. Loss of both of these functions would involve the common peroneal nerve. (**Ref. 1,** p. 615)

75. **(C)**   The cervical visceral fascia encloses the pharynx, esophagus, larynx, trachea, thyroid, and parathyroid glands. Superiorly it attaches to the hyoid bone and to the thyroid cartilage below. (**Ref. 1,** p. 194)

76. **(A)**   The buccopharyngeal fascia covers the buccinator muscle and the pharynx and is prolonged downward over the posterior surface of the esophagus. It is part of the cervical visceral fascia and borders the retropharyngeal space. (**Ref. 1,** p. 194)

77. **(D)**   The spinal cord extends to the coccyx in the fetus but at birth, due to the growth of the vertebral column, it is drawn upward to the level of L-3, and reaches only to L-2 in the adult. (**Ref. 1,** pp. 353–355)

78. **(D)**   During the maturation of the egg, four daughter cells are produced, one of which is the large, fertilizable ovum, while the others are small, rudimentary ova known as polar bodies or polocytes. (**Ref. 3,** p. 19)

79. **(B)** The foramen ovale is the bypass in the fetus that allows blood to pass from the right to the left atrium. This opening bypasses blood flowing through the nonfunctional lungs. (**Ref. 3**, p. 341)

80. **(B)** Cerebrospinal fluid returns directly to the dural venous sinuses from the subarachnoid spaces by means of the arachnoid granulations. They project into the lacunae of the venous sinuses. (**Ref. 1**, p. 324)

81. **(D)** The paramesonephric ducts develop lateral to the gonads and give rise to most of the female reproductive tract. The distal ends of the ducts fuse to form the uterovaginal primordium of the uterus and vagina. (**Ref. 3**, p. 285)

82. **(D)** The use of ribonuclease digestion and ultraviolet microscopy has shown that one of the primary components of the Nissl substance is ribonucleoprotein. (**Ref. 2**, p. 166)

83. **(B)** The facial vein anastomoses indirectly with the cavernous sinus. An infection on the nose or face can enter the facial vein, which lacks valves, and progress as an infected thrombus to the cavernous sinus. (**Ref. 11**, p. 249)

84. **(D)** The great saphenous vein begins in the medial marginal vein of the dorsum of the foot. It ascends anterior to the medial malleolus and posterior to the knee on its course to the saphenous opening. (**Ref. 1**, p. 577)

85. **(C)** The tributaries of the portal vein are the splenic, superior mesenteric, coronary (left gastric), pyloric (right gastric), cystic, and paraumbilical. The uterine veins drain into the internal iliac vein. (**Ref. 1**, p. 557)

86. **(D)** Mitochondria are involved in the production of the energy needed for chemical and mechanical work done by the cell. (**Ref. 2**, pp. 31–32)

87. **(A)** The coronary sinus, the largest vein draining the heart, opens into the right atrium. It receives the great cardiac, middle cardiac, and posterior veins of the left atrium and ventricle. (**Ref. 1**, p. 388)

88. (A)   An osteon consists of lacunae, canaliculi, concentric lamellae, and Haversian canal. It represents the structural unit of adult bone. The collagen is arranged into lamellae around a vasular canal. (**Ref. 2,** p. 145)

89. (E)   The neopallial cortex or isocortex stained by the Nissl method shows that its cell bodies are distributed in six layers, the innermost of which is the multiform or fusiform layer. (**Ref. 4,** p. 390)

90. (D)   A lesion of the otic ganglion would affect the postganglionic secretory fibers of the glossopharyngeal nerve to the parotid gland. From the otic ganglion, these fibers travel with the auriculotemporal nerve. (**Ref. 1,** p. 251)

91. (A)   Cutaneous branches of the maxillary division of the trigeminal include the inferior palpebral, external nasal, superior labial, zygomaticofacial, and zygomaticotemporal branches. (**Ref. 1,** p. 243)

92. (D)   The umbilical vein and the ductus venosus are closed off within a few days after birth; the latter becomes the ligamentum venosum and the former the ligamentum teres of the liver. (**Ref. 3,** p. 343)

93. (D)   Deep to the flexor retinaculum pass the tendons of the flexor pollicus longus, flexor digitorum superficialis and profundus. The ulnar nerve courses superficial to the retinaculum at the wrist. (**Ref. 1,** p. 152)

94. (D)   The principal sensory nerves of the face are derived from the trigeminal nerve. The ophthalmic, maxillary, and mandibular divisions supply branches to the skin of the face. (**Ref. 1,** p. 243)

95. (E)   The nasolacrimal duct, which drains the tears from the eye, opens into the inferior nasal meatus. This meatus is deep to the inferior concha. (**Ref. 1,** p. 282)

96. (C)   The cavernous sinus communicates with the pterygoid plexus of veins by means of an emissary vein in the foramen ovale. Through this vein, infections can spread from the deep face to the cranial cavity. (**Ref. 1,** p. 326)

97. **(B)** Neuroglia or gila cells are found within the central nervous system. Histologically, one can distinguish four types of neuroglia: astrocytes, oligodendrocytes, microglia, and ependymal cells. Microglia are of mesodermal origin, while the other types are ectodermal. (**Ref. 2,** pp. 170–174)

98. **(E)** The tetralogy of Fallot consists of a combination of four abnormalities: (1) a ventricular septum defect, (2) pulmonary stenosis, (3) hypertrophy of the right ventricular wall, and (4) overriding of the aorta. (**Ref. 3,** p. 334)

99. **(A)** The ventral lateral nucleus is one of the three lateral nuclei of the thalamus. This nucleus is involved in motor control circuits and receives input fibers from the cerebellum and basal ganglia that project to the motor cortex. (**Ref. 4,** p. 266)

100. **(E)** Yellow elastic fibers, called the ligamentum flavum, unite the laminae of adjacent vertebrae. They aid in returning to the erect posture after bending. (**Ref. 1,** p. 347)

101. **(E)** The metanephric diverticulum or ureteric bud develops as an outgrowth from the proximal end of the mesonephric duct. It elongates and forms the ureter, renal pelvis, major and minor calices, and the collecting tubules. (**Ref. 3,** p. 267)

102. **(C)** The sarcomere is defined as the portion of the muscle fiber between two successive Z lines. It includes an A band and half of two adjacent I bands and is the smallest subunit of the muscle cell. (**Ref. 2,** p. 197)

103. **(A)** The thoracodorsal artery is a branch of the subscapular, a branch from off the third part of the axillary. The circumflex scapular artery also branches from the subscapular artery. (**Ref. 1,** p. 117)

104. **(E)** The presence of lymphocytes is characteristic of all lymphatic organs. These lymphocytes may be diffused or organized into nodules. These cells play an important role for the immune system. (**Ref. 2,** pp. 244–245)

105. (C) The medial wall of the axilla is formed by the serratus anterior muscle and the underlying ribs. The long thoracic nerve runs on this muscle to innervate it. **(Ref. 1, p. 114)**

106. (C) The greater petrosal branch of the facial nerve supplies parasympathetic innervation to the lacrimal gland in the orbit. The other items are functions of branches of the facial nerve distal to the greater petrosal nerve. **(Ref. 1, p. 287)**

107. (B) The fertilized egg undergoes numerous mitotic divisions by the process of cleavage. The smaller daughter cells which result from cleavage are called blastomeres. **(Ref. 3, p. 35)**

108. (A) The trochlear, mandibular, maxillary, and oculomotor nerves are located in the lateral wall of the cavernous sinus. The abducens is in its lumen. The optic nerve does not enter the sinus. **(Ref. 1, p. 325)**

109. (B) The anterior division fibers of the inferior trunk contribute to the ulnar and median nerves. The median nerve also receives some fibers from the superior trunk. The ulnar and median nerves innervate the forearm and hand. **(Ref. 1, p. 119)**

110. (B) The tympanic branch of the glossopharyngeal nerve supplies parasympathetic fibers, through the otic ganglion, to the parotid gland. The tympanic nerve courses on the medial wall of the middle ear before reaching the otic ganglion. **(Ref. 1, p. 252)**

111. (A) The right and left sixth aortic arches are the last ones to develop. The proximal parts of each of these arches contribute to the right and left pulmonary arteries. The distal part of the left arch forms the ductus arteriosus. **(Ref. 3, p. 335)**

112. (A) The middle meningeal artery is the largest of the arteries supplying the dura mater. It is a branch of the maxillary artery and enters the cranium through the foramen spinosum. **(Ref. 1, p. 269)**

113. (A) The celiac trunk supplies the stomach, liver, spleen, pancreas, gallbladder, and the first portion of the duodenum. It is the most superior of the three unpaired visceral branches of the abdominal aorta. The other viscera are supplied by either the superior or inferior mesenteric arteries. (**Ref. 1,** pp. 451–454)

114. **(C)** Elastic cartilage has a very limited distribution, being found only in the auditory tube, external ear, and certain small cartilages of the larynx. (**Ref. 2,** p. 139)

115. **(C)** Stratified squamous epithelium occurs where protection is needed. It is found in the oral cavity, pharynx, esophagus, anus, vagina, and the epidermis. These surface cells retain their nuclei and are nonkeratinized. (**Ref. 2,** p. 76)

116. **(E)** Synapses may be classified on the basis of membrane specialization, organelle content, position, and variations in the quality and quantity of synaptic vesicle content of the axon terminal. The shape of the end bulb is not indicative of a type of synapse. (**Ref. 2,** pp. 169–170)

117. **(B)** The corticobulbar fibers leave the cerebral cortex and descend through the internal capsule to synapse on certain sensory nuclei and some motor nuclei of cranial nerves. These fibers end in the motor nuclei of the trigeminal, facial, and hypoglossal nuclei and the nucleus ambiguus. The Edinger–Westphal nucleus is a column of parasympathetic neurons that project to the ciliary ganglion. (**Ref. 4,** p. 144)

118. **(C)** The stylopharyngeus muscle is the only muscle derived from the third branchial arc. The muscle is innervated by the glossopharyngeal nerve as this nerve courses posterior to the muscle. (**Ref. 3,** p. 191)

119. **(B)** When the mandible is elevated from a wide-open position, the articular disc moves posteriorly. The control of this posterior movement is by the pull of the superior head of the lateral pterygoid muscle. (**Ref. 1,** p. 262)

120. **(C)** The vagal component of the pharyngeal plexus provides the innervation of the muscles of the pharynx, with the exception of stylopharyngeus and the tensor veli palatini muscle. (**Ref. 1,** p. 238)

121. (C) The internal carotid artery passes deep to the parotid gland to reach the carotid canal in the temporal bone. The facial nerve and the retromandibular vein also travel in the parotid gland. (**Ref. 1,** p. 251)

122. (A) The primary visual cortex is supplied by the calcarine branch of the posterior cerebral artery. The cortex is area 17 and receives the fibers of the geniculocalcarine tract. (**Ref. 4,** p. 406)

123. (A) The ansa cervicalis complex provides the innervation of the infrahyoid muscles and the geniohyoid muscle. It is formed by fibers from the second, third, and fourth cervical spinal nerves. (**Ref. 4,** p. 405)

124. (C) The third, fourth, and sixth cranial nerves and the ophthalmic and maxillary divisions of the trigeminal nerve are located in the wall or lumen of the sinus. Closing of the eyelids is a function of the seventh nerve and would not be affected. (**Ref. 1,** p. 325)

125. (E) Each of the structures listed course either through the scalene triangle or on the two muscles bordering the triangle. The second cervical nerve is located superior to the triangle at the level of the second cervical vertebra. (**Ref. 1,** p. 218)

126. (C) The submandibular duct has an intimate relation to the lingual nerve which crosses it twice in the submandibular region. The duct opens into the floor of the mouth at the sublingual caruncle. (**Ref. 1,** p. 215)

127. (H) The submandibular and sublingual salivary glands characteristically contain serous and mucous demilunes. The parotid gland contains only serous cells. (**Ref. 2,** p. 312)

128. (F) The trachea and much of the conducting portion of the respiratory system contain hyaline cartilage. The cartilage serves to keep the lumen open and reduces in size as the lumen diameter decreases. (**Ref. 2,** pp. 345–346)

129. (G) Tenia coli represent the three outer longitudinal muscular bands found in the muscularis externa of the large intestine. These bands extend the length of the large colon. (**Ref. 2,** p. 308)

130. (A) Kupffer cells are the phagocytic cells found lining the sinusoids of the liver. Kupffer cells are typical macrophages that metabolize products in the sinusoids. (**Ref. 2,** p. 321)

131. (B) The glands of von Ebner are the serous glands associated with the circumvallate papillae of the tongue. They drain into the V region between the anterior and posterior parts of the tongue and serve to keep the taste buds functional. (**Ref. 2,** p. 284)

132. (E) The parietal cells secretes the hydrochloric acid of the stomach. They are located in the upper part of the gastric glands. There is an abundance of mitochondria. (**Ref. 2,** p. 294)

133. (C) Transitional epithelium lines the ureter and other segments of the excretory portion of the urinary system. The superficial cells are rounded and often binucleate. A barrier membrane connects the cells. (**Ref. 2,** pp. 391–392)

134. (F) Cuneocerebellar fibers are derived from the accessory cuneate nucleus and terminate in the ipsilateral cerebellar cortex. (**Ref. 4,** p. 92)

135. (B) The corticospinal system consists of the long descending spinal tracts. They constitute the largest and most important descending fiber system in the neuroaxis. (**Ref. 4,** p. 94)

136. (C) The fibers of the reticulospinal tract descend in the anterior and anterolateral portions of the spinal cord. These fibers may function in voluntary movement, muscle tone, and respiration. (**Ref. 4,** pp. 101–103)

137. (A) The anterior spinocerebellar tract is located along the periphery of the spinal cord anterior to the posterior spinocerebellar tract and posterior to the site of emergence of the ventral root fibers. (**Ref. 4,** pp. 90–91)

138. (E) Fibers of the vestibulospinal tract descend the entire length of the spinal cord. This tract relays impulses to the spinal cord from the vestibular end organ and specific portions of the cerebellum. It is closely associated with the eighth cranial nerve. (**Ref. 4,** p. 100)

139. (C) The claustrum is a thin plate of gray matter lying in the medullary substance of the hemisphere between the lenticular nucleus and insular cortex. (**Ref. 4,** p. 279)

140. (E) The caudate nucleus is an elongated, arched, gray mass of cells related throughout its extent to the ventricular surface of the lateral ventricle. (**Ref. 4,** p. 219)

141. (A) The lenticular nucleus is closely applied to the lateral surface of the internal capsule. A layer of white matter, the lateral medullary lamina, divides the lenticular nucleus into the putamen and globus pallidus. (**Ref. 4,** p. 325)

142. (B) The fornix is a band of white fibers which comprise the primary efferent fiber system of the hippocampal formation, including commissural and projection fibers. (**Ref. 4,** p. 373)

143. (F) The ventral posterior nucleus contains cells which are among the largest in the thalamus. The nucleus is considered the largest primary somatic sensory relay nucleus of the thalamus. (**Ref. 4,** p. 270)

144. (C) The pudendal nerve, derived from S-2, S-3, and S-4, leaves the pelvis through the greater sciatic foramen to course through the gluteal region to reach the perineum. It is the primary motor and sensory innervation of this region. (**Ref. 1,** pp. 524–525)

145. (E) The saphenous nerve passes with the femoral artery through the femoral triangle and adductor canal. The nerve is a branch of the femoral nerve and is sensory from the medial side of the leg. (**Ref. 1,** p. 582)

146. (D) The sciatic nerve is derived from L-4 and L-5 and S-1, S-2, and S-3. It is the largest nerve in the body and forms the largest part of the sacral plexus. It divides into the tibial and common fibular nerve. (**Ref. 1,** pp. 580–581)

147. **(F)** The superior gluteal nerve passes through the greater sciatic foramen to supply the three abductors of the hip joint, the gluteus medius and minimus, and the tensor fasciae latae. (**Ref. 1,** p. 581)

148. **(B)** The femoral nerve lies lateral to the femoral sheath and does not enter the sheath. The nerve reaches the thigh by passing deep to the inguinal ligament. It innervates muscles that extend the leg at the knee joint. (**Ref. 1,** p. 606)

149. **(B)** The flexor carpi radialis muscle, which is innervated by the median nerve, is both an abductor and flexor of the hand at the wrist. The extensor carpi radialis longus and brevis assist in wrist abduction. (**Ref. 1,** p. 140)

150. **(C)** The biceps brachii is a ventral muscle of the arm innervated by the musculocutaneous nerve. This muscle inserts on the radial tuberosity and flexes the elbow and supinates the forearm. (**Ref. 1,** p. 125)

151. **(D)** The dorsal interossei muscles consist of four muscles located in the deep palm and innervated by the deep ulnar nerve. These muscles abduct the second, third, and fourth digits. (**Ref. 1,** p. 168)

152. **(A)** The flexor pollicis longus muscle courses from the forearm through the carpal tunnel to insert on the distal phalanx of the thumb. The tendon is enclosed by a synovial sheath (radial bursa) that wraps around the tendon. (**Ref. 1,** p. 142)

153. **(E)** The flexor digitorum profundus is the deepest of the long flexors coursing through the carpal tunnel from the forearm. The four tendons of this muscle insert on the distal phalanx and flex the distal phalanx of digits 2–5. (**Ref. 1,** p. 142)

154. **(A and C)** The duodenum receives its blood supply from two sources: the celiac artery and the superior mesenteric artery. The direct arteries are the gastroduodenal and pancreaticoduodenal. (**Ref. 1,** pp. 458–460)

155. (A) The ascending colon, cecum, two-thirds of the transverse colon, and most of the small intestine receive their blood supply from the superior mesenteric artery. The right colic artery is a direct branch of the superior mesenteric artery. (**Ref. 1,** pp. 479–481)

156. (C) The spleen receives its blood supply by way of the celiac artery. The celiac artery spirals posterior to the stomach to reach the spleen. (**Ref. 1,** pp. 457–458)

157. (B) The rectum, descending colon, and the left third of the transverse colon receive their blood supply from the inferior mesenteric artery. The superior rectal arteries supplies the upper one-third of the rectum. (**Ref. 1,** pp. 486–487)

158. (A and B) The transverse colon receives its blood supply from both the superior and inferior mesenteric arteries. The proximal part of the transverse colon is supplied by the middle colic and the distal transverse colon is provided by the left colic artery. (**Ref. 1,** pp. 484–485)

159. (E) The oculomotor nerve supplies the levator palpebrae superioris, medial rectus, superior rectus, inferior rectus, and inferior oblique muscles. The lateral rectus muscle is supplied by the abducens nerve. (**Ref. 1,** p. 295)

160. (A) The trochlear nerve courses through the lateral wall of the cavernous sinus. It then enters the orbit through the superior orbital fissure to innervate the superior oblique muscle deep to the periorbita at the roof. (**Ref. 1,** p. 325)

161. (C) The infraorbital nerve of the maxillary division of the trigeminal nerve is sensory from the upper incisor teeth, upper lip, lower eyelid, and skin of the cheek. The temporomandibular joint is innervated by the auriculotemporal nerve. (**Ref. 1,** p. 287)

162. (A) The facial nerve innervates muscles that develop from the second branchial arch, which includes the stapedius. This muscle is important in dampening loud sounds and is located in the middle ear cavity. (**Ref. 1,** p. 306)

163. **(B)** The thyrocervical arterial trunk is a branch of the subclavian artery and provides the blood supply to the muscles of the neck and shoulder and to the thyroid gland. The other branches are from the external carotid artery in the triangles of the neck. (**Ref. 1,** pp. 203–205)

164. **(A)** The posterior cord of the brachial plexus gives rise to the upper and lower subscapular, thoracodorsal, axillary, and radial nerves. The upper subscapular nerve innervates the subscapularis muscles. (**Ref. 1,** p. 121)

165. **(D)** The abductor hallucis muscle is located on the lateral side of the foot and is supplied by the medial plantar nerve. The other muscles are in the posterior thigh or posterior leg compartments and are innervated by the tibial nerve. (**Ref. 1,** p. 627)

166. **(B)** The cranial outflow of the parasympathetic division includes fibers in the oculomotor, facial, glossopharyngeal, and vagus nerves. The pelvic splanchnics form the outflow of the sacral division of the parasympathetic fibers. The trigeminal nerve is the major general somatic nerve of the head. (**Ref. 1,** p. 39)

167. **(C)** During the fourth week of development, the optic vesicle invaginates into a double-walled structure called the optic cup. The outer and inner layers of this cup form the retina. (**Ref. 3,** p. 423)

168. **(D)** The middle ear is the air-filled space of the ear that contains the promontory located on the medial wall. The other structures are found in the inner ear. (**Ref. 1,** p. 305)

169. **(E)** The foramen ovale opens into the infratemporal fossa and transmits the mandibular nerve. The other openings carry branches of the maxillary nerve in and out of the pterygopalatine fossa. (**Ref. 1,** pp. 285–288)

170. **(D)** All of the muscles listed help close the mouth except for the lateral pterygoid muscle. This muscle inserts on the neck of the mandibular condyle and the articular disk and functions in opening the mouth by pulling the mandible forward and downward. (**Ref. 1,** p. 262)

171. **(A)**   Smooth muscle is derived from mesoderm along with skeletal and cardiac muscles. Ectoderm gives rise to all other structures listed. (**Ref. 3,** p. 75)

172. **(E)**   The pancreas develops from dorsal and ventral buds of the midgut, all of which develop from endoderm. The other structures develop from mesoderm. (**Ref. 3,** p. 75)

173. **(A)**   Cartilage is an avascular tissue and nutrition of the chondrocytes within the lacunae is by materials diffusing through the matrix from capillaries outside the cartilage to the chondrocyte. (**Ref. 2,** p. 132)

174. **(A)**   All the muscles of facial expression plus the stapedius, stylohyoid, and posterior belly of the digastric are derived from the second branchial arch. (**Ref. 3,** p. 191)

175. **(D)**   Transitional epithelium is characteristic of and limited to the urinary system. It lines the urinary bladder, ureter, and proximal urethra. Large dome-like cells cover the surface and change shape with filling and emptying of the bladder. (**Ref. 2,** p. 76)

176. **(J)**   (**Ref. 5,** Fig. 2–16)

177. **(B)**   (**Ref. 5,** Fig. 2–16)

178. **(K)**   (**Ref. 5,** Fig. 2–16)

179. **(F)**   (**Ref. 5,** Fig. 2–16)

180. **(L)**   (**Ref. 5,** Fig. 2–16)

181. **(M)**   (**Ref. 5,** Fig. 2–16)

182. **(I)**   (**Ref. 5,** Fig. 2–16)

183. **(H)**   (**Ref. 5,** Fig. 2–16)

184. **(G)**   (**Ref. 5,** Fig. 2–16)

185. **(C)**   (**Ref. 5,** Fig. 2–16)

186. (A)   **(Ref. 5,** Fig. 2–16)

187. (E)   **(Ref. 5,** Fig. 2–16)

188. (D)   **(Ref. 5,** Fig. 2–16)

189. (P)   **(Ref. 5,** Fig. 1–45)

190. (O)   **(Ref. 5,** Fig. 1–45)

191. (L)   **(Ref. 5,** Fig. 1–45)

192. (M)   **(Ref. 5,** Fig. 1–45)

193. (N)   **(Ref. 5,** Fig. 1–45)

194. (E)   **(Ref. 5,** Fig. 1–45)

195. (F)   **(Ref. 5,** Fig. 1–45)

196. (G)   **(Ref. 5,** Fig. 1–45)

197. (H)   **(Ref. 5,** Fig. 1–45)

198. (Q)   **(Ref. 5,** Fig. 1–45)

199. (A)   **(Ref. 5,** Fig. 1–45)

200. (B)   **(Ref. 5,** Fig. 1–45)

201. (I)   **(Ref. 5,** Fig. 1–45)

202. (D)   **(Ref. 5,** Fig. 1–45)

203. (C)   **(Ref. 5,** Fig. 1–45)

204. (J)   **(Ref. 5,** Fig. 1–45)

205. (K)   **(Ref. 5,** Fig. 1–45)

206. (G)   **(Ref. 5,** Fig. 1–63A)

207. (F)   (**Ref. 5,** Fig. 1–63A)

208. (H)   (**Ref. 5,** Fig. 1–63A)

209. (E)   (**Ref. 5,** Fig. 1–63A)

210. (B)   (**Ref. 5,** Fig. 1–63A)

211. (C)   (**Ref. 5,** Fig. 1–63A)

212. (D)   (**Ref. 5,** Fig. 1–63A)

213. (A)   (**Ref. 5,** Fig. 1–63A)

214. (M)   (**Ref. 5,** Fig. 2–66)

215. (J)   (**Ref. 5,** Fig. 2–66)

216. (L)   (**Ref. 5,** Fig. 2–66)

217. (F)   (**Ref. 5,** Fig. 2–66)

218. (G)   (**Ref. 5,** Fig. 2–66)

219. (E)   (**Ref. 5,** Fig. 2–66)

220. (I)   (**Ref. 5,** Fig. 2–66)

221. (N)   (**Ref. 5,** Fig. 2–66)

222. (J)   (**Ref. 5,** Fig. 2–66)

223. (H)   (**Ref. 5,** Fig. 2–66)

224. (B)   (**Ref. 5,** Fig. 2–66)

225. (D)   (**Ref. 5,** Fig. 2–66)

226. (C)   (**Ref. 5,** Fig. 2–66)

227. (A)   (**Ref. 5,** Fig. 2–66)

228. (E)   **(Ref. 5,** Fig. 2–100)

229. (C)   **(Ref. 5,** Fig. 2–100)

230. (A)   **(Ref. 5,** Fig. 2–100)

231. (G)   **(Ref. 5,** Fig. 2–100)

232. (K)   **(Ref. 5,** Fig. 2–100)

233. (B)   **(Ref. 5,** Fig. 2–100)

234. (L)   **(Ref. 5,** Fig. 2–100)

235. (J)   **(Ref. 5,** Fig. 2–100)

236. (D)   **(Ref. 5,** Fig. 2–100)

237. (I)   **(Ref. 5,** Fig. 2–100)

238. (F)   **(Ref. 5,** Fig. 2–100)

239. (H)   **(Ref. 5,** Fig. 2–100)

240. (G)   **(Ref. 5,** Fig. 5–16)

241. (F)   **(Ref. 5,** Fig. 5–16)

242. (O)   **(Ref. 5,** Fig. 5–16)

243. (P)   **(Ref. 5,** Fig. 5–16)

244. (D)   **(Ref. 5,** Fig. 5–16)

245. (Q)   **(Ref. 5,** Fig. 5–16)

246. (C)   **(Ref. 5,** Fig. 5–16)

247. (B)   **(Ref. 5,** Fig. 5–16)

248. (I)   **(Ref. 5,** Fig. 5–16)

249. (M)   (**Ref. 5,** Fig. 5–16)

250. (N)   (**Ref. 5,** Fig. 5–16)

251. (T)   (**Ref. 5,** Fig. 5–16)

252. (L)   (**Ref. 5,** Fig. 5–16)

253. (S)   (**Ref. 5,** Fig. 5–16)

254. (K)   (**Ref. 5,** Fig. 5–16)

255. (H)   (**Ref. 5,** Fig. 5–16)

256. (J)   (**Ref. 5,** Fig. 5–16)

257. (E)   (**Ref. 5,** Fig. 5–16)

258. (A)   (**Ref. 5,** Fig. 5–16)

259. (R)   (**Ref. 5,** Fig. 5–16)

260. (F)   (**Ref. 5,** Fig. 7–2)

261. (H)   (**Ref. 5,** Fig. 7–2)

262. (A)   (**Ref. 5,** Fig. 7–2)

263. (C)   (**Ref. 5,** Fig. 7–2)

264. (E)   (**Ref. 5,** Fig. 7–2)

265. (O)   (**Ref. 5,** Fig. 7–2)

266. (N)   (**Ref. 5,** Fig. 7–2)

267. (M)   (**Ref. 5,** Fig. 7–2)

268. (L)   (**Ref. 5,** Fig. 7–2)

269. (D)   (**Ref. 5,** Fig. 7–2)

270. (K) (**Ref. 5,** Fig. 7–2)

271. (J) (**Ref. 5,** Fig. 7–2)

272. (B) (**Ref. 5,** Fig. 7–2)

273. (G) (**Ref. 5,** Fig. 7–2)

274. (P) (**Ref. 5,** Fig. 7–2)

275. (I) (**Ref. 5,** Fig. 7–2)

References

1. Woodburn RT: *Essentials of Human Anatomy,* 9th ed. Oxford Press, New York, 1994.
2. Junqueira LC, Carneiro J, Kelley RO: *Basic Histology,* 7th ed. Appleton & Lange, Norwalk, 1992.
3. Moore KL: *The Developing Human,* 5th ed. Saunders, Philadelphia, 1993.
4. Carpenter MB: *Core Text of Neuroanatomy,* 4th ed. Williams & Wilkins, Baltimore, 1991.
5. Agur AM: *Grant's Atlas of Anatomy,* 9th ed. Williams & Wilkins, Baltimore, 1991.

2

Biochemistry
David M. Glick

DIRECTIONS (Questions 276 through 383): Each of the questions or incomplete statements below is followed by five suggested answers or completions. Select the ONE that is best in each case.

276. The action of the antibiotic actinomycin D is in
    A. blocking electron transport
    B. blocking protein synthesis
    C. blocking bacterial cell wall synthesis
    D. blocking RNA transcription
    E. making membranes permeable to K^+

277. Phosphatidylcholine is synthesized in the liver from phosphatidylethanolamine. A metabolite essential for this conversion is
    A. phosphatidylglycerol
    B. thiamine pyrophosphate
    C. S-adenosylmethionine
    D. nicotinamide adenine dinucleotide
    E. flavin adenine dinucleotide

278. Phosphatidylcholine is synthesized from diglycerides and choline in the lung. An important intermediate in this reaction is
  A. UDP-choline
  B. choline pyrophosphate
  C. choline adenylate
  D. CDP-choline
  E. UDP-ethanolamine

279. The antibiotic streptomycin acts by
  A. transferring its acetyl group to elongation factor EF-2
  B. binding to hydroxymethyl cytosine residues of viral DNA
  C. preventing processing to tRNA by a pyrimidine N-methyl transferase
  D. interfering with cell wall biosynthesis of gram-positive bacteria
  E. interfering with protein chain initiation by binding to 30S ribosomes

280. Cholera toxin acts by
  A. preventing release of a guanine nucleotide from a protein associated with adenylate cyclase of intestinal cells, thus keeping the enzyme in a stimulated state
  B. competitively inhibiting vasopressin's action on its target cells
  C. complexing with, and thus inhibiting, aldosterone
  D. combining with the regulatory subunit of, and thus relieving the inhibition on, a prostaglandin synthetase
  E. glycosylating, and thus inhibiting, the Na^+ resorption sites in the distal tubules

281. One physiological activity of caffeine is to inhibit
  A. adenylate cyclase
  B. guanylate cyclase
  C. cyclic nucleotide diesterase
  D. the cyclooxygenase pathway
  E. dissociation of GTP from a G-protein

282. Diisopropylfluorophosphate (DFP) is an effective inhibitor for trypsin, chymotrypsin, and elastase because
   A. all three enzymes recognize the isopropyl side chain
   B. it is a transition state analog
   C. it reacts with a histidine residue at the active site
   D. it reacts with a cysteine residue at the active site
   E. it reacts with a serine at the active site

283. The pK_a values of phosphoric acid are 2.1, 7.2, and 12.3. What is the ratio $[HPO_4^{2-}]/[H_2PO_4^-]$ in a phosphate solution at pH 6.2?
   A. 0.1
   B. 0.5
   C. 1.0
   D. 5.0
   E. 10.0

284. The Watanabe hyperlipidemic rabbit and patients with type IIa hypercholesterolemia both share a deficiency of
   A. HDL receptors
   B. apoprotein E
   C. LDL receptors
   D. VLDL
   E. beta-lipoprotein

285. Patients with severe renal disease may not be able to make use of the normal dietary sources of
   A. vitamin A
   B. vitamin B_6
   C. vitamin C
   D. vitamin D
   E. vitamin E

286. The iron in oxyhemoglobin
   A. has six ligands, four of them being the pyrrole nitrogen atoms of protoporphyrin IX
   B. has six ligands, one of them being the sulfhydryl sulfur atom of a cysteine residue
   C. has four ligands, these being the pyrrole nitrogen atoms of protoporphyrin IX

D. has six ligands, two of them being the two oxygen atoms of the O_2 molecule

E. has 8 ligands, two of them being the two oxygen atoms of the O_2 molecule

287. The primary effect of a light impulse in the retina is
   A. isomerization of *trans*-retinol to *cis*-retinol
   B. reduction of 11-*cis*-retinal to *cis*-retinol
   C. isomerization of *cis*-retinol to *trans*-retinol
   D. reduction of *trans*-retinal to *trans*-retinol
   E. isomerization of 11-*cis*-retinal to *trans*-retinal

288. A coenzyme required in various carboxylations is
   A. NADP
   B. biotin
   C. coenzyme A
   D. pantotheine
   E. thiamine pyrophosphate

289. Catalase promotes which reaction?
   A. $H_2O_2 + AH_2 \rightarrow 2H_2O + A$
   B. $O_2^- + 2H_2O + 2H^+ \rightarrow O_2 + H_2O_2$
   C. $2H_2O_2 \rightarrow 2H_2O + O_2$
   D. $O_2 + RH + NADPH \rightarrow ROH + NADP^+ + OH^-$
   E. $4 \text{ cyt } a/a_3^{2+} + O_2 + 4H^+ \rightarrow 4 \text{ cyt } a/a_3^{3+} + 2H_2O$

290. Trypsin will cleave the tripeptide
   A. alanyl-arginyl-leucine
   B. phenylalanyl-prolyl-serine
   C. glycyl-threonyl-valine
   D. asparaginyl-tyrosyl-lysine
   E. isoleucyl-aspartyl-glutamine

291. A competitive inhibitor alters an enzyme's kinetics by
   A. increasing the apparent Km
   B. decreasing the apparent Km
   C. increasing the apparent Vmax
   D. decreasing the apparent Vmax
   E. decreasing both the apparent Km and the apparent Vmax

292. In a typical anabolic pathway (eg, pyrimidine biosynthesis) the end product regulates the rate of metabolite flux through the pathway by

    A. allosteric stimulation of the first committed step in the pathway

    B. allosteric inhibition of the first committed step

    C. allosteric stimulation of the final committed step

    D. allosteric inhibition of the final committed step

    E. product inhibition of that enzymatic step which forms it

293. Binding of cAMP to its receptor protein in *E. coli* results in increased synthesis of β-galactosidase because the cyclic nucleotide-receptor protein complex is bound to

    A. the operator

    B. the repressor

    C. the activator

    D. the promotor

    E. the polymerase

294. The control exercised over β-galactosidase production in *E. coli* by the cAMP-receptor protein complex is called

    A. positive translational control

    B. negative transcriptional control

    C. positive transcriptional control

    D. posttranscriptional modification

    E. posttranslational modification

295. Factor XIII stabilizes blood clots by cross-linking

    A. α-amino groups of one fibrin chain with α-carboxyl groups of another

    B. α-amino groups of one fibrin chain with β-carboxyl groups of another

    C. α-amino groups of one fibrin chain with γ-carboxyl groups of another

    D. ε-amino groups of one fibrin chain with β-carboxyl groups of another

    E. ε-amino groups of one fibrin chain with γ-carboxyl groups of another

296. Collagen is held in its characteristic fibrous form by
   A. α-helix structure
   B. α-pleated sheet structure
   C. disulfide bridges
   D. interchain hydrogen bonds
   E. salt bridges to hyaluronic acid

297. The V, D, J, and C genes *all* recombine to form
   A. immunoglobulin light chains only
   B. immunoglobulin heavy chains only
   C. immunoglobulin light chains and heavy chains
   D. IgG only
   E. IgG and IgM

298. Satellite DNA renatures from single strands to double strands at very low concentrations. This is consistent with the fact that it is
   A. highly repetitive
   B. coding for ribosomal RNA
   C. coding for histones
   D. composed of introns
   E. composed of unique sequences

299. Normal immunoglobulin IgG
   A. has two heavy chains and two light chains, both types containing variable and constant segments
   B. has one heavy chain with the variable segment and two light chains with the constant segments
   C. has two heavy chains and two light chains, only the former having the variable segment
   D. has two heavy chains and two light chains, only the latter having the variable segment
   E. has two heavy chains, which are polypeptides, and two light chains, which are oligosaccharides

300. If a native globular protein contains equal numbers of residues of each of the following amino acids, which one can be expected to have the most side chains in the interior of the molecule?
   A. arginine
   B. glutamine
   C. glycine
   D. histidine
   E. valine

301. The glycogen branching enzyme is
   A. a glycogen synthetase
   B. an amylo(1,4)-transglycosylase
   C. an amylo(1,4 → 1,6)-transglycosylase
   D. an α-amylase
   E. a β-amylase

302. In humans, the tricarboxylic acid cycle intermediates, α-ketoglutarate and oxaloacetate, give rise to the amino acids
   A. threonine and arginine, respectively
   B. arginine and threonine, respectively
   C. proline and asparagine, respectively
   D. argine and valine, respectively
   E. tyrosine and aspartate, respectively

303. A compound that is NOT an obligatory intermediate in the glycolytic metabolism of glucose is
   A. 1,3-diphosphoglyceric acid
   B. fructose-1,6-diphosphate
   C. fructose-6-phosphate
   D. glucose-1-phosphate
   E. glucose-6-phosphate

304. Glucose-6-phosphate dehydrogenase deficiency is often benign until primaquine or other similar drugs puts heavy pressure on the erythrocyte's
   A. ATP reserves
   B. reduced glutathione pool
   C. glucose transport
   D. 2,3-diphosphoglycerate reserves
   E. methemoglobin stores

305. The route for synthesis of phosphoenolpyruvate from pyruvate is
- **A.** pyruvate → oxaloacetate → malate → phosphoenolpyruvate
- **B.** pyruvate → lactate → oxaloacetate → phosphoenolpyruvate
- **C.** pyruvate → malate → fumarate → phosphoenolpyruvate
- **D.** pyruvate → oxaloacetate → fumarate → phosphoenolpyruvate
- **E.** pyruvate → oxaloacetate → phosphoenolpyruvate

306. A cofactor in the conversion of glucose-1-phosphate to glucose-6-phosphate is
- **A.** AMP
- **B.** 3′,5′-cAMP
- **C.** glucose-1,6-diphosphate
- **D.** NAD^+
- **E.** pyridoxal phosphate

307. Radiologists can now identify sites of myocardial ischemia by visualizing regions which fail to metabolize a substrate adequately to sustain ATP production. One such substrate which cannot be used by ischemic myocardium for maintaining ATP production is
- **A.** glucose
- **B.** galactose
- **C.** fructose
- **D.** palmitate
- **E.** glycerol

308. Inhibitors of ornithine decarboxylase have been developed as antineoplastic agents. Which class of molecules important in regulation of the cell cycle would be affected by such drugs?
- **A.** purines
- **B.** pyrimidines
- **C.** histones
- **D.** polyamines
- **E.** ribonucleotides

309. Which compound exerts a key control over liver gluconeogenesis by positive modulation of the pyruvate carboxylase reaction?
- **A.** acetyl-CoA
- **B.** N-acetylglutamic acid
- **C.** biotin
- **D.** carnitine
- **E.** citric acid

310. Lactose intolerance is due to
   A. a lack of β-galactosidase
   B. a lack of galactose-1-phosphate
   C. very low levels of galactose-1-phosphate uridyl transferase in the liver
   D. an unusually rapid reaction of galactose-1-phosphate with uridine
   E. deficiency in UDP-glucose epimerase

311. Alkaptonuria and albinism are both defects associated with the metabolism of
   A. tryptophan
   B. tyrosine
   C. cysteine
   D. proline
   E. taurine

312. Phosphofructokinase is
   A. stimulated by ATP and inhibited by citrate and by glucose-6-phosphate
   B. stimulated by long-chain fatty acyl-CoA esters
   C. stimulated by fructose-6-phosphate and inhibited by fructose-1,6-diphosphate
   D. inhibited by AMP
   E. stimulated by AMP and inhibited by citrate and by ATP

313. Glycogen is synthesized by the reaction of
   A. UDP-glucose with the reducing end of a glycogen primer
   B. UDP-glucose with the nonreducing end of a glycogen primer
   C. glucose-1-phosphate with the reducing end of a glycogen primer
   D. glucose-6-phosphate with the nonreducing end of a glycogen primer
   E. glucose-6-phosphate with the reducing end of a glycogen primer

314. The oligosaccharide attached to an asparagine residue of a glycoprotein is donated to the polypeptide by
   A. UDP-monosaccharides, one residue at a time
   B. UDP-oligosaccharides

    C. dolichol pyrophosphoryl-monosaccharides, one residue at a time
    D. dolichol pyrophosphoryl-oligosaccharide
    E. oligosaccharide-bearing oligosaccharide carrier protein

315. An uncoupler of oxidative phosphorylation causes
    A. increased respiration and synthesis of ATP
    B. decreased respiration and increased synthesis of ATP
    C. increased respiration and decreased synthesis of ATP
    D. decreased respiration and synthesis of ATP
    E. lowered body heat production

316. Marfan's syndrome is associated with a defect in the structure of
    A. dynein
    B. collagen
    C. keratin
    D. glycosaminoglycans
    E. myosin

317. Malonate inhibits the tricarboxylic acid cycle because it blocks
    A. fatty acid oxidation
    B. further metabolism of *cis*-aconitic acid
    C. further metabolism of succinic acid
    D. formation of ATP
    E. condensation of acetyl-CoA oxaloacetic acid

318. The substrates for the two enzymatic reactions in the tricarboxylic acid cycle in which CO_2 is liberated are
    A. citrate and α-ketoglutarate
    B. isocitrate and α-ketoglutarate
    C. *cis*-aconitate and α-ketoglutarate
    D. citrate and oxaloacetate
    E. isocitrate and oxaloacetate

319. The chemiosmotic theory explains the action of a major class of uncouplers of oxidative phosphorylation as

    A. hydrolysis of a high-energy phosphate intermediate, possibly imidazole phosphate

    B. dissipation of a proton gradient across the mitochondrial membrane

    C. dissipation of the charge across the mitochondrial membrane

    D. permitting K^+ to pass across the mitochondrial membrane

    E. the uncoupler acting as an alternative electron acceptor from reduced cytochrome

320. Cyanide blocks the electron transport system by combining with

    A. cytochrome b

    B. cytochrome c

    C. cytochrome oxidase

    D. the nonheme iron protein

    E. ubiquinone

321. Cholesterol synthesis in human cells is inhibited by the interaction of

    A. lanosterol with mevalonic kinase

    B. squalene with HMG-CoA reductase

    C. cholesterol with HMG-CoA reductase

    D. lanosterol with squalene synthetase

    E. cholesterol with mevalonic kinase

322. The lipoprotein that is increased most immediately following ingestion of fat is

    A. very low-density lipoprotein

    B. low-density lipoprotein

    C. high-density lipoprotein

    D. very high-density lipoprotein

    E. chylomicron

323. Lecithin-cholesterol acyl transferase

    A. transfers cholesterol from the interior of LDL to the exterior of HDL

    B. transfers the choline side chain from cholesterol to lecithin

    C. converts free cholesterol from cell membranes to cholesterol esters in HDL

D. converts cholesterol esters in LDL to free cholesterol in cell membranes

E. transfers an acyl side chain to lecithin to permit its cyclization to the steroid ring system of cholesterol

324. In the uptake of fatty acids into mitochondria, there is involvement of
  A. agmantine
  B. carnitine
  C. carnosine
  D. lipoic acid
  E. pantothenic acid

325. In protein biosynthesis
  A. each amino acid recognizes its codon on the mRNA template because of a structural complementarity between amino acid and codon
  B. reliability of translation is assured by traces of DNA in the ribosome
  C. each amino acid is first attached to an anticodon specific for the amino acid
  D. a given codon–anticodon pair must have identical base sequences to avoid formation of "degenerate" proteins
  E. the recognition of each amino acid and its codon on the mRNA is achieved through specific tRNA molecules

326. During cell division, the double-stranded DNA is segregated so that
  A. both old strands are in one daughter cell and both new strands are in the other
  B. one strand of the old and one of the new strands are in each daughter cell
  C. the old and new strands segregate among the cells at random
  D. all old strands remain in the parent cell and all new strands are in the daughter cells
  E. all new strands remain in the parent cell and all old strands are in the daughter cells

327. The first step in incorporating an amino acid into a growing protein molecule involves
    A. the formation of an ester bond between the amino acid carboxyl group and the 2'-hydroxyl group of tRNA
    B. the formation of a peptide bond between the amino acid carboxyl group and the N-terminal amino group of the growing peptide
    C. the expenditure of energy as GTP for the formation of an aminoacyl-tRNA
    D. the formation of an anhydride of the amino acid carboxyl group and adenylic acid
    E. transfer of the amino acid from an aminoacyl-CoA to tRNA

328. The correct flow of metabolites through the urea cycle is
    A. citrulline → ornithine → homoarginine → arginine → urea
    B. ornithine → arginine → argininosuccinate → citrulline → urea
    C. citrulline → arginine → argininosuccinate → ornithine → urea
    D. citrulline → ornithine → arginine → argininosuccinate → urea
    E. ornithine → citrulline → argininosuccinate → arginine → urea

329. Methionine is formed by
    A. cleavage of S-adenosylmethionine
    B. methylation of cysteine by 5'-methyltetrahydrofolate
    C. methylation of homocysteine by 5'-methyltetrahydrofolate
    D. reduction of methionine sulfoxide
    E. cleavage of cystathionine

330. The vitamin whose product participates in the conversion of serine to glycine is
    A. biotin
    B. folic acid
    C. pantothenic acid
    D. thiamine
    E. α-tocopherol

331. Phenylketonuria is due to the absence of the enzyme that
  A. deaminates tyrosine
  B. hydroxylates phenylalanine
  C. oxidizes homogentisic acid
  D. converts tyrosine to dopa
  E. iodinates tyrosine

332. The nutritional role of the carotenoids lies in their conversion in vivo to
  A. ascorbic acid
  B. cobalamin
  C. folic acid
  D. prostaglandins
  E. vitamin A

333. The biosynthesis of coenzyme A requires dietary
  A. biotin
  B. folic acid
  C. intrinsic factor
  D. pantothenic acid
  E. thiamine

334. Pernicious anemia is
  A. a dietary vitamin B_{12} deficiency
  B. a deficiency of a vitamin B_{12}-requiring enzyme
  C. an inability to absorb vitamin B_{12}
  D. an inability to convert vitamin B_{12} to cyanocobalamin
  E. an inability to convert vitamin B_{12} to adenosylcobalamin

335. Kwashiorkor is a condition caused by a diet
  A. deficient in protein
  B. deficient in calories
  C. deficient in niacin
  D. deficient in thiamine
  E. deficient in riboflavin

336. Vitamin K plays an essential role in
  A. dissolving blood clots
  B. postribosomal modification of some proteins
  C. maintenance of the retina's integrity
  D. preventing bile stasis
  E. biosynthesis of factor XI

337. An animal is in negative nitrogen balance when
  A. dietary nitrogen and extracted nitrogen are equal
  B. dietary nitrogen exceeds excreted nitrogen
  C. excreted nitrogen exceeds dietary nitrogen
  D. the urine is free of nitrogen
  E. new tissue is being synthesized

338. How does 3′,5′-cAMP increase the rate of glycogenolysis?
  A. it promotes the formation of a phosphorylated form of glycogen phosphorylase
  B. it serves as a cofactor for glycogen phosphorylase
  C. it serves as a precursor of 5′-AMP, which is a cofactor for glycogen phosphorylase
  D. it furnishes phosphates for the phosphorolysis of glycogen
  E. it relieves the inhibition of glycogen phosphorylase due to glucose-6-phosphate

339. Which of the following statements concerning DNA is INCORRECT?
  A. the base composition of DNA is characteristic of a given species
  B. closely related organisms exhibit similar base compositions
  C. the two strands of double helical DNA run in the same direction (3′ to 5′)
  D. the ratio of the sum of the bases A plus T to G plus C is unity
  E. different tissues of any given organism have the same weight of DNA per diploid nucleus

340. In man the primary excretion product of purines is
  A. allantoin
  B. hypoxanthine

C. inosine
D. uric acid
E. urea

341. Purine salvage pathways feature a reaction that
   A. replaces the ribose of a purine nucleoside with ribose-5-phosphate
   B. replaces the ribose-5-phosphate of a purine nucleotide with ribose
   C. converts a free purine base to a purine nucleoside
   D. converts a free purine base to a purine nucleotide
   E. oxidizes purines to uric acid

342. The compound shown in Figure 2.1 is an intermediate in the synthesis of
   A. a prosthetic group of the pyruvic dehydrogenase complex
   B. a prosthetic group of cytochrome oxidase
   C. histidine
   D. proline
   E. tryptophan

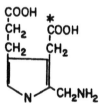

Figure 2.1

343. The starred carboxyl group (see Figure 2.1) is derived from
   A. the carboxyl group of indoleacetic acid
   B. the carboxyl group of glycine
   C. the carboxyl group of proline
   D. the free carboxyl group of succinyl-CoA
   E. a carboxyl group of isocitric acid

344. From a knowledge of the standard oxidation-reduction potential it is possible, for a redox reaction, to calculate
   A. the reaction rate
   B. the standard free energy
   C. the activation energy
   D. the pH
   E. none of the above

345. NADH reduces coenzyme Q through the mediation of an enzyme complex containing
   A. cytochrome
   B. lipoic acid
   C. heme
   D. flavin mononucleotide
   E. cytochrome b

346. The P:O ratio observed upon conversion of succinate to fumarate in a system carrying out oxidative phosphorylation is
   A. 0
   B. 1
   C. 2
   D. 3
   E. 4

347. Which of the following membrane lipids has NO charged groups?
   A. phosphatidyl choline
   B. phosphatidyl serine
   C. ceramide
   D. ganglioside
   E. phosphatidyl inositol

348. Acetoacetate and β-hydroxybutyrate (standard redox potential −0.35V) and fumarate and succinate (standard redox potential +0.03V) are mixed together at concentrations of 1 M each at pH 7.0 and the reaction permitted to go to equilibrium. What is the $\Delta\mathscr{E}'$ for the spontaneous reaction when the components are first mixed?
   A. −0.32V
   B. +0.38V
   C. −0.38V
   D. +0.32V
   E. none of these

349. The mechanisms of activation of trypsin, chymotrypsin, and elastase all involve
   A. movement of the residues in the active site induced by binding of substrate
   B. critical alignment of the side chains of residues in the catalytic site upon selective cleavage of certain peptide bonds in the inactive zymogens
   C. distortion of the substrate upon binding to the active site
   D. a significant refolding of the polypeptide chain into a new conformation upon selective proteolysis
   E. a key participatory role of a bound metal ion

350. Which statement about inhibitors is true?
   A. addition of a competitive inhibitor to a mixture of enzyme and substrate should reduce the rate of production formation by 50% if the concentration of inhibitor is equal to K_I
   B. the value of K_I for a competitive inhibitor is dependent upon the substrate concentration
   C. in the case of noncompetitive inhibition, no difference can be detected in the dissociation constant for substrate, regardless of the inhibitor concentration
   D. the apparent dissociation constant for substrate increases upon addition of an uncompetitive inhibitor
   E. most noncompetitive inhibitors are substrate analogs which combine reversibly with the enzyme

351. When K_s and Km for an enzyme are found to be very different, then
   A. the catalytic step is probably much slower than the binding and dissociation of substrate to and from the enzyme
   B. the enzyme is probably displaying marked negative cooperativity
   C. there are different amino acids involved in binding and catalysis
   D. there is probably an allosteric effector present
   E. the steady-state concentration of the enzyme–substrate complex may be far from equilibrium

352. From the graph (Figure 2.2), the Km for this enzyme may be estimated to be approximately

   A. $\dfrac{1}{50}$ μM

   B. $\dfrac{1}{250}$ μM

   C. 50 μM
   D. 100 μM
   E. 250 μM

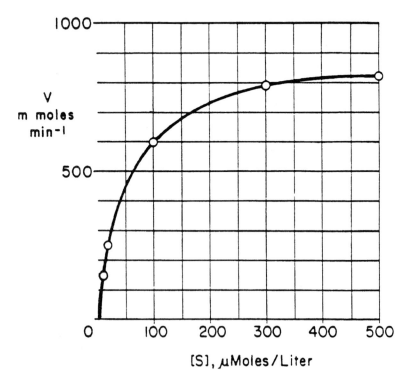

Figure 2.2

353. The Lineweaver–Burke plots in Figure 2.3 for enzymatic transformation of the two substrates glucose and mannose indicate that
 A. the k_{cat} for glucose is higher than that for mannose
 B. the two substrates are bound with equal affinities but the values of k_{cat} are different
 C. mannose is bound to the enzyme less tightly than glucose
 D. the Km for glucose is greater than the Km for mannose
 E. the two substrates are probably bound at different catalytic sites on the enzyme

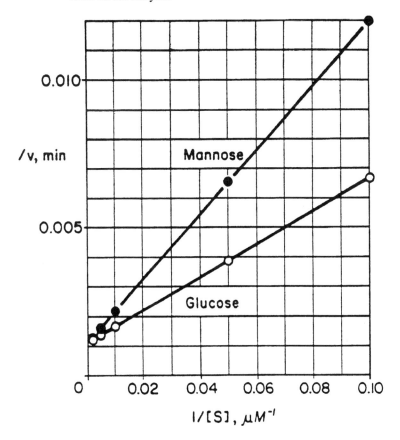

Figure 2.3

354. GTP does NOT participate in
  A. biosynthesis of AMP
  B. biosynthesis of phosphoenolpyruvate
  C. polypeptide chain elongation
  D. biosynthesis of isopentenyl pyrophosphate
  E. activation of the β-adrenergic receptor

355. An enzyme that uses the thiamine pyrophosphate prosthetic group is
  A. pyruvate carboxylase
  B. glucose-6-phosphate dehydrogenase
  C. α-ketoglutarate dehydrogenase
  D. transaldolase
  E. 6-phosphogluconate dehydrogenase

356. A carboxylation that requires biotin is formation of
  A. γ-carboxyglutamate residues from glutamate residues
  B. malate from pyruvate
  C. methylmalonyl-CoA from propionyl-CoA
  D. succinyl-CoA from propionyl-CoA
  E. oxaloacetate from phosphoenolpyruvate

357. Patients with α_1-antiproteinase deficiency may develop emphysema because they cannot
  A. inhibit the plasmin-catalyzed digestion of the lung's connective tissue, which accompanies activation of neutrophils in pulmonary inflammation
  B. inhibit thrombic digestion which accompanies activation of neutrophils' inflammatory reactions
  C. activate the repair of lung tissue mediated by α_1-antiproteinase after inflammatory damage
  D. block the action of leukocyte elastase released by activated neutrophils in the lung
  E. inhibit thrombin that normally controls any incipient hemorrhages

358. Bile acids aid digestion by
  A. donating conjugated glycine and taurine groups to long-chain fatty acids
  B. neutralizing the alkaline pancreatic juice
  C. acting as cofactors for pancreatic amylase

   D.   forming micelles with products of lipase action
   E.   protecting the gastric lining from the damaging effects of
         gastric HCl

359. A role NOT played by porphyrin-containing proteins is
   A.   conversion of phenylalanine to tyrosine
   B.   steroid hydroxylation
   C. CO_2 transport in the blood
   D.   detoxification of amphetamines
   E.   detoxification of H_2O_2

360. Carbamoyl phosphate is involved in synthesis of
   A.   anserine
   B.   glycine
   C.   uric acid
   D.   uracil
   E.   methionine

361. The development of symptoms of pellagra may be due to
   A.   a malabsorption syndrome associated with inadequate secre-
         tion of bile acids into the duodenum
   B.   a malabsorption of tyrosine
   C.   alkaptonuria associated with severe undernourishment
   D.   a severely inadequate intake of niacin
   E.   a failure of the gastric mucosa to secrete a glycoprotein that
         normally assists absorption of a dietary factor

362. Among the roles of succinyl-CoA is assisting in
   A.   choline biosynthesis
   B.   catabolism of ketone bodies
   C.   activation of β-adrenergic receptors
   D.   ketogenesis
   E.   steroidogenesis

363. A pentapeptide of the composition alanine, glycine, lysine, phenylalanine, tryptophan has an N-terminal alanine. After chymotryptic digestion, the product shows both N-terminal alanine and N-terminal glycine. This is compatible with the sequence
   A. Ala-Gly-Phe-Lys-Trp
   B. Ala-Phe-Gly-Lys-Trp
   C. Ala-Trp-Phe-Lys-Gly
   D. Ala-Lys-Gly-Trp-Phe
   E. Ala-Lys-Gly-Phe-Trp

364. A protein will reveal its N-terminal amino acid when treated with the Sanger reagent (fluoro-2,4-dinitrobenzene) if it has an N-terminal
   A. N-acetylated amino acid
   B. proline
   C. pyroglutamic acid
   D. cysteamine
   E. myristyl-glycine

365. Prostaglandin endoperoxidase synthase
   A. is responsible for production of both prostaglandins and leukotrienes
   B. is responsible for production of both prostaglandins and prostacyclin
   C. acts exclusively upon arachidonate
   D. is irreversibly activated by aspirin
   E. is responsible for production of prostaglandins G_2 and H_2

366. The 5-carbon skeletons of ornithine and citrulline can be derived most directly from
   A. orotic acid
   B. aspartic acid
   C. succinic acid
   D. proline
   E. methionine

367. The modified amino acid, 3-methyl-histidine, occurs in
   A. keratin
   B. collagen

    C. resilin
    D. elastin
    E. myosin

368. An amino acid that is wholly or partially ketogenic is
    A. glycine
    B. phenylalanine
    C. cysteine
    D. valine
    E. proline

369. The closest biosynthetic precursor of pyruvate is
    A. threonine
    B. methionine
    C. citrate
    D. cysteine
    E. α-ketoglutarate

370. A distinctive biochemical feature of brown adipose tissue is
    A. an abundance of mitochondria
    B. high levels of myoglobin
    C. hormonal control of cortisol
    D. high levels of prostaglandin synthesis and release
    E. production of melanin

371. The intrinsic and extrinsic pathways of blood coagulation and the pathways of complement activation are all examples of
    A. G-protein-dependent activations
    B. protein kinase-dependent amplification
    C. protease-dependent amplification
    D. coupled phosphorylation–dephosphorylation systems
    E. lipoxygenase-dependent pathways

372. A pharmacological action of lithium ion (Li^+) is inhibition of
    A. monoamine oxidase
    B. re-uptake of norepinephrine across the presynaptic membrane
    C. acetylcholinesterase
    D. inositol monophosphate hydrolysis
    E. cyclic nucleotide phosphodiesterase

373. Besides xanthine, xanthine oxidase acts on
  A. guanine
  B. inosine
  C. uric acid
  D. hypoxanthine
  E. superoxide (O_2^-)

374. Inositol triphosphate
  A. activates protein kinase C by lowering its requirement for Ca^{2+}
  B. complexes with Ca^{2+} and activates protein kinase C
  C. serves as the precursor of an activator of protein kinase C
  D. releases Ca^{2+} from the endoplasmic reticulum
  E. activates phospholipase C

375. A modification of mRNA that occurs after its synthesis on a template is
  A. addition of poly-ADP-ribose
  B. transport across the mitochondrial membrane
  C. addition of CCA sequence to the 3'-end
  D. addition of CCA sequence to the 5'-end
  E. removal of internal polynucleotide sequences

376. Components of the nucleosome include
  A. one copy of spermine
  B. histones H2A, H2B, H3, and H4
  C. about 2000 base pairs of DNA
  D. one molecule of RNase H
  E. one molecule of polymerase III

377. Erythrocyte membrane proteins include
  A. spectrin
  B. dermatan sulfate
  C. cytochrome oxidase
  D. Na^+-H^+ transporter
  E. β-galactosidase

378. DNA biosynthesis in normal mammalian cells can
  A. occur on an RNA template, catalyzed by reverse transcriptase
  B. occur only in the nucleus

C. involve ribonucleotide triphosphates of adenine, guanine, cytosine, and thymine as substrates

D. involve the addition of mononucleotides to the 3′ end of an RNA primer

E. involve the addition of mononucleotides to the 5′ end of an RNA primer

379. Genetic recombination experiments depend upon the action of restriction endonucleases that act on DNA
A. to cleave at palindromic sequences
B. to generate . . . pCpCpA 3′ termini
C. in non-coding regions
D. which must be single-stranded
E. excise introns and splice exons

380. An activity NOT supported by mitochondria is
A. oxidative cleavage of catecholamines
B. protein synthesis
C. fatty acid oxidation
D. glycolysis
E. ketone body synthesis

381. A component of mitochondrial electron transport that does not accept hydrogen atoms is
A. non-heme iron
B. NAD
C. ubiquinone
D. FMN
E. menadione

382. An essentially irreversible enzymatic reaction of glycolysis is that catalyzed by
A. phosphofructokinase
B. glyceraldehyde-3-phosphate dehydrogenase
C. glycerokinase
D. lactate dehydrogenase
E. phosphoglyceromutase

383. An essentially irreversible enzymatic reaction of gluconeogenesis is that catalyzed by
  A. malate dehydrogenase
  B. glycerophosphate dehydrogenase
  C. enolase
  D. fructose diphosphate phosphatase
  E. phosphoenolpyruvate carboxykinase

DIRECTIONS (Questions 384 and 385): This section consists of a situation, followed by a series of questions. Study the situation, and select the ONE best answer to each question following it.

CASE HISTORY (Questions 384 and 385)   You have been asked to purify a tripeptide, aspartyl-aspartyl-arginine (asp-asp-arg), from some contaminant precursors. It has been suggested that electrophoresis in a buffer at a pH in which the tripeptide moves neither to the anode nor to the cathode will be effective as a purification procedure.

384. You should adjust the pH of the buffer to
  A. above the pK of the side chain of arg
  B. the pK of the side chain of arg
  C. a pH midway between the pK of arg and the pK of asp
  D. the pK of the side chain of asp
  E. a pH midway between the main chain carboxyl and the α-amino groups

385. At the pH you have selected, the main chain carboxyl and the α-amino groups
  A. will be each 50% charged and 50% uncharged
  B. will both be charged
  C. will both be uncharged
  D. will both be protonated
  E. will both be unprotonated

DIRECTIONS (386 through 425): Each group of questions below consists of lettered headings followed by a list of numbered words, phrases, or statements. For each numbered word, phrase, or statement, select the ONE lettered heading that is most closely associated with it. Each lettered heading may be used once, more than once, or not at all.

Questions 386 through 390

A. high glycine content
B. lysine–glucose condensation product
C. ε-lysine–pyridoxal phosphate condensation product
D. desmosine residue
E. γ-carboxyglutamate residue

386. Collagen

387. Hemoglobin A_{1c}

388. Elastin

389. Prothrombin

390. Glycogen phosphorylase

Questions 391 through 395

A. mRNA
B. tRNA
C. rRNA
D. nuclear DNA
E. mitochondrial DNA

391. CCA 3′-terminus

392. Organized into nucleosomes

393. Circular molecule

394. Poly A sequences

395. Pseudo-U bases

Questions 396 through 400

    A. ketogenesis
    B. fatty acid oxidation
    C. fatty acid synthesis
    D. cholesterol biosynthesis
    E. phospholipid biosynthesis

396. Hydroxymethylglutaryl-CoA reductase

397. Hydroxymethylglutaryl-CoA lyase

398. Acetyl-CoA carboxylase

399. Fatty acyl-CoA dehydrogenase (FAD-dependent)

400. S-Adenosylmethionine transferase

Questions 401 through 405

    A. glycolysis
    B. glyoxylate shunt
    C. anapleurosis
    D. tricarboxylic acid cycle
    E. pentose phosphate pathway

401. Pyruvate kinase

402. Pyruvate carboxylase

403. Enolase

404. Aconitase

405. Transaldolase

Questions 406 through 410

    A. serine
    B. lysine
    C. tryptophan
    D. phenylalanine
    E. histidine

406. Dehydratase

407. Dioxygenase

408. Deaminase

409. Hydroxylase

410. Dehydrogenase

Questions 411 through 415

    A. pK_a 4
    B. pK_a 6
    C. pK_a 8
    D. pK_a 10
    E. pK_a 12

411. β-Carboxyl group (aspartate)

412. Guanidino (arginine)

413. Sulfhydryl (cysteine)

414. Imidazole (histidine)

415. Phenol (tyrosine)

Questions 416 through 420

    A. enolase
    B. fatty acid-activating enzyme
    C. hexokinase
    D. ribonuclease A
    E. UDPG epimerase

416. Hydrolase

417. Isomerase

418. Ligase

419. Lyase

420. Transferase

Questions 421 through 425

    A. circular dichroism (CD)
    B. nuclear magnetic resonance (NMR)
    C. ultracentrifugation
    D. ultraviolet spectroscopy
    E. x-ray diffraction

421. Detect the ionization of a tyrosine residue

422. Detect an α-helix

423. Detect interatomic distances in solution

424. Determine molecular weight

425. Determine crystal structure

Biochemistry

Answers and Comments

276. (D) Actinomysin D intercalates with the bases in a DNA double helix, preventing its correct transcription. (**Ref. 2,** pp. 864–865; **Ref. 3,** pp. 516–517; **Ref. 5,** p. 412)

277. (C) S-Adenosyl methionine is the donor of methyl groups for synthesis of choline from ethanolamine as it is for most other biological methylations. (**Ref. 1,** p. 434; **Ref. 2,** p. 665; **Ref. 3,** p. 610; **Ref. 5,** p. 549)

278. (D) The type II pneumocyte forms phosphatidyl choline for surfactant synthesis by condensation of CDP-choline with diglycerides derived from phospholipids. (**Ref. 1,** pp. 432–434; **Ref. 2,** p. 665; **Ref. 3,** p. 609; **Ref. 4,** p. 242; **Ref. 5,** p. 550)

279. (E) Streptomycin interferes with recognition of codon and anticodon in prokaryotes, and allows a high level of incorrect pairings, leading to many incorrectly synthesized proteins. (**Ref. 1,** p. 744; **Ref. 2,** p. 928; **Ref. 3,** p. 987; **Ref. 5,** p. 759)

280. (A) The abnormally high levels of cyclic-AMP in the cells causes their continuous activation, with the resultant massive loss of fluid. (**Ref. 1,** p. 1065; **Ref. 2,** p. 774; **Ref. 3,** p. 800; **Ref. 4,** pp. 759–760; **Ref. 5,** pp. 982–983)

281. **(C)** Caffeine inhibits the breakdown of cyclic-AMP, thus elevating its levels in tissues and magnifying the effect of hormones that use cyclic-AMP as a second messenger. (**Ref. 3**, p. 774; **Ref. 4**, p. 263; **Ref. 5**, p. 464)

282. **(E)** The serine proteases all cleave peptide bonds by a common mechanism, in which a catalytic triad participates in a charge transfer system to relay the attraction of a proton from aspartate through the histidine to the hydroxyl group of serine, making that group exceptionally reactive toward the carbonyl group of a peptide bond, but also toward DFP and similar organophosphates. (**Ref. 1**, pp. 102–105, 175–177; **Ref. 3**, p. 386; **Ref. 4**, pp. 87–88; **Ref. 5**, p. 192)

283. **(A)** The Henderson–Hasselbalch equation applies: $pH = pK_a + \log([\text{salt}]/[\text{acid}])$. (**Ref. 1**, pp. 10–11; **Ref. 2**, p. 94; **Ref. 3**, p. 43; **Ref. 5**, pp. 41–42)

284. **(C)** There are several causes of the insufficiency of functional LDL receptors that is recognized as familial hypercholesterolemia, a group of autosomally dominant inherited disorders. Receptor synthesis may be defective, the receptor may fail to be inserted into the plasma membrane, or the receptor may be physically present but functionally inoperative. In the Watanabe hyperlipidemic rabbit, a deletion in the LDL receptor gene results in its failure to insert into the membrane. (**Ref. 1**, pp. 445–446; **Ref. 2**, p. 679; **Ref. 3**, pp. 628–629; **Ref. 4**, p. 256; **Ref. 5**, pp. 562–563)

285. **(D)** Vitamin D_3 (cholecalciferol, CC) is synthesized in the skin upon exposure to UV light, but is not biologically active until hydroxylated to the 25-hydroxy compound (25-HCC) in the liver, then again to the dihydroxy form, 1,25-DHCC, in the kidney. (**Ref. 1**, pp. 1121–1124; **Ref. 2**, p. 752; **Ref. 3**, p. 635; **Ref. 4**, p. 520; **Ref. 5**, p. 569)

286. **(A)** The Fe^{2+} ion in hemoglobin is coordinated by the four porphyrin pyrrole nitrogen atoms in one plane, and by a histidine imidazole nitrogen on one side of the porphyrin ring, leaving space for another ligand on the other side of the ring, which can be occupied by O_2 or CO. (**Ref. 3**, pp. 217–218; **Ref. 4**, pp. 50–51; **Ref. 5**, pp. 159–160)

287. **(E)** The conformational change associated with isomerization of opsin-bound 11-*cis*-retinal to all-*trans*-retinal causes it to dissociate from the protein, opsin. (**Ref. 1,** pp. 945–948; **Ref. 2,** p. 259; **Ref. 3,** p. 1051; **Ref. 4,** p. 589; **Ref. 5,** pp. 1031–1032)

288. **(B)** At the expense of the chemical energy of ATP, the biotin moiety of some carboxylases is carboxylated, and the carboxylate can then be transferred to an acceptor substrate. (**Ref. 2,** pp. 466–467; **Ref. 3,** p. 489; **Ref. 4,** pp. 212–213; **Ref. 5,** pp. 440–441)

289. **(C)** Catalase converts hydrogen peroxide to molecular oxygen and water. Peroxidases, on the other hand, catalyze the oxidation of substrates by hydrogen peroxide: $XH_2 + H_2O_2 \rightarrow 2\,H_2O + X$. (**Ref. 1,** p. 21; **Ref. 2,** p. 35; **Ref. 3,** pp. 368–369; **Ref. 4,** pp. 114–115; **Ref. 5,** p. 422)

290. **(A)** Trypsin is an endopeptidase—ie, unlike carboxypeptidases and aminopeptidases, which are exopeptidases (it cleaves internal peptide bonds of a polypeptide chain)—that cleaves arginyl- and lysyl- bonds in proteins, as well as in model compounds. Because the bonds it cleaves are of amino residues that are found on the surface of globular proteins, trypsin is quite active against native (un-denatured) protein substrates. (**Ref. 1,** p. 1074; **Ref. 2,** p. 510; **Ref. 3,** p. 146; **Ref. 4,** pp. 36–37; **Ref. 5,** p. 178)

291. **(A)** When the substrate and inhibitor compete for the same binding site, very high substrate concentrations may overcome the effect of the inhibitor. (**Ref. 1,** pp. 157–158; **Ref. 2,** p. 221; **Ref. 3,** pp. 382–383; **Ref. 4,** p. 83; **Ref. 5,** pp. 193–194)

292. **(B)** Typically, the first or committed step of a pathway (eg, carbamoyl phosphate synthetase) is regulated by a product of the pathway (eg, CTP). (**Ref. 1,** pp. 188–189; **Ref. 2,** p. 723; **Ref. 3,** pp. 390–392; **Ref. 4,** p. 99; **Ref. 5,** p. 609)

293. **(D)** For prokaryotic RNA polymerase to initiate transcription of a DNA template, it must bind at a region of the gene called the promoter. Binding of the polymerase to the promoter of the β-galactosidase gene is facilitated when a cyclic-AMP acceptor protein (CAP) is also present at this region of the DNA. (**Ref. 1,** pp. 813–815; **Ref. 2,** pp. 954–956; **Ref. 3,** p. 930; **Ref. 4,** pp. 435–437; **Ref. 5,** pp. 803–805)

294. **(C)** Regulation of RNA synthesis on a DNA template is considered to be control at the transcriptional level. The facilitation of RNA transcription, mediated by the cyclic-AMP/CAP complex at the promoter, is an example of positive transcriptional control. (**Ref. 1,** pp. 813–815; **Ref. 2,** pp. 954–956; **Ref. 3,** p. 930; **Ref. 4,** pp. 435–437; **Ref. 5,** pp. 803–805)

295. **(E)** An ε-lysine amino group of one chain displaces ammonia from the γ-carboxamide of a glutamine residue on a neighboring chain and forms an interchain lysyl-glutamate isopeptide crosslink. (**Ref. 1,** p. 968; **Ref. 4,** p. 681; **Ref. 5,** p. 250)

296. **(D)** The >C=O··HN< hydrogen bonds and restricted motion around prolyl and hydroxyprolyl residues lock collagen into its characteristic structure. (**Ref. 1,** pp. 62–65; **Ref. 3,** p. 183; **Ref. 4,** pp. 634–635; **Ref. 5,** p. 265)

297. **(B)** The assembly of gene segments to form immunoglobulin genes occurs uniquely in B lymphocytes. The genes for light chains of immunoglobulins are formed from V (variable), J (joining), and C (constant) segments. A separate set of V, D (diversity), J and C segments are assembled to encode heavy chains. (**Ref. 2,** pp. 848–850; **Ref. 3,** 884–886; **Ref. 5,** pp. 904–907)

298. **(A)** The rate of renaturation of double-strand DNA from its separated single strands depends on the degree of repetition of the nucleotide sequences. Highly repetitive single-strand DNA renatures most rapidly and at the lowest concentration. Because of its unusual composition, the highly repetitive DNA which is associated with the centromeres of chromosomes can be separated from the bulk of the genomic DNA and is called satellite DNA. (**Ref. 1,** p. 647; **Ref. 3,** p. 998; **Ref. 5,** p. 836)

299. **(A)** The light chain has one variable and one constant region; the heavy chain has one variable and three constant domains. (**Ref. 1,** pp. 93–95; **Ref. 2,** p. 848; **Ref. 3,** pp. 251–253; **Ref. 4,** pp. 672–673; **Ref. 5,** p. 900)

300. **(E)** Side chains that would otherwise decrease the entropy of the bulk water phase are segregated to the interior of the molecule, and the more polar groups are found on the exterior, where they interact with the bulk water phase by electrostatic, dipolar, and hydrogen bonding. (**Ref. 1,** pp. 30–31; **Ref. 2,** p. 163; **Ref. 3,** pp. 192–193; **Ref. 4,** p. 44; **Ref. 5,** p. 30)

301. **(C)** The enzyme transfers glycosyl bonds from a 4-hydroxyl group of one glucose residue to a 6-hydroxyl group of a neighboring glucose residue of glycogen. (**Ref. 1,** p. 344; **Ref. 2,** p. 613; **Ref. 3,** p. 551; **Ref. 4,** pp. 181–182; **Ref. 5,** p. 457)

302. **(C)** Transamination of α-ketoglutarate gives rise to glutamate, and the other 5-carbon amino acids, glutamine, proline, and arginine are all synthesized from it. Transamination of oxaloacetate yields aspartate, which can be amidated to form asparagine. Note that threonine and valine are essential amino acids in man, and that tyrosine is synthesized only by hydroxylation of phenylalanine, another essential amino acid. (**Ref. 2,** p. 697; **Ref. 3,** p. 705; **Ref. 4,** pp. 287–289; **Ref. 5,** p. 579)

303. **(D)** Glucose-1-P is a metabolite of the pathways of glycogen synthesis and breakdown; glucose-6-phosphate is a metabolite of the pathways of glycolysis and gluconeogenesis. The two glucose-phosphates are interconverted by phosphoglucomutase. (**Ref. 1,** pp. 298–303; **Ref. 2,** p. 402; **Ref. 3,** pp. 438–441; **Ref. 4,** p. 174; **Ref. 5,** pp. 356–357)

304. **(B)** Peroxide generated by metabolism of the drug consumes reduced glutathione, which is needed for maintenance of the normal reducing atmosphere in the cell. When the dehydrogenase is defective, normal activities of the cell are impaired. (**Ref. 1,** p. 362; **Ref. 3,** pp. 500–501; **Ref. 4,** p. 692; **Ref. 5,** pp. 436–437)

305. **(E)** Mitochondrial pyruvate is carboxylated to oxaloacetate, which passes into the cytosol by being first reduced to malate (which crosses the mitochondrial membrane) then being reoxidized. Finally, oxaloacetate is converted to phosphoenolpyruvate in the PEP carboxykinase reaction. (**Ref. 1,** pp. 327–328; **Ref. 2,** p. 603; **Ref. 3,** pp. 488–490; **Ref. 4,** pp. 190–191; **Ref. 5,** p. 439)

306. (C) The reaction proceeds by transfer of one phosphate from glucose diphosphate to a serine residue on the enzyme, forming one of the monophosphate products. The phosphoenzyme then transfers its phosphate to the glucose monophosphate substrate, reforming the diphosphate and completing the catalytic cycle. **(Ref. 1,** pp. 340–341; **Ref. 2,** p. 422; **Ref. 3,** pp. 461–462; **Ref. 4,** p. 181; **Ref. 5,** p. 454)

307. (D) In myocardial ischemia, perfusion, hence oxygenation of cardiac tissue, is inadequate. Under these conditions, generation of ATP by aerobic metabolism comes to a halt, and further ATP synthesis by anaerobic glycolysis may only very briefly support the energy needs of the heart. Glucose, galactose, fructose, and glycerol can all be catabolized via anaerobic glycolysis, but fatty acids can be used as sources of ATP only when the electron transport pathway of the mitochondria carries out oxidative phosphorylation. **(Ref. 2,** pp. 485–486; **Ref. 3,** pp. 578–584; **Ref. 4,** pp. 221–223; **Ref. 5,** pp. 475–476)

308. (D) Polyamines, such as spermine, spermidine, and putrescine, interact strongly with nucleic acids by Coulombic forces, and have been implicated in a number of nucleic acid regulatory reactions. **(Ref. 1,** pp. 503–504; **Ref. 2,** p. 715; **Ref. 3,** p. 714; **Ref. 4,** p. 328)

309. (A) Elevated levels of acetyl-CoA stimulate synthesis of oxaloacetate, which is oxidized via the tricarboxylic acid cycle, or is converted to phosphoenolpyruvate via anapleurotic reactions. **(Ref. 1,** p. 335; **Ref. 2,** p. 465; **Ref. 3,** p. 548; **Ref. 4,** p. 193; **Ref. 5,** p. 441)

310. (A) Several forms of the deficiency have been described, the partial deficiency being especially prominent among non-Caucasians. The undigested lactose becomes a substrate for bacterial fermentation in the lumen of the intestines, which causes many of the symptoms of lactose intolerance. **(Ref. 1,** p. 1079; **Ref. 2,** p. 424; **Ref. 3,** pp. 457–458; **Ref. 4,** p. 619)

311. (B) The symptoms of alkaptonuria are due to the failure to catabolize tyrosine beyond the intermediate, homogentisic acid, as a result of a deficiency of a dioxygenase. Albinism is due to the failure to convert tyrosine to melanin as a result of a deficiency of the enzyme tyrosinase. (**Ref. 1**, p. 508; **Ref. 2**, p. 531; **Ref. 3**, p. 725; **Ref. 4**, pp. 310–311; **Ref. 5**, p. 513)

312. **(E)** Citrate signals a sufficient rate of formation of Ac-CoA and limits the rate of glycolysis. Similarly, AMP signals an inadequate level of phosphorylation (of ADP), and by stimulating phosphofructokinase, provides the substrates of the tricarboxylic acid cycle and oxidative phosphorylation. In a parallel example, a sufficiency of CTP limits the activity of the carbamoyl synthetase that initiates the pyrimidine biosynthetic pathway. (**Ref. 1**, pp. 312–313; **Ref. 2**, pp. 407, 568; **Ref. 3**, p. 452; **Ref. 4**, p. 194; **Ref. 5**, pp. 359–360)

313. **(B)** Glycogen is extended by the UDP-glucose donation of its glucosyl group to the free C-4 hydroxyl group of the non-reducing end of the primer. (**Ref. 1**, pp. 343–344; **Ref. 2**, pp. 612–613; **Ref. 3**, pp. 550–551; **Ref. 4**, p. 181; **Ref. 5**, p. 455)

314. **(D)** The oligosaccharide is assembled on a dolichol pyrophosphate carrier in the endoplasmic reticulum, then transferred to the protein. The glycocalyx is further refined (monosaccharide groups removed and added) in the Golgi apparatus. (**Ref. 1**, pp. 376–378; **Ref. 2**, p. 931; **Ref. 3**, pp. 560–561; **Ref. 4**, pp. 626–630; **Ref. 5**, pp. 773–774)

315. **(C)** When electron transport is not restrained by the availability of ADP and phosphate, oxidation (ie, electron transport) is, by definition, uncoupled from phosphorylation. (**Ref. 1**, p. 283; **Ref. 2**, p. 556; **Ref. 3**, p. 524; **Ref. 4**, p. 127; **Ref. 5**, pp. 421–422)

316. **(B)** Marfan's disease, a disorder of connective tissue, is due to a defect in collagen synthesis at the level of processing of the procollagen chains. (**Ref. 1**, p. 761; **Ref. 4**, pp. 637–638)

317. **(C)** Malonate, the 3-carbon dicarboxylic acid, is a competitive inhibitor of succinic dehydrogenase, differing from the normal substrate by having only one methylene group. (**Ref. 1**, p. 259; **Ref. 2**, pp. 457–458; **Ref. 3**, p. 471; **Ref. 4**, p. 124; **Ref. 5**, pp. 192–193)

318. **(B)** Both CO_2 molecules are formed in dehydrogenase steps, the first by a β-oxidative decarboxylation, the second by an α-oxidative decarboxylation. (**Ref. 1**, pp. 256–257; **Ref. 2**, p. 453; **Ref. 3**, pp. 481–483; **Ref. 4**, pp. 166–167; **Ref. 5**, pp. 375–376)

319. **(B)** During electron transport, separation of the transfer of hydrogen atoms from the transfer of electrons down the electron transport chain generates a proton gradient, which is used to drive the phosphorylation of ADP. (**Ref. 1**, p. 285; **Ref. 2**, p. 560; **Ref. 3**, p. 528; **Ref. 4**, p. 127; **Ref. 5**, p. 421)

320. **(C)** Cyanide, by complexing with the heme iron of reduced cytochrome oxidase, prevents its reoxidation by oxygen. Azide (N_3^-) acts in the same way. (**Ref. 1**, p. 281; **Ref. 2**, p. 556; **Ref. 3**, p. 517; **Ref. 4**, p. 124; **Ref. 5**, p. 413)

321. **(C)** Cholesterol, or a closely related metabolite, blocks the first committed step in its own biosynthetic pathway, the formation of mevalonic acid from hydroxymethyl-glutaryl-CoA. (**Ref. 1**, p. 441; **Ref. 2**, p. 679; **Ref. 3**, p. 626; **Ref. 4**, pp. 269–270; **Ref. 5**, p. 560)

322. **(E)** The chylomicrons contain triglycerides, resynthesized from partially digested dietary lipid components after they have passed across the intestinal mucosa. (**Ref. 1**, p. 1087; **Ref. 2**, p. 481; **Ref. 4**, pp. 253–254; **Ref. 5**, pp. 560–561)

323. **(C)** Lecithin-cholesterol acyl transferase (LCAT) facilitates "reverse transport of cholesterol," ie, from peripheral tissues to liver, by transferring a long-chain fatty acyl group from HDL phosphatidyl-choline (lecithin) to free cholesterol. The resulting cholesterol ester enters the interior of the HDL particle, in which form it is transported to the liver for further processing, eg, to bile acids. (**Ref. 1**, pp. 446–447; **Ref. 2**, p. 677; **Ref. 3**, p. 627; **Ref. 4**, pp. 270–271)

324. **(B)** Transesterification allows fatty acyl groups to traverse the mitochondrial membrane as carnitine esters; carnitine being exchanged for CoA before transport, and CoA for carnitine after transport. (**Ref. 1**, pp. 408–409; **Ref. 2**, p. 485; **Ref. 3**, p. 580; **Ref. 4**, p. 221; **Ref. 5**, pp. 473–475)

325. **(E)** An activating enzyme and the tRNA it recognizes are specific for only one amino acid, ensuring that the correct amino acid is matched to a tRNA that bears the correct codon. (**Ref. 1,** pp. 687–688; **Ref. 2,** pp. 910–913; **Ref. 3,** pp. 962–963; **Ref. 4,** pp. 421–422; **Ref. 5,** pp. 743–744)

326. **(B)** This is called semi-conservative replication. Each double helix is composed of the template and the product of a polymerase reaction. (**Ref. 1,** pp. 663–664; **Ref. 2,** p. 817; **Ref. 3,** pp. 819–821; **Ref. 5,** pp. 79–81)

327. **(D)** An amino acid activating enzyme forms an amino acyl-AMP and then transfers the amino acyl moiety to the cognate tRNA. Because the acyl-AMP intermediate is so reactive, it can exist only in a protected (from water) pocket on the surface of the enzyme. (**Ref. 1,** pp. 682–688; **Ref. 2,** p. 913; **Ref. 3,** pp. 962–963; **Ref. 4,** pp. 421–422; **Ref. 5,** pp. 734–735)

328. **(E)** Ornithine condenses with carbamoyl phosphate to form citrulline, which then combines with aspartic acid to form argininosuccinate. This is cleaved to arginine, which is then hydrolyzed to urea and ornithine. (**Ref. 1,** pp. 481–485; **Ref. 2,** p. 518; **Ref. 3,** p. 689; **Ref. 4,** pp. 299–300; **Ref. 5,** pp. 500–502)

329. **(C)** De novo methylation of methionine involves (a) reduction of the one-carbon tetrahydrofolate species to the level of methyl tetrahydrofolate and (b) vitamin B_{12} catalyzed transfer of the methyl group to the sulfur of homocysteine. (**Ref. 1,** pp. 501–504; **Ref. 2,** p. 702; **Ref. 3,** p. 697; **Ref. 5,** pp. 582–583)

330. **(B)** Serine donates its hydroxymethyl group to tetrahydrofolic acid, its C-1, C-2, and N becoming glycine. (**Ref. 1,** pp. 516–518; **Ref. 2,** p. 524; **Ref. 3,** pp. 696–699; **Ref. 4,** p. 302; **Ref. 5,** p. 580)

331. **(B)** The disease is due to a hereditary deficiency of phenylalanine hydroxylase activity or to the metabolism of the biopterin cofactor. (**Ref. 1,** pp. 506–507; **Ref. 2,** p. 529; **Ref. 3,** pp. 722–723; **Ref. 4,** p. 312; **Ref. 5,** p. 513)

332. **(E)** The carotenes can be cleaved to yield retinal, vitamin A alcohol, which is phosphorylated and converted to other related metabolites. (**Ref. 1**, pp. 1118–1119; **Ref. 2**, pp. 259–260; **Ref. 3**, p. 635; **Ref. 4**, p. 588; **Ref. 5**, pp. 324, 571)

333. **(D)** Coenzyme A is composed of adenosine-3,5-diphosphate, β-alanine, cysteamine, and phosphopantothenic acid. It is in a thioester linkage to the sulfhydryl group of the pantetheine moiety that carboxylic acids are activated. (**Ref. 1**, p. 1132; **Ref. 2**, p. 448; **Ref. 3**, p. 470; **Ref. 4**, pp. 577–578; **Ref. 5**, p. 323)

334. **(C)** A glycoprotein, intrinsic factor which normally aids absorption, is absent in pernicious anemia, so vitamin B_{12} cannot be absorbed by the gut. (**Ref. 1**, pp. 1134–1135; **Ref. 2**, p. 496; **Ref. 3**, p. 700; **Ref. 4**, pp. 581–583; **Ref. 5**, p. 509)

335. **(A)** This severe protein deficiency appears in parts of the world where the diet is almost exclusively cereal or other starchy food. The specific symptoms of kwashiorkor develop rapidly in the malnourished state, and may be due to an inability to withstand normal oxidative stresses. (**Ref. 1**, p. 557; **Ref. 4**, pp. 758–759)

336. **(B)** The final stage in the synthesis of calcium-binding proteins, notably blood-clotting factors II, VII, IX, and X, is the vitamin K-dependent carboxylation of several glutamic acid side chains. (**Ref. 1**, p. 1125; **Ref. 2**, p. 926; **Ref. 3**, pp. 636; **Ref. 4**, pp. 594–596; **Ref. 5**, pp. 251–252)

337. **(C)** Nitrogen balance is the relation of dietary to excreted nitrogen, being positive when there is a net retention of nitrogen, and negative when there is a net loss. (**Ref. 1**, p. 477; **Ref. 3**, p. 680; **Ref. 4**, p. 293; **Ref. 5**, p. 578)

338. **(A)** Cyclic-AMP relieves the inhibition of a protein kinase that when activated, phosphorylates glycogen phosphorylase kinase. This in turn, activates glycogen phosphorylase by phosphorylating it. (**Ref. 1**, pp. 353–355; **Ref. 2**, pp. 765–766; **Ref. 3**, pp. 552–555; **Ref. 4**, pp. 183–184; **Ref. 5**, p. 459)

339. **(C)** The DNA double helix has polydeoxynucleotide strands that run anti-parallel to each other, ie, in the direction that one strand has 5′ to 3′ diester linkages, the other has 3′ to 5′ linkages.

(**Ref. 1,** p. 618; **Ref. 2,** pp. 334–335; **Ref. 3,** pp. 101, 104; **Ref. 4,** pp. 378–379; **Ref. 5,** pp. 76–77)

340. (D) The most oxidized purine, uric acid, cannot be further catabolized by primates. Although of limited solubility, it is normally excreted in the urine. (**Ref. 1,** p. 544; **Ref. 2,** 727–728; **Ref. 3,** p. 751; **Ref. 4,** p. 379; **Ref. 5,** pp. 618–619)

341. (D) A purine is returned to the pool of metabolites able to participate in biosynthetic and other reactions, by accepting a ribose moiety from ribose-1-P to yield a nucleoside and phosphate; eg, guanidine + ribose-1-P → guanosine + phosphate. (**Ref. 1,** pp. 544–545; **Ref. 2,** p. 729; **Ref. 3,** pp. 744–745; **Ref. 4,** pp. 367, 373; **Ref. 5,** p. 606)

342. (B), 343. (D) Succinyl-CoA condenses with glycine to form δ-amino levulinic acid, two molecules of which condense to form the pyrrole compound shown, porphobilinogen, an intermediate in the biosynthesis of porphyrins. (**Ref. 1,** pp. 1009–1010; **Ref. 2,** pp. 710–711; **Ref. 3,** pp. 731–733; **Ref. 4,** pp. 339–340; **Ref. 5,** pp. 594–595)

344. (B) The standard redox potential, $\mathscr{E}°$, is related to the standard free energy, $\Delta G°'$, by the equation $\Delta G°' = -n\mathscr{F}\Delta\mathscr{E}°'$, where n is the number of electrons and $\mathscr{F}$ is the Faraday constant, 96,500 J/mol/V. (**Ref. 1,** pp. 270–272; **Ref. 2,** pp. 387–389; **Ref. 3,** pp. 508–510; **Ref. 5,** pp. 399–400)

345. (D) The mitochondrial NADH dehydrogenase is a multi-subunit complex of polypeptides containing both FMN and non-heme iron (NHI) protein. Electrons flow from NADH to FMN to NHI to coenzyme Q. The hydrogen atoms themselves do not pass from FMN to NHI, nor from NHI to CoQ. (**Ref. 1,** pp. 277–281; **Ref. 2,** pp. 545–546; **Ref. 3,** pp. 510–512; **Ref. 4,** p. 121; **Ref. 5,** pp. 402–403)

346. (C) Because the electrons from the oxidation of succinate enter the electron transport chain at the level of coenzyme Q, only two ATPs, not three, are synthesized per atom of oxygen consumed. (**Ref. 1,** pp. 279–284; **Ref. 2,** pp. 565–566; **Ref. 3,** pp. 520–521; **Ref. 4,** p. 123; **Ref. 5,** p. 412)

347. **(C)** Phosphatidyl serine, phosphatidyl inositol, and gangliosides are all negatively charged phospholipids, due to the phosphate group; phosphatidyl choline is a zwitterion. Ceramide is N-acyl sphingosine, neutral lipid. (**Ref. 1**, pp. 450–451; **Ref. 2**, p. 250; **Ref. 3**, p. 305; **Ref. 4**, p. 148; **Ref. 5**, p. 552)

348. **(B)** Under these conditions (1 M, pH 7, etc.) $\mathscr{E}' = \mathscr{E}^{o\prime}$. The $\Delta\mathscr{E}^{o\prime}$ is $(+0.03) - (-0.35) = +0.38$ V, so fumarate will oxidize β-hydroxybutyrate to acetoacetate. (**Ref. 1**, pp. 272, 280; **Ref. 2**, pp. 387–388; **Ref. 3**, pp. 508–510; **Ref. 4**, pp. 112–113; **Ref. 5**, pp. 399–401)

349. **(B)** At the active site of the serine proteases is a serine residue, which in the first phase of catalysis is poised to displace the nascent N-terminal amino group of the substrate and form an ester with the emerging C-terminal group. The serine hydroxyl group is polarized by an aspartate β-carboxylate group, whose negative charge is relayed through an imidazole. The three residues at the active site, serine, histidine, and aspartate, are termed the catalytic triad. (**Ref. 1**, pp. 102–105; **Ref. 2**, p. 510; **Ref. 3**, pp. 395–396; **Ref. 4**, p. 611; **Ref. 5**, p. 246)

350. **(C)** Classical non-competitive inhibition is achieved via interference with catalysis alone while substrate binding is unaffected. Unlike in competitive inhibition, the inhibitor does not occupy the substrate-binding site. (**Ref. 1**, p. 158; **Ref. 2**, p. 220; **Ref. 3**, p. 384; **Ref. 4**, p. 83; **Ref. 5**, pp. 193–194)

351. **(E)** The dissociation constant for a substrate from an enzyme, K_s, is a true equilibrium constant. The Michaelis constant, K_m, is a ratio of kinetic constants for the synthesis and breakdown (forward to products or backward to reactants) of the enzyme–substrate complex: when the steady-state concentration of the ES complex is far from its equilibrium value, K_s and K_m are significantly different. (**Ref. 1**, pp. 146–147; **Ref. 2**, p. 216; **Ref. 3**, pp. 358–360; **Ref. 4**, p. 81; **Ref. 5**, pp. 190–191)

352. **(C)** K_m may be evaluated as the value of the substrate concentration at which the velocity is equal to half its limiting maximum value (V_{max}). (**Ref. 1**, pp. 146–148; **Ref. 2**, p. 214; **Ref. 3**, p. 362; **Ref. 4**, pp. 80–81; **Ref. 5**, p. 189)

353. (C) In the Lineweaver–Burk plot (1/v vs. 1/S), the slope is K_m/V_{max}, and the x-intercept is $-1/K_m$. The K_m for mannose is greater than that for glucose, suggesting that mannose is bound to the enzyme less tightly. (**Ref. 1**, pp. 146–148; **Ref. 2**, pp. 215–216; **Ref. 3**, p. 362; **Ref. 4**, pp. 80–81; **Ref. 5**, p. 189)

354. (D) Formation of the biosynthetic isoprene unit, isopentenyl pyrophosphate, proceeds from HMG-CoA by reduction to mevalonic acid, then the expenditure of 3 ATPs to add to it 2 phosphate groups and to extract from it the elements of H_2O and CO_2. (**Ref. 1**, pp. 440–442; **Ref. 2**, p. 670–672; **Ref. 3**, p. 624; **Ref. 4**, pp. 266–268; **Ref. 5**, pp. 555–556)

355. (C) α-Ketoglutarate dehydrogenase is very similar to pyruvate dehydrogenase. It decarboxylates the substrate and attaches the remainder, which is on the oxidation level of an aldehyde, to TPP, before transferring it to oxidized lipoic acid and then to the sulfhydryl groups of coenzyme A. (**Ref. 1**, p. 362; **Ref. 2**, pp. 455–456; **Ref. 3**, pp. 482–483; **Ref. 4**, p. 166; **Ref. 5**, pp. 382–383)

356. (C) The carboxylation of the α carbon of propionyl-CoA, like that of acetyl-CoA, requires a biotin cofactor. Energy for the reaction is supplied by the ATP, required in the prior carboxylation of biotin. (**Ref. 1**, p. 494; **Ref. 2**, p. 493; **Ref. 3**, p. 586; **Ref. 4**, p. 192; **Ref. 5**, p. 506)

357. (D) Normally, small amounts of elastase are kept in check by circulating inhibitors. In the case of the hereditary deficiency of α_1-antiproteinase, there is no such protection, and the elastin of the connective tissue, especially in the lung, is destroyed by elastase. (**Ref. 2**, p. 235; **Ref. 4**, p. 671; **Ref. 5**, pp. 247–248)

358. (D) Bile acids are amphipathic molecules, having polar and non-polar sides. As such, they form an interface between the polar globules of dietary triglycerides and the aqueous digestive fluid. (**Ref. 1**, pp. 1083–1085; **Ref. 2**, pp. 480–481; **Ref. 3**, p. 574; **Ref. 4**, p. 611; **Ref. 5**, p. 559)

359. (A) Phenylalanine hydroxylase is a mixed function oxygenase. The two substrates that are oxidized are phenylalanine, becoming tyrosine, and a tetrahydrobiopterin cofactor, which must be reduced (by NADPH) to continue the catalytic cycle. (**Ref. 1**, p. 506; **Ref. 2**, pp. 529–530; **Ref. 3**, p. 722; **Ref. 4**, p. 291; **Ref. 5**, p. 511)

360. (D) The carbamoyl phosphate synthetase of pyrimidine biosynthesis is distinct from the one involved in urea biosynthesis. The remaining atoms of the pyrimidine ring are furnished by aspartate. (**Ref. 1**, pp. 547–549; **Ref. 2**, p. 722; **Ref. 3**, pp. 679–680; **Ref. 4**, pp. 369–370; **Ref. 5**, pp. 607–609)

361. (D) Pellagra is a dietary niacin deficiency. The vitamin is incorporated into pyrimidine nucleotides, which serve as cofactors in dehydrogenase and mixed function oxygenase reactions. Another source of the pyrimidine nucleus is tryptophan, but the rate of conversion of tryptophan to niacin is quite slow. In any case, a diet deficient in niacin is unlikely to be adequate in tryptophan. (**Ref. 1**, p. 1129; **Ref. 3**, p. 726; **Ref. 4**, p. 577; **Ref. 5**, p. 617)

362. (B) For activation of acetoacetate, ie, conversion to acetoacetyl-CoA, there is a transfer of the CoA moiety from the succinyl group of succinyl-CoA to acetoacetate, yielding succinate and acetoacetyl-CoA. (**Ref. 1**, p. 416; **Ref. 2**, p. 500; **Ref. 3**, p. 589; **Ref. 4**, pp. 226–227; **Ref. 5**, p. 479)

363. (B) Chymotrypsin cleaves peptide bonds involving aromatic amino acids, ie, phenylalanyl-, tryptophanyl-, and tyrosyl-bonds. As the new *N*-terminal amino acid is glycine, there must have been a phe-gly or trp-gly peptide bond in the pentapeptide. (**Ref. 1**, p. 46; **Ref. 2**, p. 510; **Ref. 3**, p. 146; **Ref. 4**, p. 611; **Ref. 5**, pp. 220–221)

364. (B) FDNB, the Sanger reagent, will react with the free (secondary) amino group of proline. Other options are *N*-blocked. Cystamine has no carboxyl group and therefore cannot be an *N*-terminal residue. (**Ref. 2**, pp. 148–149; **Ref. 3**, p. 164; **Ref. 4**, p. 36; **Ref. 5**, pp. 52–53)

365. (E) The enzyme has two activities. It first converts arachidonic acid (or some closely similar 20-carbon multiply-unsaturated acids) to prostaglandin G_2, which possesses an endoperoxidase bridge across the cyclopentane nucleus, and a peroxide function on C-15. In the second activity, it converts prostaglandin G_2 to prostaglandin H_2, which has a hydroxyl in place of the peroxide at C-15. (**Ref. 1,** pp. 462–464; **Ref. 2,** pp. 656–657; **Ref. 3,** pp. 639–641; **Ref. 4,** pp. 236–237; **Ref. 5,** pp. 990–991)

366. **(D)** Proline may be oxidized and the ring opened to form glutamic semi-aldehyde. This can be transaminated to ornithine, which condenses with carbamoyl phosphate to form citrulline. (**Ref. 1,** pp. 498–500; **Ref. 2,** pp. 518–519, 532; **Ref. 4,** pp. 300, 306; **Ref. 5,** pp. 505, 579)

367. **(E)** Myosin and actin contain 3-methyl histidine. As it is not catabolized, its appearance in the urine can be used as a measure of the turnover of muscle protein. (**Ref. 1,** p. 959; **Ref. 4,** p. 661)

368. **(B)** The 3-carbon fragment of phenylalanine is shortened, and the aromatic ring of phenylalanine is oxidized and opened to form fumaroyl acetoacetate. When cleaved, it yields the ketone, acetoacetate, and fumarate, which is glucogenic. (**Ref. 1,** pp. 506–507; **Ref. 2,** pp. 529, 537; **Ref. 3,** p. 687; **Ref. 4,** pp. 312–313; **Ref. 5,** p. 503)

369. **(D)** Cysteine may have the elements of H_2S abstracted from it to form pyruvate. The reaction is analogous to the abstraction of H_2O from serine. (**Ref. 1,** p. 504; **Ref. 2,** p. 526; **Ref. 3,** p. 716; **Ref. 4,** pp. 307–308; **Ref. 5,** p. 504)

370. **(A)** Brown adipose tissue is characterized by a high level of mitochondria, whose cytochromes give it its characteristic color. Uncoupled electron transport generates heat (rather than chemical energy) and so the tissue is thermogenic. (**Ref. 1,** pp. 1101–1102; **Ref. 2,** pp. 566–567; **Ref. 3,** p. 525; **Ref. 4,** pp. 264–265; **Ref. 5,** pp. 421–422)

371. **(C)** Typical intermediates are protease zymogens, which upon limited proteolysis by an activated protease higher in the hierarchy of factors, itself becomes an active protease and can act upon a factor lower in the hierarchy. Because the actions of the factors are catalytic, there is an amplification of the effect at each stage.

(**Ref. 1,** pp. 96, 966–973; **Ref. 3,** p. 399; **Ref. 4,** pp. 678–679; **Ref. 5,** pp. 248, 899)

372. (**D**)   Unless inositol is recycled into inositol phosphatephospholipids, hormone sensitive cells become depleted of the precursor of inositol triphosphate and diacylglycerol second messengers. Li^+ prevents this recycling and reduces the ability of such cells to respond to stimuli. (**Ref. 1,** pp. 873–875; **Ref. 3,** p. 805; **Ref. 5,** p. 987)

373. (**D**)   The enzyme oxidizes inosinic acid (formed by deamination of adenine) to hypoxanthine (which is also formed by deamination of guanine) and oxidizes hypoxanthine to uric acid. In humans, uric acid is not metabolized further. (**Ref. 1,** p. 546; **Ref. 2,** p. 728; **Ref. 3,** p. 751; **Ref. 4,** p. 372; **Ref. 5,** p. 619)

374. (**D**)   Hormone stimulation of some cells activates a phospholipase C (PLC), which hydrolyzes phosphatidyl inositol diphosphate, generating inositol triphosphate (IP_3) and diacyl glycerol (DAG). IP_3 can cause the release of sequestered Ca^{2+} into the cytosol, and DAG activates a Ca^{2+}-dependent protein kinase. The synergistic action of the two products of PLC promotes phosphorylation of proteins that are responsible for the physiological response for which the cell has been programmed. (**Ref. 1,** pp. 873–875; **Ref. 2,** p. 771; **Ref. 3,** pp. 494–497; **Ref. 4,** pp. 684–685; **Ref. 5,** pp. 985–987)

375. (**E**)   Non-coding regions (introns) are excised from primary transcripts, as the remaining expressed sequences (exons) are spliced together. (**Ref. 1,** pp. 715–716; **Ref. 2,** p. 866; **Ref. 3,** pp. 1020–1022; **Ref. 4,** pp. 413–414; **Ref. 5,** pp. 722–723)

376. (**B**)   The nucleosome is a packaging of DNA into compact structures. The double helix is wound one and a half times around a complex of histones, which being basic, neutralize the charge of the phosphate groups. The string of nucleosomes may, itself, be wound into a higher order packaging unit by being turned into wide loops that are stacked in a large coil. (**Ref. 1,** pp. 638–640; **Ref. 2,** pp. 806–807; **Ref. 3,** pp. 1003–1005; **Ref. 4,** pp. 388–389; **Ref. 5,** pp. 827–829)

377. (A) Spectrin is a tetramer of two dissimilar subunits. Its ends can associate with each other intermolecularly and form a flexible webbing underneath the membrane of the erythrocyte. (**Ref. 1,** p. 212; **Ref. 2,** p. 281; **Ref. 3,** pp. 314–316; **Ref. 4,** pp. 694–695; **Ref. 5,** pp. 305–307)

378. (D) The 3′-hydroxyl group of the growing polynucleotide displaces a pyrophosphate from each added deoxyribonucleotide triphosphate. (**Ref. 1,** p. 665; **Ref. 2,** p. 820; **Ref. 3,** p. 840; **Ref. 4,** p. 397; **Ref. 5,** p. 672)

379. (A) Restriction endonucleases cleave at regions of symmetry, 4 to 8 base pairs long, in a DNA molecule. The requirement for symmetry means the sequence of one strand (3′ to 5′) must be the same as the antiparallel strand (also read 3′ to 5′). (**Ref. 1,** pp. 642–643; **Ref. 2,** pp. 986–987; **Ref. 3,** pp. 863–867; **Ref. 4,** pp. 452–453; **Ref. 5,** pp. 858–859)

380. (D) Glycolysis is a cytosolic function. It generates pyruvate that can be reduced to lactate, or transported into mitochondria for oxidation. (**Ref. 1,** p. 188; **Ref. 2,** p. 544; **Ref. 3,** p. 436; **Ref. 4,** p. 9)

381. (A) Non-heme iron undergoes oxidation-reduction cycles by changing the valence state of the iron atom, as do the cytochromes. Other electron carriers attach one (eg, NAD^+ to NADH) or two (FAD to $FADH_2$) hydrogen atoms. (**Ref. 1,** pp. 275–276; **Ref. 2,** pp. 547–548; **Ref. 3,** p. 511; **Ref. 4,** pp. 121–122; **Ref. 5,** p. 403)

382. (A) Phosphofructokinase converts fructose-6-phosphate to fructose-1,6-diphosphate. A high energy bond of ATP is consumed to form the phosphate ester bond, the remaining energy appearing as heat. As humans, for example, homeotherms, ie, we exist at a constant temperature. We have no possibility of storing heat energy, and have no way to reverse the reaction such as this. (**Ref. 1,** pp. 299–300; **Ref. 2,** pp. 407, 604; **Ref. 3,** p. 440; **Ref. 4,** p. 121; **Ref. 5,** p. 359)

383. (B) The conversion of fructose-1,6-diphosphate to fructose-6-phosphate is not a reverse of the kinase reaction. The phosphate is not incorporated into ATP, but is released as inorganic phosphate. (**Ref. 1,** pp. 317–322; **Ref. 2,** p. 604; **Ref. 3,** p. 542; **Ref. 4,** pp. 190–192; **Ref. 5,** pp. 439–440)

384. (D), 385. (B) The tripeptide asp-asp-arg will be at its isoelectric point when it has two negative charges and two positive charges. This condition is achieved by adjusting the pH so that the guanidinium and main chain carboxyl and amino groups are both charged and half the aspartic side chains are charged, ie, the pH = pK_a of the aspartic acid β-carboxyl group. (**Ref. 1,** pp. 36–38; **Ref. 3,** pp. 48–49; **Ref. 4,** pp. 22–25; **Ref. 5,** pp. 21, 41–42)

386. (A), 387. (B), 388. (D), 389. (E), 390. (C) The lettered amino acid modifications or secondary structures are characteristic of the numbered proteins. As the side chain of every third residue of each collagen chain in a triple helix is directed inward, only glycine, with a hydrogen atom side chain, is compatible with this requirement. Blood glucose slowly condenses, non-enzymatically, with the *N*-terminal lysines of hemoglobin A. Elastin is cross-linked into a resilient network by conversion of some lysine side chain amino groups to aldehyde functions and condensation with the amino groups of other lysine side chains. The vitamin K-dependent addition of carboxylate groups to glutamate side chains is characteristic of several Ca^{2+}-binding proteins. Glycogen phosphorylase has a covalently bound pyridoxal phosphate, which participates in catalysis. (**Ref. 1,** pp. 61–66, 971–972, 1030–1031; **Ref. 2,** pp. 118, 172, 175, 422; **Ref. 4,** pp. 58, 579, 596–597, 634–635, 637; **Ref. 5,** pp. 251–252, 262, 275, 452, 642; **Ref. 5,** pp. 252, 262, 274–275, 452, 642)

391. (B), 392. (D), 393. (E), 394. (A), 395. (B) The numbered characteristics apply to the various types of lettered nucleic acids. Primary transcripts are modified in several ways before becoming mature mRNA, among them addition of poly-A tails to the 5′-end. tRNA is also modified, notably in the formation of several unusual bases and the formation of a pCpCpA sequence at the 3′-end. Mitochondrial DNA resembles bacterial DNA in several respects, among them its circular structure. Nuclear DNA is condensed into nucleosomes, which are packed in a solenoidal array into chromosomes. (**Ref. 1,** pp. 638–641, 687–695; **Ref. 2,**

pp. 795, 807, 872, 876–877; **Ref. 3,** pp. 853, 948, 960, 1004, 1019–1020; **Ref. 4,** pp. 388–389, 413–415, 745; **Ref. 5,** pp. 713, 721, 739–742, 826–829, 833)

396. (D), **397.** (A), **398.** (C), **399.** (B), **400.** (E) These numbered enzymes are characteristic of the lettered metabolic pathways. HMG-CoA is reduced for the synthesis of mevalonic acid in the formation of isopentenyl-pyrophosphate, the biosynthetic isoprene unit of terpene (sterol) synthesis, or it is cleaved to acetoacetate and acetyl-CoA for ketogenesis. Acetyl-CoA is carboxylated for formation of malonyl units for extension of growing fatty acyl chains. Desaturation of fatty acyl-CoA is effected by an FAD-linked dehydrogenase. Conversion of phosphatidyl ethanolamine to phosphatidyl choline depends upon the addition of methyl groups from S-adenosyl methionine. (**Ref. 1,** pp. 393, 409, 415, 434, 441; **Ref. 2,** pp. 486, 500, 643, 665, 670; **Ref. 3,** pp. 582, 589, 591, 610, 624; **Ref. 4,** pp. 212, 222, 225, 244, 266; **Ref. 5,** pp. 475, 481, 549, 556)

401. (A), **402.** (C), **403.** (A), **404.** (D), **405.** (E) The numbered enzymes are characteristic of the lettered metabolic pathways. Pyruvate kinase is one of the irreversible steps of glycolysis, forming pyruvate and ATP from phosphoenolpyruvate and ADP. Pyruvate carboxylase forms a 4-carbon dicarboxylic acid (oxaloacetate) to replenish the TCA cycle when it becomes depleted of intermediates, removed for gluconeogenesis or amino acid synthesis. Enolase forms phosphoenolpyruvate from 2-phosphoglycerate. Aconitase interconverts citrate, *iso*-citrate and *cis*-aconitate. Transaldolase transfers a 2-carbon fragment between aldose-phosphates in the pentose-phosphate pathway. (**Ref. 1,** pp. 256, 303, 327–328, 363; **Ref. 2,** pp. 413, 437, 454–455, 465; **Ref. 3,** pp. 445, 479, 496–497, 540; **Ref. 4,** pp. 166, 176, 190, 203; **Ref. 5,** pp. 357, 378, 388, 429)

406. (A), **407.** (C), **408.** (E), **409.** (D), **410.** (B) The lettered amino acids are metabolized by enzymes of the numbered category. Serine is dehydrated to form pyruvate; one route of threonine catabolism is dehydrogenation to α-amino ketobutyrate; the pyrrole ring of tryptophan is opened by a dioxygenase; phenylalanine is hydroxylated to form tyrosine; and histidine is deaminated to form urocanic acid; lysine condenses with α-ketoglutarate and

the Schiff's base adduct is reduced, then oxidized by a dehydrogenase to rearrange the double bond and allow cleavage to glutamate and aminoadipate semialdehyde. (**Ref. 1**, pp. 497, 499, 507,
511, 513; **Ref. 2**, pp. 526–533; **Ref. 3**, pp. 722, 725–727, 731;
Ref. 4, pp. 305, 312, 316, 317)

411. (A), **412.** (E), **413.** (C), **414.** (B), **415.** (D) The most
acidic protein functional groups are the carboxyls; the most basic
are the guanidino groups of arginine. The imidazole group of histidine has a pK_a near neutrality. Sulfhydryl (cysteine) and pheno-
lic hydroxyl (tyrosine) groups have somewhat alkaline pk_a values.
(**Ref. 1**, p. 35; **Ref. 2**, p. 113; **Ref. 3**, pp. 137; **Ref. 5**, p. 21)

416. (D), **417.** (E), **418.** (B), **419.** (A), **420.** (C) Enzymes are
classified according to their mechanisms. Ribonuclease hydrolyzes the phosphodiester bonds of RNA; epimerases reverse
the orientation about an asymmetric center (in this case convert-
ing UDP-glucose to UDP-galactose); the fatty acid activating enzyme, a synthetase, uses the energy of ATP to attach a fatty acyl
group to the sulfhydryl of coenzyme A; enolase abstracts the elements of water from 2-phosphoglycerate; and hexokinase transfers the terminal phosphate of ATP to C-6 of glucose. (**Ref. 1**,
p. 141; **Ref. 2**, p. 201; **Ref. 3**, pp. 340–341)

421. (D), **422.** (A), **423.** (B), **424.** (C), **425.** (E) Physical
methods are used to determine aspects of protein structure. The
tyrosine residues have a characteristic UV absorbance, which becomes stronger and shifts to longer wavelengths upon deprotona-
tion; the wavelength dependence of optical rotation (CD) gives
evidence of secondary structure (eg, α-helix); NMR allows identification of distances between paramagnetic nuclei (^{13}C, ^{15}N, ^{17}O,
^{31}P, etc.); rate of sedimentation in a strong gravitational field is a
measure of molecular weight; and x-ray diffraction locates the
positions of atoms in a crystal. (**Ref. 1**, pp. 78–85; **Ref. 3**,
pp. 128–132, 156–157, 205–212; **Ref. 5**, pp. 50, 59–62, 326–328)

References

1. Devlin TE (ed.): *Textbook of Biochemistry; With Clinical Correlations,* 3rd ed. Wiley–Liss, New York, 1992.
2. Lehninger AL, Nelson DL & Cox MM: *Principles of Biochemistry,* 2nd ed. Worth, New York, 1993.
3. Matthews CK, van Holde KE: *Biochemistry.* Benjamin/Cumings, Redwood City, 1990.
4. Murray RK, Granner DK, Mayes PA, Rodwell VW: *Harper's Biochemistry,* 23rd ed. Appleton & Lange, Norwalk, 1993.
5. Stryer L: *Biochemistry,* 3rd ed. Freeman, New York, 1988.

3

Microbiology
Charles W. Kim

DIRECTIONS (Questions 426 through 525): Each of the numbered items or incomplete statements in this section is followed by answers or by completions of the statement. Select the ONE lettered answer or completion that is best in each case.

---

426. The most significant cytopathic effect induced by HIV is in
   A. T4 lymphocytes
   B. macrophages
   C. B cells
   D. monocytes
   E. neural cells

427. Human herpesvirus type 6 (HHV-6)
   A. is genetically identical to other herpesviruses
   B. is morphologically dissimilar to other herpesviruses
   C. is now recognized as the etiologic agent of roseola infantum
   D. has been shown to exhibit low infection rate in young children
   E. is not cytopathic for T lymphocytes in cell culture

428. The following statements accurately describe *Moraxella catarrhalis* EXCEPT
    A. it was previously known as *Branhamella catarrhalis*
    B. it was originally named *Neisseria catarrhalis*
    C. it is a member of the normal flora of many (40 to 50%) normal school children
    D. it is incapable of causing infection
    E. it can be differentiated from other *Neisseria* by its lack of carbohydrate fermentation

429. *Helicobacter pylori* is
    A. rodlike but not curved
    B. associated with chronic gastritis
    C. synonymous with *Campylobacter* species
    D. nonmotile
    E. Gram-positive in tissue

430. Regarding *Mycobacterium avium-intracellulare* complex
    A. it is of insignificance in the frequency of the disease it causes in humans
    B. the organisms in this group are not resistant to antituberculous drugs
    C. disseminated infections remain rare
    D. disseminated infections are now the most common systemic bacterial infection in AIDS patients
    E. it rarely causes cavitary pulmonary disease

431. Which of the following statements regarding the Hantaan virus is LEAST likely to be correct?
    A. the virus can cause hemorrhagic fever that can lead to renal insufficiency and failure
    B. the virus has been classified as a bunyavirus
    C. the virus had been recovered from a rodent, *Apodemus agrarius,* in Korea
    D. hemorrhagic fever caused by this virus has not been observed in the Western Hemisphere
    E. the virus was isolated only in 1976

432. A young woman develops fever during menstruation, accompanied by sore throat and muscle pain. Within 48 hours, the condition has progressed to severe shock. Blood culture is negative. The patient claims to use tampons. The likely diagnosis is

    A. toxic shock syndrome associated with *Streptococcus pyogenes*

    B. toxic shock syndrome associated with *Staphylococcus aureus*

    C. toxic shock syndrome associated with *Streptococcus agalactiae*

    D. toxic shock syndrome due to the release of tissue necrosis factor

    E. toxic shock syndrome due to the release of interleukin 1 (IL-1)

433. A young adult male was examined by the doctor because of a cough that was accompanied by fever, headache, and malaise. Upon examination, there was pleural effusion. It was clinically diagnosed as pneumonia. There was no bacteria in the Gram-stained smear. A high titer of cold agglutinins to the I antigen was demonstrated in the patient's serum. The most likely etiology is

    A. *Mycobacterium avium* complex

    B. *Mycobacterium tuberculosis*

    C. *Mycoplasma pneumoniae*

    D. *Mycoplasma fermentans*

    E. *Streptococcus pneumoniae*

434. The immunoglobulin that constitutes approximately 75% of the total serum immunoglobulin in normal adults and crosses the placenta is of the class

    A. IgA

    B. IgD

    C. IgE

    D. IgG

    E. IgM

435. A young man in his mid-twenties presented with mucosal lesions in his mouth. Based on his low T4 cell count and other signs during the past few months, he was diagnosed as having AIDS. The most likely etiology of the lesions is

A. *Aspergillus*
B. *Mucor*
C. *Candida*
D. *Rhizopus*
E. *Geotrichum*

436. An enzyme elaborated by group A streptococci that catalyzes the lysis of fibrin is

A. hyaluronidase
B. coagulase
C. streptokinase
D. collagenase
E. hemolysin

437. The capsule of the organism appears swollen and becomes more refractile in the presence of the specific antiserum in

A. *Staphylococcus aureus*
B. *Streptococcus pyogenes*
C. *Streptococcus viridans*
D. *Streptococcus pneumoniae*
E. *Enterococcus faecalis*

438. Following inhalation of tubercle bacilli, the characteristic nodule that appears in the lung parenchyma ia referred to as

A. tubercle
B. caseation necrosis
C. cavity
D. primary complex
E. Ghon complex

439. Subacute bacterial endocarditis occurs most commonly with

A. group A streptococci
B. group B streptococci
C. viridans streptococci
D. pneumococci
E. staphylococci

440. All of the statements refer to herpesvirus type 2 (HSV-2) EXCEPT
  A. it is usually sexually transmitted
  B. it may be transmitted to the newborn during birth from an active lesion in the mother's birth canal
  C. it has been found in cervical and vulvar carcinomas
  D. fever blister is the most common manifestation
  E. the virus remains latent in lumbar and sacral ganglia

441. Individuals with defects in the later-acting components of complement, such as C5, C6, C7, and C8 have a higher than normal frequency of
  A. recurrent pyogenic infections
  B. recurrent disseminated neisserial infections
  C. glomerulonephritis
  D. leukocytosis
  E. fulminant meningococcemia

442. Allergic bronchopulmonary aspergillosis
  A. is an allergic disease that requires both IgE and IgG antibodies to *Aspergillus*
  B. does not cause any long damage
  C. does not occur in infants and children
  D. is known to have a specific genetic predilection
  E. does not induce high levels of IgE

443. The following statements describe Lyme disease EXCEPT
  A. it is caused by *Borrelia burgdorferi*
  B. the etiologic agent contains 2 major surface proteins, OspA and OspB
  C. the etiologic agent is transmitted exclusively by nymphal tick of the genus *Ixodes*
  D. it commonly presents 3 consecutive stages of illness
  E. IgG response to the infection persists for years if untreated

444. A member of the U.S. military personnel returned from Somalia after serving for five months. While in Somalia, he experienced fever, chills, and headache. He had been stationed in a southern riverine in Somalia. Blood films revealed only rings, many with

double chromatin dots. There were no schizonts. The most likely diagnosis is
  A. tertian malaria
  B. quartan malaria
  C. malignant tertian malaria
  D. ovale malaria
  E. babesiosis

445. *Legionella pneumophila*
  A. is Gram-positive
  B. can be recovered from lung biopsies
  C. is commonly isolated from urine
  D. is easily transmitted from person to person
  E. is not susceptible to any antibiotic

446. Which one of the following statements concerning meningococcal disease is INCORRECT?
  A. passive immunity from mother to infants does not occur
  B. the incidence of healthy carriers is considerably higher than that of cases
  C. fatigue may contribute to increased susceptibility
  D. the organism is initially present in the nasopharynx
  E. the infection remains confined to the nasopharynx in healthy carriers

447. *Clostridium difficile*
  A. is never found in healthy adults
  B. produces toxin A, which is a highly potent cytotoxin
  C. is a fast-growing organism
  D. produces toxins A and B that can be detected in the stool
  E. can easily establish itself in adult healthy colon

448. The following statements describe systemic anaphylaxis in humans EXCEPT
  A. it occurs within seconds or minutes after exposure to the allergin
  B. there is urticaria and wheezing dyspnea
  C. the cytotropic antibody, IgE, plays a major role
  D. it never results in death
  E. usual causative allergens are drugs, insect venom, and foods

449. In order to prevent neonatal transmission of hepatitis B, a pregnant woman suspected of being infected
  A. should be immediately treated with antibiotics
  B. should receive corticosteroid therapy
  C. should be screened for the presence of anti-HBe
  D. should receive both active and passive immunization
  E. should receive only hyperimmune globulin (HBIG)

450. The methicillin-resistant *Staphylococcus aureus* (MRSA) strains
  A. have not shown resistance to penicillinase-resistant penicillins
  B. have not shown resistance to cephalosporins
  C. do not develop resistance to antimicrobics due to penicillinase production
  D. develop resistance to antimicrobics that is chromosomally mediated
  E. have caused only minor endemics of hospital infections

451. All of the following statements describe interferons for viral disease EXCEPT
  A. they are virus inhibitors produced by intact animals when infected with viruses
  B. they are produced by cells in tissue culture when stimulated with viruses or synthetic double-stranded RNA
  C. they fall into 3 groups, IFN-α, IFN-β, IFN-γ
  D. the different interferons are antigenically distinct
  E. the different interferons are produced by all cell types

452. Which one of the following rickettsial diseases does NOT give a positive Weil–Felix reaction?
  A. epidemic typhus
  B. endemic typhus
  C. scrub typhus
  D. Q fever
  E. Rocky Mountain spotted fever

453. In EBV infection
  A. Epstein–Barr virus is acquired on initial contact with an infected person
  B. antibodies to EBV are found in 10% of adults

C. the lymphocyte count is not markedly raised

D. EBV cannot be isolated from throat washings during acute disease

E. there is not good correlation between heterophile antibody titer and severity of illness

454. A 50-year-old male resident of eastern Long Island with fever and weakness consulted his physician. He related that he enjoyed the outdoors and spent many hours walking in the woods. Blood films revealed red blood cells that contained small rings and a few cells that contained x-shaped forms. The most likely diagnosis is

A. malaria

B. pneumocystosis

C. babesiosis

D. toxoplasmosis

E. American trypanosomiasis

455. The rash of Rocky Mountain spotted fever

A. never involves the palms and soles

B. may become hemorrhagic

C. first appears on the face

D. usually appears on the tenth day after onset

E. begins over the trunk

456. Each of the following statements refer to streptococcal M protein EXCEPT

A. it is located on the surface of group A streptococci

B. it is an antiphagocytic fibrillar molecule

C. more than 70 antigenically distinct serotypes have been described

D. it has no relationship to virulence

E. its activity is nullified with appearance of type-specific antibodies

457. Meningococcal vaccines
  A. are recommended for children as part of routine immunization
  B. provoke immediate antibody response in the first year of life
  C. are currently used for populations at high risk, such as military recruits
  D. are not recommended for children even with predisposing factors
  E. are effective in preventing disease in a major susceptible group because of good antibody response

458. In addition to the Lancefield antigen, the following streptococcus possesses polysaccharide capsular type antigens designated Ia, Ib, Ic, II, and III. It causes pneumonia, sepsis, and meningitis during the first 2 months of life with a high mortality rate. It is most likely
  A. group A streptococcus
  B. group B streptococcus
  C. group D streptococcus
  D. viridans streptococcus
  E. pneumococcus

459. The gravid females of which one of the following parasites migrate from the anus to the perianal and perineal regions for oviposition?
  A. *Enterobius vermicularis*
  B. *Strongyloides stercoralis*
  C. *Trichinella spiralis*
  D. *Necator americanus*
  E. *Ascaris lumbricoides*

460. The species most frequently responsible for *Salmonella* gastroenteritis worldwide is
  A. *S. choleraesuis*
  B. *S. schottmuelleri*
  C. *S. hirschfeldii*
  D. *S. newport*
  E. *S. typhimurium*

461. An example of immunization with attenuated living bacterium in humans is
   A. BCG vaccine
   B. pertussis vaccine
   C. Salk vaccine
   D. cholera vaccine
   E. TAB vaccine

462. The IgA class of immunoglobulins in humans
   A. is the most abundant of the immunoglobulins in serum
   B. accounts for less than 10% of the total immunoglobulin in serum
   C. is produced in relatively low concentrations in the gastrointestinal, respiratory, and genitourinary tracts
   D. is uniformly a monomer
   E. is present in only trace amount (0.2% of total immunoglobulin) in serum

463. Major clinical syndrome caused by herpes simplex virus type 2 (HSV-2) is
   A. genital herpes
   B. recurrent oral–labial lesions
   C. pharyngitis
   D. keratitis
   E. herpes encephalitis

464. The purified PRP vaccine produced from type b polysaccharide capsule of *Haemophilus influenzae*
   A. is recommended for children beyond 36 months of age
   B. has been highly immunogenic
   C. is being coupled to a protein carrier to enhance immunogenicity
   D. is known to be immunogenic for very young children of 18 months of age
   E. has shown efficacy in all clinical trials

465. The following statements refer to hepatitis B virus EXCEPT
   A. it is a double-stranded enveloped DNA virus
   B. the envelope of the virus contains the hepatitis B surface antigen (HBsAg)
   C. there are two major subtypes of hepatitis B surface antigen
   D. aggregates of HBsAg are found in serum during infection
   E. the presence of hepatitis B DNA in serum is an indication that infectious virions are present

466. Tuberculate chlamydospores (thick-walled spores covered with finger-like projections) are characteristic and diagnostic of
   A. *Sporothrix schenckii*
   B. *Blastomyces dermatitidis*
   C. *Paracoccidioides brasiliensis*
   D. *Histoplasma capsulatum*
   E. *Geotrichum candidum*

467. The following extracellular metabolites of streptococci are antigenic EXCEPT
   A. streptolysin S
   B. streptolysin O
   C. erythrogenic toxin
   D. streptokinase
   E. streptodornase

468. The genitourinary tract is NOT the site for the following organism
   A. *Mycoplasma fermentans*
   B. *Mycoplasma hominis*
   C. *Mycoplasma genitalium*
   D. *Mycoplasma pneumoniae*
   E. *Ureaplasma urealyticum*

469. In the double diffusion precipitin reactions in agar gel, a solution of antigen (A) is placed in two adjacent wells and the homologous antibody anti-A (a-A) is placed in the center well. Two precipitin bands form and eventually join at their contiguous ends and fuse (Fig. 3.1). This pattern is known as
   A. reaction of partial identity
   B. cross reaction
   C. reaction of nonidentity

D. reaction of identity
E. partial cross reaction

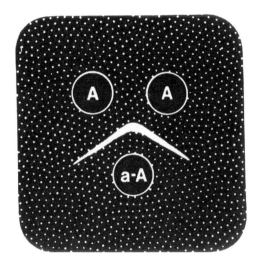

Figure 3.1

470. The following statements refer to *Enterococcus faecalis* EXCEPT
    A. it is able to grow at 45°C
    B. it is a member of group D streptococci
    C. it is frequently associated with urinary tract infections
    D. it cannot be distinguished from *Enterococcus faecium*
    E. it grows in the presence of 40% bile and hydrolyzes esculin

471. Each one of the following statements concerning hepatitis D is correct EXCEPT
    A. it causes delta hepatitis
    B. it is a small single-stranded RNA virus
    C. it requires the presence of hepatitis B surface antigens for its transmission
    D. it requires the presence of hepatitis B surface antigens for its replication
    E. the protein RNA complex is surrounded by hepatitis B surface antigen

472. In the equivalence zone of the precipitin reaction of a monospecific system, the supernatants
- **A.** contain both unreacted antibodies and unreacted antigen
- **B.** contain both excess antibodies and excess antigen
- **C.** contain free antibody
- **D.** contain free antigen
- **E.** are usually devoid of both detectable antibody and detectable antigen

473. All the following statements are true regarding viral lipids EXCEPT
- **A.** a number of different viruses contain lipids as part of their structure
- **B.** lipid-containing viruses are sensitive to ether
- **C.** distribution or loss of lipid results in loss of infectivity
- **D.** lipid-containing viruses are resistant to ether
- **E.** lipid-containing viruses are sensitive to organic solvents

474. In the replication of a RNA virus, eg, poliovirus, the single-stranded RNA can serve as its own messenger RNA for the synthesis of RNA polymerase. This step is preceded by
- **A.** formation of replicative intermediate
- **B.** synthesis of viral RNA
- **C.** maturation of virus particles
- **D.** uncoating of viral RNA
- **E.** release of virus particles

475. The chlamydiae differ from true viruses in the following important characteristics EXCEPT
- **A.** they possess both RNA and DNA
- **B.** they possess bacterial-type cell wall
- **C.** they possess ribosomes
- **D.** they multiply by binary fission
- **E.** their growth cannot be inhibited by antimicrobial drugs

476. Tissue graft from one region to another within the same individual is known as
- **A.** allograft
- **B.** isograft
- **C.** autograft
- **D.** xenograft
- **E.** homograft

477. A young man who works as a landscaper had a small localized wound on his foot that resulted from a splinter. The small but deep wound became necrotic. Organisms shown in Figure 3.2 were observed on a smear made after the wound was cleaned. The organisms shown in Figure 3.2 are

A. *Clostridium perfringens*
B. *Clostridium tetani*
C. *Clostridium botulinum*
D. *Clostridium difficile*
E. *Bacteroides fragilis*

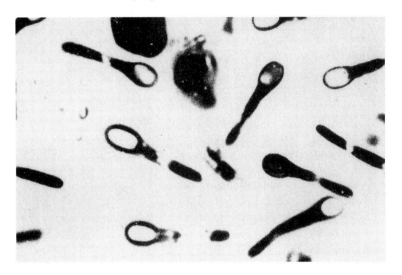

Figure 3.2

478. In the agglutination reaction some sera give effective agglutination reactions only when diluted several hundred- or thousand-fold; they do not visibly react with the antigen when undiluted or slightly diluted. This region of the titration in which this occurs is called

A. prozone
B. postzone
C. equivalence zone
D. agglutination
E. antigen-excess zone

479. The following statements are correct concerning interleukin 2 (IL-2) EXCEPT
   A. it was initially referred to as T cell growth factor
   B. it is elaborated by antigen-activated T cells
   C. it promotes T cell differentiation
   D. it does not augment natural killer (NK) cell activity
   E. recombinant IL-2 is as active as natural IL-2

480. The most prevalent type of dermatomycosis in humans known popularly as "athlete's foot" is usually caused by
   A. *Microsporum* sp. or *Epidermophyton floccosum*
   B. *M. audouinii* or *M. canis*
   C. *Trichophyton violaceum* or *Candida albicans*
   D. *M. gypseum* or *M. audouinii*
   E. *Trichophyton* sp. or *E. floccusum*

481. All the statements refer to transformation EXCEPT
   A. the recipient cell takes up soluble DNA released from donor cell
   B. it can be the most important mechanism of genetic exchange for certain bacteria
   C. it was originally found in the pneumococcus
   D. it occurs in both Gram-positive and Gram-negative bacteria
   E. it is a one-step occurrence

482. Which of the following is an example of naturally transmitted passive immunity?
   A. transfer of immunity by means of cells
   B. transmission of antibodies from mother to fetus *in utero*
   C. immunization in which the material injected causes the production of antibodies
   D. production of immunity resulting from an inapparent infection
   E. transfer of immunity by means of injections of serum

483. In a tuberculin test
   A. a positive test reveals active disease
   B. reactivity persists for only a short time after infection
   C. specificity is high for the tubercle bacillus but not for closely related mycobacteria
   D. a positive test reveals previous mycobacterial infection
   E. the reaction is not a very useful diagnostic feature

484. Which of the following fragments of complement is involved in immune adherence and opsonization?
   A. C3a
   B. C5a
   C. C3b
   D. C8
   E. C9

485. Human cysticercosis is due to *Cysticercus cellulosae,* the larval form of
   A. *Hymenolepis nana*
   B. *H. diminuta*
   C. *Taenia saginata*
   D. *T. solium*
   E. *Echinococcus granulosus*

486. Although pathogenic strains of *Clostridium perfringens* produce various metabolites, which toxin is of primary importance?
   A. hyaluronidase
   B. collagenase
   C. lecithinase C
   D. proteinase
   E. deoxyribonuclease

487. Exotoxins are
   A. heat-stable
   B. lipopolysaccharide in nature
   C. part of the cell wall of bacteria
   D. protein in nature
   E. less potent than endotoxins

488. Compared to the primary antibody response, which one of the following is LEAST likely to be correct regarding secondary antibody response?
   A. it is more rapid
   B. it rises to higher levels
   C. much more IgG is produced
   D. much more IgM is produced
   E. level of IgG persists longer

489. A young man from Puerto Rico was referred to a hospital in New York City because of abdominal pain. He had lived in Puerto Rico for 25 years until his recent arrival in the U.S. He had experienced ascites and hepatomegaly. Stool examination revealed a large egg (150 μm in length) as seen below in Figure 3.3. Based on the egg and the case history, the most likely diagnosis is

   A. fasciolopsiasis
   B. schistosomiasis
   C. ascariasis
   D. trichuriasis
   E. hookworm infection

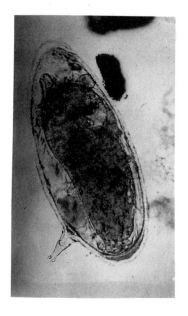

Figure 3.3

490. The following statements describe herpes simplex virus EXCEPT

   A. it has a special pattern of latency
   B. it has a special pattern of recurrence
   C. the initial infection ordinarily occurs in children between 6 and 18 months of age

D. it persists following initial infection
E. cell-mediated immunity plays no role following initial infection

491. Regarding pneumococci
  A. specific sera against pneumococci have no effect on the rate of phagocytosis
  B. the capsular polysaccharide protects the pneumococcus from phagocytosis
  C. with the loss of the capsule, the organism loses type specificity but retains its pathogenicity
  D. antibodies against the bacterial capsule produce an agglutination reaction but show no protective power
  E. antibodies to the whole somatic portion of pneumococcal cells show high protective power

492. The adult worms of *Schistosoma haematobium* usually reside in the
  A. tributaries of the inferior mesenteric vein
  B. cutaneous venules
  C. intrahepatic portal blood
  D. pelvic veins
  E. pulmonary arterioles

493. The specific effect of antinomycin D on eukaryotic and prokaryotic cells is it
  A. binds to the small subunit of ribosomes
  B. binds to the large subunit of ribosomes
  C. causes release of polypeptide chain
  D. binds to DNA
  E. binds to RNA

494. The following considerations are correct for delayed-type hypersensitivity EXCEPT
  A. an antigenic stimulus is necessary for the induction of the hypersensitive state
  B. a reaction occurs only on exposure to the specific inciting antigen
  C. the induction period is much longer than that required for antibody production
  D. it is mediated by T cells
  E. specificity is carrier-specific

495. The primary lesion or chancre of syphilis usually develops within
  A. 24 hours
  B. 2 to 4 days
  C. 5 to 8 days
  D. 10 to 30 days
  E. 6 months

496. All the following statements describe the polioviruses EXCEPT
  A. they are composed of a central core of single-stranded RNA
  B. there are three antigenic types
  C. they grow poorly in simian cell line cultures
  D. they are 28 nm in diameter
  E. they are inactivated by ultraviolet light

497. Which ONE of the following toxins is formed only by certain strains of coagulase-positive staphylococci and cause acute gastrointestinal upset in humans following ingestion?
  A. staphylolysin
  B. staphylokinase
  C. leukocidin
  D. enterotoxin
  E. dermonecrotoxin

498. The virus group responsible for acute respiratory disease and epidemic keratoconjunctivitis is
  A. echoviruses
  B. coxsackieviruses
  C. adenoviruses
  D. influenza viruses
  E. rhinoviruses

499. The description LEAST likely to be correct pertaining to staphylococcal infections of the skin is
  A. staphylococcal infection of the skin is the most common bacterial infection in humans
  B. carbuncles are limited to the neck and upper back
  C. carbuncle is essentially the same as furuncle
  D. most furuncles evolve in 3 to 5 days
  E. secondary and satellite lesions result from autoinoculation

500. Living spirochetes are used in serodiagnostic tests for syphilis in
   A. TPCF (*Treponema pallidum* complement fixation)
   B. TPCP (*T. pallidum* cryolysis complement fixation)
   C. TPI (treponema immobilization test)
   D. RPCF (Reiter protein complement fixation)
   E. VDRL (Venereal Disease Research Laboratory)

501. All the following statements describe diphtheria toxin EXCEPT
   A. it is produced by strains of *C. diphtheriae* infected with a temperate bacteriophage carrying structural gene for toxin production
   B. different strains of *C. diphtheriae* vary greatly in their capacity for toxin production when infected by the specific bacteriophage gene
   C. its toxicity is the same for humans and animals
   D. its yield is markedly influenced by inorganic iron content of the medium
   E. it is produced at maximal levels only when iron becomes the growth-rate limiting substrate

502. Which ONE of the following classes or subclasses of immunoglobulin does NOT activate complement via the classical pathway?
   A. IgG1
   B. IgG2
   C. IgG3
   D. IgG4
   E. IgM

503. In most individuals with herpes zoster, the chief site of involvement is the
   A. genitals
   B. lumbar region
   C. trunk
   D. buccal mucosa
   E. extremities

504. Which ONE of the following descriptions of amebic liver abscess is LEAST likely to be correct?
   A. it results from establishment and multiplication of trophozoites in the liver
   B. it occurs more frequently in the right lobe than in the left
   C. it may be a sequela of chronic intestinal amebiasis
   D. it may be a sequela of acute amebic dysentery
   E. it does not occur without symptomatic intestinal amebiasis

505. In addition to endotoxin, which ONE of the following members of the enteric bacilli also produces an exotoxin?
   A. *Shigella dysenteriae*
   B. *S. flexneri*
   C. *S. boydii*
   D. *S. sonnei*
   E. *Salmonella typhi*

506. *Yersinia pestis*
   A. is a Gram-positive coccobacillus
   B. has a single antigenic type
   C. is not enveloped even when freshly isolated
   D. virulence is dependent on V and W antigens, as well as other factors
   E. is an extracellular parasite

507. All of the statements refer to primary genital herpes EXCEPT
   A. it is a sexually transmitted exogenous infection
   B. it is generally caused by HSV-2
   C. tender inguinal adenopathy is common
   D. there are no systemic symptoms
   E. multiple vesicles develop that are painful

508. The current inactivated influenza vaccines
   A. induce antibodies that persists for more than 6 months
   B. induce high level of IgA in the respiratory tract
   C. induce low level of IgA in the respiratory tract
   D. in a single subcutaneous infection will confer immunity within 10 days
   E. are not recommended for children with chronic heart disease

509. The clinical manifestation of cholera is due to
   A. ulceration of the mucosa
   B. invasion of the mucosa by the organism
   C. peritonitis
   D. loss of fluid
   E. invasion of the blood

510. The spirochetes
   A. are nonmotile
   B. are seen best in the living state by dark-field illumination
   C. are strictly aerobic
   D. form endospores
   E. are not very susceptible to chemotherapeutic agents

511. The principal mode of transmission for infectious hepatitis virus A is
   A. from infected blood
   B. from infected plasma
   C. by ingestion
   D. by an insect bite
   E. from nonsterile syringes

512. A 40-year-old man who was originally from a rural region in Greece consulted a physician because of a protuberant abdomen. He had experienced a dull right upper quadrant abdominal pain. As a child he lived on the second floor of a home, the first floor being occupied by domestic animals, such as sheep, goats, and dogs. He often played on the ground floor with the dogs. The history highly suggests
   A. echinococcosis
   B. amebiasis
   C. toxoplasmosis
   D. schistosomiasis mansoni
   E. opisthorchiasis

513. All the following statements refer to endospores EXCEPT
   A. they are formed under conditions of inadequate nutrition
   B. the surrounding mother cell is called a sporangium
   C. they are formed within certain Gram-positive organisms
   D. they are cryptobiotic
   E. they are less resistant than the parental cells to lethal effects of heat, drying, and freezing

514. *Rhodococcus equi*
  A. is motile
  B. is Gram-negative
  C. is anaerobic
  D. can cause necrotizing pneumonia in immunocompromised patients
  E. is not pathogenic for humans

515. *Microsporidium* spp.
  A. are transmitted via inhalation of oocysts
  B. cause pneumonia in immunosuppressed patients
  C. cause hemolytic anemia in immunosuppressed patients
  D. cause diarrhea in immunosuppressed patients
  E. invade primarily the brain in immunosuppressed patients

516. Pili or fimbriae
  A. are found in Gram-positive bacilli
  B. are longer than flagella
  C. consist of polysaccharides
  D. function as adhesins
  E. arise from outside the cytoplasmic membrane

517. The following statements are correct concerning hepatitis B (HBV) EXCEPT
  A. there is a wide range of extrahepatic manifestations
  B. there are chronic forms of hepatitis B lasting longer than 6 months
  C. a patient with hepatitis B may continue for a long time as a carrier of the whole virus or HBsAg
  D. most patients continue only for a very short time as carriers
  E. cirrhosis and primary hepatocellular carcinoma are probable sequelae of hepatitis B

518. Tufts of flagella along the cylinder of the bacterial cell are described as being
  A. monotrichous
  B. lophotrichous
  C. amphitrichous
  D. peritrichous
  E. trichous

519. The portal of entry for the following protozoa is through the mouth EXCEPT

   A. *Microsporidium* spp.
   B. *Cryptosporidium parvum*
   C. *Isospora belli*
   D. *Babesia microti*
   E. *Dientamoeba fragilis*

520. An adult male presenting a draining lesion on his jaw consulted a physician. The face appeared to be swollen. Samples of the pus, crushed between two slides and stained, revealed Gram-positive branching rods. The etiology is most likely

   A. *Actinomyces*
   B. *Mycobacterium*
   C. *Corynebacterium*
   D. *Streptomyces*
   E. *Candida*

521. Thayer–Martin medium is a selective medium for

   A. *Pseudomonas*
   B. *Neisseria*
   C. *Salmonella* and *Shigella*
   D. *Haemophilus*
   E. *Pasteurella*

522. Concerning *Pseudomonas aeruginosa:*

   A. opportunistic infection with *P. aeruginosa* is rare
   B. *P. aeruginosa* pneumonia is generally very mild
   C. it is most consistently resistant to antimicrobics
   D. it can cause otitis externa ("swimmer's ear") but is uncommon
   E. it plays a minor role in cystic fibrosis complications

523. Of the *Bacteroides fragilis* complex

   A. *B. fragilis* predominates among Gram-negative infections in the abdominal cavity
   B. *B. fragilis* is sensitive to penicillin and many other β-lactams
   C. plasmids that carry resistance determinants have not been demonstrated for *B. fragilis*
   D. *B. fragilis* is Gram-positive
   E. *B. fragilis* lacks a capsule

524. A dishwasher came into the doctor's office because of lesions on his hands that consisted of erythematous papules with tenderness and erythema. The nail beds (paronychia) were also affected. Scraping from the lesion in potassium hydroxide preparation revealed pseudohyphae, as well as budding yeast cells. The etiology is most likely
  A. *Aspergillus fumigatus*
  B. *Candida albicans*
  C. *Candida parapsilosis*
  D. *Candida krusei*
  E. *Torulopsis glabrata*

525. The catalase test is useful in the differentiation of
  A. one group of streptococci from another group
  B. staphylococci from streptococci
  C. one group of enterobacteria from another group
  D. *Shigella* from *Salmonella*
  E. Enterobacteriaceae from *Pseudomonas*

DIRECTIONS (Questions 526 through 575): Each set of matching questions in this section consists of a list of five to ten lettered options (some of which may be figures) followed by several numbered items. For each numbered item, select the ONE lettered option that is most closely associated with it. Each lettered option may be selected once, more than once, or not at all.

Questions 526 and 527

  A. erythromycin
  B. chloramphenicol
  C. streptomycin
  D. tetracycline
  E. spectinomycin

For each mechanism of action, select the associated drug.

526. This aminoglycoside inhibits protein synthesis of bacteria by attaching to and inhibiting the function of the 30S ribosomal subunit

527. This macrolide inhibits growth of bacteria by interfering with protein synthesis by binding to the 50S subunit

Questions 528 and 529

    A. *Haemophilus influenzae*
    B. *Staphylococcus aureus*
    C. *Legionella pneumophila*
    D. *Streptococcus pneumoniae*
    E. *Mycoplasma pneumoniae*

For each type of pneumonia, select the most appropriate etiologic agent.

528. Necrotizing and multiple pneumonia caused by a Gram-negative rod

529. A walking pneumonia caused by pleomorphic bacteria

Questions 530 and 531

    A. HBsAg
    B. HBcAg
    C. HBeAg
    D. anti-HBs
    E. anti-Hbc

For each description of antigen and function of antibody, select the most appropriate hepatitis B antigen and antibody

530. A glycoprotein that is associated with the core antigen

531. Antibody that is correlated with protection against the disease

Questions 532 and 533

  A. *Legionella pneumophila*
  B. *Mycobacterium avium*
  C. *Mycoplasma pneumoniae*
  D. *Chlamydia psittaci*
  E. *Coxiella burnetii*

For each mode of transmission, select the appropriate etiologic agent.

532. The usual mode of transmission to humans for this intracellular organism is via contaminated dust and aerosols from sheep and cattle

533. The transmission of this obligate intracellular organism to humans is via dust or droplet from droppings of infected birds

Questions 534 and 535

  A. exotoxin A
  B. streptodornase
  C. erythrogenic toxin
  D. streptolysin S
  E. streptolysin O

For each source of toxin and enzyme, select the associated toxin or enzyme.

534. A toxin that is elaborated only by lysogenic streptococci

535. An enzyme elaborated by many streptococci that is responsible for hemolytic zones on blood agar plate

Questions 536 and 537

    A. measles
    B. mumps
    C. rubella
    D. varicella
    E. shingles

For each clinical description, select the corresponding disease.

536. Vesicular eruption from reactivation of latent virus

537. The appearance of Koplik's spots on mucous membranes

Questions 538 and 539

    A. *Plasmodium vivax*
    B. *Plasmodium malariae*
    C. *Trypanosoma cruzi*
    D. *Trypanosoma gambiense*
    E. *Babesia microti*

For each diagnostic description in a stained blood smear, select the most likely blood-borne protozoa.

538. In a stained blood smear, the protozoa usually appears in U- or S-shape.

539. In a stained blood smear, the mature schizont resembles a "rosette."

Questions 540 and 541

    A. Lancefield serogroup A
    B. Lancefield serogroup B
    C. Lancefield serogroup C
    D. Lancefield serogroup D
    E. Lancefield serogroup G

For each clinical syndrome, select the responsible serogroup.

540. The serogroup of streptococci that are a leading cause of pneumonia, sepsis, and meningitis in the first 2 months of life

541. The serogroup of streptococci that produces a toxin responsible for the rash seen in scarlet fever

Questions 542 and 543

    A. toxoplasmosis
    B. pneumocystosis
    C. cryptococcosis
    D. candidiasis
    E. disseminated varicella-zoster

For each described condition in AIDS patients, select the associated opportunistic infection.

542. The most common opportunistic infection seen in AIDS patients

543. Eosphagitis as an opportunistic infection in AIDS patients

Questions 544 and 545

    A. cell conjugation
    B. mutation
    C. transduction
    D. translation
    E. transformation
    F. transcription

For each means of genetic transfer, select the appropriate type of transfer.

544. Genetic transfer by uptake of naked DNA

545. Genetic transfer by viral infection

Questions 546 and 547

    A. *Sporothrix schenckii*
    B. *Aspergillus fumigatus*
    C. *Blastomyces dermatitidis*
    D. *Coccidioides immits*
    E. *Cryptococcus neoformans*
    F. *Paracoccidioides brasiliensis*

For each pathognomonic feature, select the appropriate fungus.

546. Produces subcutaneous nodules along the lymphatics

547. Multiple buds may be observed in sputum and in tissue

Questions 548 and 549

    A. Lyme disease
    B. rickettsialpox
    C. relapsing fever (borreliosis)
    D. Q fever
    E. Rocky Mountain spotted fever

For each vector that is responsible for transmitting the etiologic agent, select the associated disease.

548. Transmitted primarily by *Ixodes* hard tick

549. Transmitted primarily by *Dermacentor* hard tick

Questions 550 and 551

    A. erythromycin
    B. tetracycline
    C. ketoconazole
    D. metronidazole
    E. clindamycin

For each effective treatment, select the appropriate drug.

550. Antibiotic that is effective against fungi

551. Antibiotic that is effective against several protozoa

Questions 552 and 553

    A. *Necator americanus*
    B. *Enterobius vermicularis*
    C. *Trichinella spiralis*
    D. *Schistosoma mansoni*
    E. *Trichuris trichiura*

For each stage responsible for transmission, select the appropriate parasite.

552. Nematode infective in the egg stage following extrinsic development

553. Nematode infective in the larval stage following extrinsic development

Questions 554 and 555

    A. *Trichophyton mentagrophytes*
    B. *Microsporum audouinii*
    C. *Epidermophyton floccosum*
    D. *Histoplasma capsulatum*
    E. *Trichophyton rubrum*

For each clinical condition, select the appropriate fungus.

554. Causes infection of the skin but not the nails

555. Causes pulmonary infection

Questions 556 through 560

    A. methisazone
    B. enviroxime
    C. amantadine
    D. ribavirin
    E. azidothymidine
    F. acyclovir
    G. ganciclovir

For each action, select the associated drug.

556. Prophylactically effective against influenza A strains

557. Strong inhibition of herpes simplex virus

558. Inhibition of replication of HIV

559. Inhibition of replication of poxvirus

560. Effective against syncytial virus infections

Questions 561 through 565

    A. cholera
    B. meningococcal infection
    C. mumps
    D. pneumococcal infection
    E. poliomyelitis
    F. rabies
    G. tuberculosis
    H. yellow fever

For each type of vaccine, select the disease for which it is used.

561. Purified capsular polysaccharide vaccine used in military recruits

562. Live attenuated virus vaccine to protect international travelers

563. Capsular polysaccharide vaccine prepared from 23 types of the microorganism most commonly encountered

564. Inactivated vaccine that is indicated for those who have been exposed to the virus or prophylactically for those at high risk

565. Live attenuated vaccine given routinely to children and susceptible seronegative male patients

Questions 566 through 570

- **A.** *Neisseria gonorrhoeae*
- **B.** *Chlamydia trachomatis*
- **C.** *Treponema pallidum*
- **D.** *Haemophilus ducreyi*
- **E.** *Calymmatobacterium granulomatis*
- **F.** HIV
- **G.** herpes simplex virus
- **H.** hepatitis B virus
- **I.** *Trichomonas vaginalis*
- **J.** *Candida albicans*

For each description of a sexually transmitted infection, select the most likely etiologic agent.

566. An uncommon disease with persistent genital papules or ulcers caused by a Gram-negative bacillus that is morphologically and antigenically similar to *Klebsiella*

567. A painful and tender chancroid ulcer that may involve inguinal lymph nodes and develop into an abscess within a node (bubo) caused by a Gram-negative bacillus

568. Urethritis with purulent discharge seen in males, and discharge and pain associated with infection of the cervix caused by Gram-negative intracellular diplococci

569. Vaginitis and urethritis caused by a flagellate

570. Lymphogranuloma venereum caused by an obligate intracellular bacteria

Questions 571 through 575: Refer to Figure 3.4A, B, C, D, E to answer the questions.

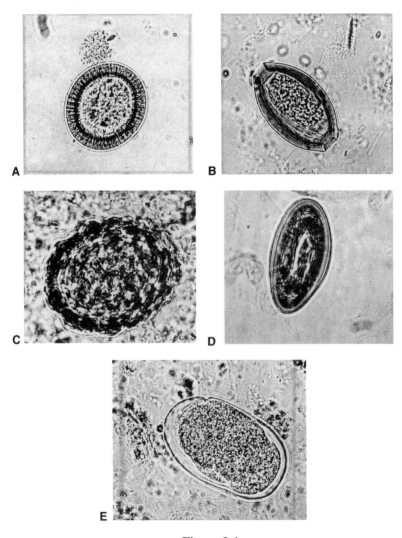

Figure 3.4

For each description, select the appropriate egg.

571. Egg that is evacuated in the stool in an unembryonated condition and possessing a transparent prominence at each end

572. Thin-shelled and transparent egg that is laid in an early stage of cleavage

573. Egg that is characterized by broad radial striations in the shell

574. Large egg, measuring 45 to 70 × 35 to 50 μm, with an outermost, coarsely mammillated layer

575. Embryonated egg flattened on one side with colorless double shell

Microbiology

Answers and Comments

426. **(A)** The consequences of HIV infection of T4 cells are most significant. Infected T4 cells express a high level of HIV gp120 on their surface which leads to their depletion. The consequences are devastating because the T4 lymphocytes play a critical role in the human immune response. HIV does not induce as significant a cytopathic effect in monocytes as it does in T4 cells. (**Ref. 2,** pp. 574–575)

427. **(C)** The new human herpesvirus, designated human herpesvirus type 6, appears to be the etiologic agent of roseola infantum or exanthem subitum, which is a common disease of infants and children 6 months to 4 years of age. Serologic studies have indicated that almost all children acquire the infection by 5 years of age. (**Ref. 6,** pp. 529, 575)

428. **(D)** Although *Moraxella catarrhalis* is a member of the normal flora in 40 to 50% of normal school children, it can cause bronchitis, pneumonia, sinusitis, otitis media, and conjunctivitis. Immunocompromised patients are also at risk to infections caused by this member of the normal flora. (**Ref. 2,** p. 255)

429. **(B)** *Helicobacter pylori* was first observed on the surface of gastric antral epithelium in patients with active chronic gastritis.

It is highly motile and is closely associated with gastric mucus-secreting cells. In tissue it is curved and stain Gram-negative, but in culture it is more rodlike. (**Ref. 4,** pp. 679–680)

430. (D) *Mycobacterium avium-intracellulare* complex infections, which were once considered rare, are now the most common systemic bacterial infection in AIDS patients. The infection usually develops with the decline of the patient's general clinical condition and helper T4(CD4+) lymphocyte concentrations. Clinically the patient experiences progressive weight loss and intermittent fever, chills, night sweats, and diarrhea. The organisms are resistant to antituberculous drugs, and prognosis is grave. (**Ref. 6,** pp. 456–457)

431. (D) Hemorrhagic fever with renal syndrome caused by Hantaan virus has been recognized in the Western Hemisphere, such as in different areas of France. The virus has been isolated in the domestic rat, *Rattus norwegicus,* in the U.S., suggesting that there is an increased risk of human exposure. (**Ref. 2,** pp. 502–503)

432. (B) Toxic shock syndrome associated with *Staphylococcus aureus* seen during or immediately after menstruation is related to the use of highly absorbent intravaginal tampons with the liberation of toxic shock syndrome toxin 1 (TSST1) by large numbers of *S. aureus* in and around the tampon. The toxin induces the production of interleukin and tumor necrosis factor (TNF) by macrophages. To what extent the syndrome is a response to IL1 and TNF production or to other effects of the toxin is uncertain. Following removal of high-absorbancy tampons from sales, the incidence of toxic shock syndrome has declined. (**Ref. 6,** pp. 280, 284)

433. (C) *Mycoplasma pneumoniae* accounts for approximately 20% of all cases of pneumonia. Pulmonary symptoms usually consist of a nonproductive cough. X-ray reveals a lobar pneumonia and pleural effusions are seen in 25% of cases. *M. pneumoniae* is not detectable by Gram stain. The most common nonspecific response involves the production of high titers of cold hemagglutinins (IgM antibodies) to I antigen of human RBCs in more than two-thirds of patients with symptomatic *M. pneumoniae* infection. (**Ref. 6,** pp. 417–418)

434. (D) IgG constitutes approximately 75% of the total serum immunoglobulin in normal adults. IgG is the only class of immunoglobulin that is able to cross the placenta, thereby offering protection to the newborn during the first few months of life. (**Ref. 7,** pp. 116–117)

435. (C) AIDS patients are highly susceptible to candidiasis, especially involving the mucosal surfaces of the oropharynx and esophagus. Oral candidiasis is one of the criteria for the diagnosis of AIDS and AIDS-related complex. The depression of cell-mediated immunity is manifested by an abnormally low T4 cell count and high (50 to 70%) mucosal candidiasis, oral thrush, esophagitis, or both. (**Ref. 4,** p. 1140)

436. (C) Group A streptococcus produces two different streptokinases. These are antigenically distinct from the streptokinase of the group C streptococcus, which is the source for the commercial production of streptokinase for use as thrombolytic agent in humans. Streptokinase forms a complex with plasminogen activator and catalyzes the conversion of plasminogen to plasmin, leading to the digestion of fibrin. (**Ref. 4,** p. 423)

437. (D) In the presence of the specific antiserum the capsule of *S. pneumoniae* appears greatly swollen and more refractile, indicating a positive reaction. This is the Neufeld quellung or capsular precipitation reaction which not only identifies an organism but also its specific type of pneumococcus. (**Ref. 4,** p. 434)

438. (A) The characteristic tubercle develops in the lung parenchyma after inhalation of tubercle bacilli and development of delayed hypersensitivity. The meaning of tubercle comes from the Latin, *tuberculum,* which means small lump. (**Ref. 3,** p. 653)

439. (C) The viridans group of streptococci can cause subacute bacterial endocarditis when they reach previously damaged heart valves as in the case of transient bacteria from tooth extraction. These α-streptococci are protected by fibrin and platelets as they multiply on the valve. (**Ref. 6,** p. 312)

440. (D) Fever blisters or cold sores are lesions that usually recur from an initial infection of the buccal mucosa, tongue, gums, and pharynx with herpesvirus type 1 (HSV-1). The virus becomes latent within the sensory nerve root ganglia of the trigeminal nerve and may be reactivated to cause the recurrent blisters. (**Ref. 6,** p. 562)

441. **(B)** Patients with defects in the later-acting components of complement, C5, C6, C7, and C8, have a much higher than normal frequency of disseminated meningococcal and gonococcal (neisserial) infections. The lytic function of the late-acting components is believed to be required to defend adequately against these highly encapsulated organisms. (**Ref. 7,** p. 363)

442. **(A)** Allergic bronchopulmonary aspergillosis (ABPA) is caused by a concomitant IgE and IgG antibody response to the fungus, *Aspergillus fumigatus.* It causes bronchiectasis and other destructive lung changes. There is no known genetic predilection other than that related to atopy. The total serum IgE level is characteristically high. (**Ref. 7,** pp. 412–413)

443. **(C)** The spirochete, *Borrelia burgdorferi,* which causes Lyme disease, is transmitted through the bite of a tick. The ticks include *Ixodes pacificus* on the West Coast, *I. dammini* on the East Coast and the Midwest, and *I. ricinus* in Europe. The Lone Star tick, *Amblyomma americanum,* which transmits tularemia and Rocky Mountain spotted fever agents, can also transmit *B. burgdorferi.* (**Ref. 4,** p. 670)

444. **(C)** Malaria due to *Plasmodium falciparum* is known as malignant tertain malaria. Double chromatin dots are frequently found in the ring forms of *P. falciparum;* they are only occasionally found in the rings of other species. The late stages of *P. falciparum* sequester in visceral capillaries; only the ring forms and gametocytes are found in the peripheral blood. (**Ref. 5,** pp. 82, 90, 92)

445. **(B)** *Legionella pneumophila* can be recovered from lung biopsy specimens, as well as from bronchial washings, pleural fluid, or blood. It is more difficult to recover from sputum due to the predominance of bacteria of the normal flora. Fortunately, it is not communicable from infected patients to others, although it is ubiquitous in the environment. (**Ref. 2,** pp. 264–265)

446. (A) Infants may have passive immunity to meningococcal disease through IgG antibodies from immune mothers. Immunity is associated with specific, complement-dependent bactericidal antibodies in the serum. These antibodies develop after subclinical infections, which the mothers may have had. (**Ref. 2,** p. 255)

447. (D) *Clostridium difficile* strains that are medically important produce two distinct large polypeptide toxins, A and B. Toxin A is primarily an enterotoxin, while toxin B is a highly potent cytotoxin. Both toxins may be detected in the stool, toxin A with antibody-based tests and toxin B by tissue culture assays. In fact, the detection of toxins A and/or B in the stool of a patient with antimicrobic-associated diarrhea (AAD) establishes this organism as the likely etiologic agent. (**Ref. 6,** pp. 336–337)

448. (D) Systemic anaphylaxis is the occurrence of IgE-mediated reaction simultaneously in multiple organs. It is evoked by a minute quantity of allergin. It can be potentially fatal, death being attributed to asphyxiation from upper airway edema and congestion, irreversible shock, or a combination of these factors. Death that occurs after many hours of shock may be from the late phase effect of IgE allergic reaction or secondary to the failure of other organs. (**Ref. 7,** p. 400)

449. (D) A combination of active and passive immunization is the most effective approach to prevent neonatal transmission of hepatitis B. Two types of inactivated subunit hepatitis B vaccine are available; one has been developed by purification and inactivation of HBsAg from the blood of chronic carriers, and the other is recombinant surface antigen prepared in yeast. Hyperimmune globulin is prepared from sera of subjects who have high titer antibody to HBsAg but do not harbor the antigen itself. (**Ref. 6,** pp. 555–556)

450. (D) The methicillin-resistant *Staphylococcus aureus* (MRSA) strains develop resistance that is chromosomally mediated. It is probably mutational in origin, involving production of a particular penicillin-binding protein, PBP-2′, which is believed to be a peptodoglycan transpeptidase with a low affinity for β-lactam antimicrobics. (**Ref. 6,** p. 281)

451. (E) Interferons are of multiple species and fall into 3 general groups, IFN-α, IFN-β, IFN-γ, that are similar in size but antigenically distinct. The different classes are produced by different cell types. IFN-α is synthesized predominantly by leukocytes, IFN-β mainly by fibroblasts, and IFN-γ only by lymphocytes. (**Ref. 2,** pp. 401–402)

452. (D) *Coxiella burnetii,* the etiologic agent for Q fever, does not elicit antibodies for *Proteus* polysaccharide O antigen; hence, the Weil–Felix reaction is negative. Since the Weil–Felix reaction is based on the cross-reaction between rickettsial antigens and *Proteus* O antigen, it has limited clinical use. (**Ref. 4,** pp. 704, 713)

453. (E) Infection with EBV induces synthesis of circulating antibodies against viral antigens and against unrelated antigens found in sheep, horse, and some beef red blood cells. These heterophile antibodies do not cross-react with antibodies specific for EBV, and there is no good correlation between heterophile antibody titer and severity of illness. (**Ref. 6,** p. 573)

454. (C) Babesiosis appears to be endemic to the eastern seacoast, including Long Island where the tick, *Ixodes dammini,* that transmits *Babesia microti* is prevalent. *B. microti* appears as small rings within the red blood cell. Some are x-shaped like a Maltese cross. Clinical manifestations mimic malaria, such as fever, weakness, jaundice, and hepatomegaly. (**Ref. 5,** p. 102)

455. (B) The rash in Rocky Mountain spotted fever appears from the second to the fourth day after the onset, first on the peripheral parts of the body. It is usually maculopapular early in the disease but may later become petechial or hemorrhagic. (**Ref. 4,** p. 706)

456. (D) The M protein is the major virulence factor of group A streptococci and renders them resistant to phagocytosis. The antiphagocytic activity of the M protein is attributed to an interference with the deposition of the complement component C3b onto the streptococcal cell surface. Hence, activation of the alternative complement pathway and opsonization of the organism are inhibited. (**Ref. 4,** pp. 420–421)

457. (C) The polysaccharide meningococcal vaccines are currently used in populations at high risk, such as military recruits, and in control of epidemics. However, they are not recommended for routine immunization of children unless there are predisposing factors. The quadrivalent vaccine containing A, C, Y, and W-135 polysaccharides does not provoke good antibody response in the first year of life. (**Ref. 6,** p. 348)

458. (B) Group B streptococci are a leading cause of pneumonia, sepsis, and meningitis during the first 2 months of life. The mortality rate is between 30 to 60% of infected cases. Most cases result from contamination of the infant from the mother's genital tract. In addition to their Lancefield antigen, they possess polysaccharide capsular antigens which form the serologic typing system for strains within the group. The type antigens have been designated Ia, Ib, Ic, II, and III. (**Ref. 6,** p. 305)

459. (A) The gravid females of *E. vermicularis,* containing more than 11,000 eggs, migrate to the perianal and perineal regions where the eggs are expelled in masses by contractions of the uterus and vagina under the stimulus of a lower temperature and aerobic environment. (**Ref. 5,** p. 136)

460. (E) Gastroenteritis, so-called food poisoning, is the most common clinical manifestation of *Salmonella* infection. The most common agent for *Salmonella* gastroenteritis worldwide is *S. typhimurium.* (**Ref. 3,** p. 576)

461. (A) Various living avirulent tubercle bacilli, particularly BCG (an attenuated bovine organism), have been used to induce a certain degree of resistance in those individuals heavily exposed to infection. Immunization with these organisms is a substitute for primary infection with virulent tubercle bacilli which have inherent danger. In the United States, the use of BCG is suggested only for tuberculin-negative persons who are heavily exposed. (**Ref. 2,** p. 277)

462. (B) IgA normally accounts for less than 10% of the total immunoglobulin in human serum. However, it is the principal immunoglobulin in external secretions, such as colostrum, respiratory and intestinal mucin, saliva, tears, and genitourinary tract mucin. It plays a major role in protecting mucosal surfaces from invasion by infectious agents. Its presence in colostrum helps to protect the suckling newborn from infection. (**Ref. 3,** p. 289)

463. (**A**) In the United States, 70% of first episodes of genital HSV infection are caused by HSV-2, although HSV-1 can also cause it. Genital HSV-2 disease is more likely to recur than genital HSV-1 infection. (**Ref. 6,** p. 563)

464. (**C**) The PRP vaccine of type b *Haemophilus influenzae* has failed to show efficacy in occasional clinical trials in certain geographic areas. Thus, a new class of polysaccharide-protein conjugate vaccines is being explored to enhance the immune response. These include conjugates of PRP with diphtheria toxoid, tetanus toxiod, and an outer membrane protein from group B *Neisseria meningitidis.* (**Ref. 6,** p. 407)

465. (**C**) The hepatitis B surface antigen (HBsAg) has been shown to possess a group-specific determinant, *a,* and two sets of mutually exclusive subtype determinants, *d* and *y* and *w* and *r*. Therefore, there are four major subtypes of hepatitis B surface antigen. There is antigenic cross-reactivity and cross-protection between subtypes. (**Ref. 6,** p. 551)

466. (**D**) In older cultures of *Histoplasma capsulatum* on Sabouraud glucose agar, there are numerous round to pyriform, thick-walled macroconidia (8 to 16 μm) which are covered with finger-like projections known as tuberculate spores; these tuberculate chlamydospores are characteristic and diagnostic for *H. capsulatum.* (**Ref. 4,** p. 1098)

467. (**A**) Streptolysin S (SLS) is an oxygen-stable nonantigenic toxin. It consists of a polypeptide attached to an oligonucleotide. It is lytic for red and white blood cells. Most strains of group A streptococci produce SLS, which is responsible for the surface hemolysis seen on blood agar plates. (**Ref. 4,** p. 422)

468. (**D**) *Mycoplasma pneumoniae* is an important pathogen of the respiratory tract. In general, *M. pneumoniae* accounts for approximately 20% of all cases of pneumonia. The infection caused by *M. pneumoniae* is occasionally associated with arthritis, meningoencephalitis, hemolytic anemia, and rash. *M. fermentans, M. hominis, M. genitalium,* and *Ureaplasma urealyticum* are inhabitants of the genitourinary tract. (**Ref. 6,** pp. 416–417, 419)

469. (D)   If a solution of antigen is placed in two adjacent wells and the homologous antibody is placed in the center well, the two precipitin bands will eventually join at their contiguous end and fuse. This pattern is known as the reaction of identity. This is seen whenever indistinguishable antigen–antibody systems react in adjacent fields. (**Ref. 3,** pp. 320–321)

470. (D)   The enterococcal species within the group D antigen may be separated on the basis of biochemical reactions, eg, *E. faecalis* ferments sorbitol, whereas *E. faecium* does not. Also, variations in peptidoglycan structure exist between the species. For example, *E. faecalis* contains only glutamic acid, lysine, and alanine, while *E. faecium* contains also aspartic acid. (**Ref. 4,** pp. 427–428)

471. (D)   Although the hepatitis D virus requires the presence of hepatitis B surface antigens for its transmission, it does not require B for its replication. The delta virus produces its own antigens, but it does co-opt the hepatitis B surface antigen in assembling its coat. (**Ref. 6,** p. 556)

472. (E)   In the equivalence zone or equivalence point, the precipitation is maximum. Hence, the supernatants are usually devoid of both detectable antibody and detectable antigen, and the amount of antibody in the corresponding precipitate represents the total amount of antibody in the volume of serum tested. (**Ref. 3,** p. 258)

473. (D)   There are many lipid-containing viruses, eg, herpesviruses and myxoviruses, that are sensitive to treatment with ether and other organic solvents, indicating that disruption or loss of lipid results in loss of infectivity. Non-lipid-containing viruses are generally resistant to the action of ether. (**Ref. 2,** pp. 374–375)

474. (D)   The viral RNA is uncoated before the single-stranded RNA can serve as its own messenger RNA. This messenger RNA is translated, resulting in the formation of RNA polymerase. (**Ref. 2,** pp. 380–381)

475. (E) The growth of chlamydiae, unlike viruses, can be inhibited by many antimicrobial drugs, including tetracyclines and erythromycins. (**Ref. 2,** p. 300)

476. (C) Transplanted tissues are defined in terms of genetic identity. Hence, when there is a transplant of tissues from one site to another in the same individual, it is referred to as an autograft. (**Ref. 3,** p. 463)

477. (B) *Clostridium tetani* has a typical round terminal spore that gives it a drumstick appearance. Spores are formed readily in nature and remain viable in soil for many years. Spores may be introduced into wounds with contaminated soil. A puncture wound containing a splinter is typical and is ideal for germination of spores in the wound, causing tetanus. (**Ref. 6,** p. 332)

478. (A) It can be shown that unagglutinated cells in the prozone actually have antibodies adsorbed on their surfaces. The prozone phenomenon is not due simply to antibody excess, but often involves special blocking or incomplete antibodies. (**Ref. 3,** p. 267)

479. (D) IL-2 not only stimulates proliferation and lymphokine production by T cells and B cells but also by NK cells. Large granular lymphocytes (LGL) can be stimulated by IL-2 to proliferate, to produce other lymphokines, and to exhibit enhanced NK activity. (**Ref. 7,** pp. 86, 89)

480. (E) The most prevalent type of human dermatophytosis is what is popularly referred to as "athlete's foot." It usually is caused by *Trichophyton rubrum, T. mentagrophytes,* or *E. floccosum.* (**Ref. 2,** p. 315)

481. (E) Transformation may be considered to occur in three steps: binding of exogenous DNA to the cell surface, uptake or transport of the bound DNA through the cell membrane, and integration or recombination of the donor DNA fragment with the recipient genome. (**Ref. 4,** p. 137)

482. (B) Passive immunity occurs without active participation of the recipient host (fetus) and results from antibody transfer from an immune host (mother) *in utero.* Since there is no stimulus for continued synthesis of antibody, its duration of effect is transitory. This passive transfer may be reinforced by antibodies taken up by the child in mother's milk, but the immunity wanes at 4 to 6 months of age. (**Ref. 2,** p. 145)

483. (**D**) Delayed-type hypersensitivity to tuberculin is highly specific for the tubercle bacillus and various closely related mycobacteria. A positive test indicates previous mycobacterial infection; it does not establish the presence of active disease. It is a useful diagnostic and epidemiological tool. Conversion of negative to positive reaction is good evidence for a recent infection. (**Ref. 3,** p. 655)

484. (**C**) The binding of C3b to antibody–antigen aggregates and to antibody-sensitized cells causes them to adhere to polymorphonuclear leukocytes, macrophages, and certain other cells. This adherence of C3b has powerful opsonic activity because it greatly increases the cell's susceptibility to phagocytosis. (**Ref. 3,** p. 390)

485. (**D**) Human cysticercosis is due to *Cysticercus cellulosae,* the larval form of *Taenia solium.* Human infection with the larval stage occurs either by ingestion of food or water contaminated with human feces containing *T. solium* eggs or by autoinfection with unclean hands of unsuspecting carriers of the adult worm. It can also occur when eggs from gravid proglottids are transferred by reverse peristalsis into more proximal parts of the small intestine of the individual infected with *T. solium.* (**Ref. 5,** pp. 207–208; **Ref. 4,** p. 1209)

486. (**C**) The toxin, which is hemolytic, necrotizing, and lethal, has been identified as lecithinase C. It is produced by the pathogenic strains of *Clostridium perfringens* and is of primary importance. It acts on lecithin-containing lipoprotein complexes in cell membranes. (**Ref. 4,** p. 639)

487. (**D**) Exotoxins are proteins elaborated by bacteria as extracellular products, which possess enzymatic activity and are toxic for target cells. Diphtheria, tetanus, and botulinum toxins are examples of exotoxins. (**Ref. 4,** pp. 390–391)

488. (D) In the secondary response, the amount of IgM produced is similar to that in primary response after the first contact with antigen. However, much more IgG is produced and the level of IgG tends to persist much longer than in the primary response. (**Ref. 2,** p. 111)

489. (B) Schistosomiasis mansoni is present in Puerto Rico. The main manifestation of the disease is hepatosplenic enlargement with ascites. Diagnosis can be made in the laboratory by demonstrating the typical egg that measures 115 to 175 μm in length with a conspicuous lateral spine. (**Ref. 4,** pp. 1213, 1214)

490. (E) Cell-mediated immunity develops after primary infection with herpes simplex and probably is a major immunologic factor in maintaining a latent state. Impairment of cellular immunity is correlated with episodic recurrences. In immunosuppressed patients the herpes simplex virus is commonly activated and disseminated, leading to acute disease. (**Ref. 3,** p. 932)

491. (B) The capsular polysaccharide of pneumococcus protects the organism from phagocytosis. Removal of the capsule with an enzyme specific for the polysaccharide renders the organism nonpathogenic and readily susceptible to phagocytosis. (**Ref. 4,** p. 435)

492. (D) The adult worms of *Schistosoma haematobium* live primarily in the pelvic veins. The eggs are deposited in the vesicle plexuses, producing lesions in the urinary bladder, genitalia, and, to some extent, in the rectum. (**Ref. 5,** p. 251)

493. (D) Actinomycin forms complexes specifically with DNA, thereby impairing DNA function. This binding is dependent upon guanine residues and helical secondary structure. (**Ref. 4,** p. 167)

494. (C) The time required for induction of delayed-type hypersensitivity (DTH) is generally about the same as for the induction of effector lymphocytes from resting precursor cells, such as cytotoxic T lymphocytes (CTLs) from precursor cells (pre-CTLs) and antibody-secreting B cells from resting B cells. That time period is about 1 week after antigen is first administered. (**Ref. 3,** p. 434)

495. (D) The median incubation period from contact until the appearance of the primary syphilitic chancre is about 21 days, the period being proportional to the size of the infecting inoculum. The chancre develops at the site of infection. (**Ref. 6,** p. 898)

496. (C) The growth of polioviruses can be readily obtained in primary or continuous cells line cultures derived from various tissues of humans and monkey kidney, testis, or muscle cells. However, they do not grow in cells of lower animals. (**Ref. 2,** p. 471)

497. (D) Enterotoxins appear to be formed only by coagulase-positive staphylococci, but not by all such strains. Those strains of phage groups III and IV produce such enterotoxins that cause in humans an acute gastrointestinal upset within 2 to 5 hours of ingestion. The toxins act on neural receptors in the upper gastrointestinal tract, stimulating the vomiting center in the brain. (**Ref. 6,** p. 279)

498. (C) Knowledge of human adenovirus infections is derived primarily from clinical observations and from experiments on volunteers. The data show that the diseases predominantly involve the respiratory tract and the eye. Type 3 or 7 has been isolated from a number of fatal cases of nonbacterial pneumonia in infants. Types 8, 19, and 37 are associated with epidemic keratoconjunctivitis. (**Ref. 3,** p. 923)

499. (C) A carbuncle is similar to a furuncle but has multiple foci and extends into the deeper layers of fibrous tissue. Carbuncles are limited to the neck and upper back, where the skin is thick and elastic. (**Ref. 4,** p. 410)

500. (C) In the treponema immobilization test (TPI), living motile spirochetes are immobilized in the presence of reagenic antibody and complement. This test requires living organisms. It is also positive in non-venereal treponematoses, bejel, yaws, and pinta. (**Ref. 4,** p. 664)

501. (C) The toxicity of the diphtheria toxin varies in different hosts. Doses as low as 160 ng/kg of body weight are lethal for humans, rabbits, guinea pigs, and birds. On the other hand, rats and mice are highly resistant unless the toxin is administered intracerebrally. (**Ref. 4,** p. 490)

502. (**D**) Important biologic distinctions have been correlated with the various classes and subclasses of immunoglobulin. For example, IgG4 does not activate complement via the classical pathway, whereas the other three IgG subclasses (IgG1, IgG2, IgG3) and IgM do. IgM antibodies are more efficient than IgG antibodies by virtue of their higher valence, which permits the development of large complexes with antigen. (**Ref. 7,** p. 134)

503. (**C**) The crop of vesicles in zoster appears over the skin supplied by the affected nerves. The eruption is usually unilateral with the trunk, head, and neck most commonly involved. The duration and severity of cutaneous eruption are generally proportionate to the age of the patient. (**Ref. 2,** p. 429)

504. (**E**) Amebic liver abscess may arise from subclinical, as well as from symptomatic intestinal amebiasis. Hence, symptomatic amebiasis is not always evident. Amebas have not been demonstrated in the stool of all cases of hepatic amebiasis. Approximately, only one third of the patients with hepatic amebiasis have amebas that are detectable in the stool. (**Ref. 5,** p. 28)

505. (**A**) The Shiga bacillus is apparently unique among the dysentery bacilli in that in addition to the endotoxin, which is a polysaccharide–lipid–polypeptide complex similar to the endotoxins of other enteric bacilli, it also produces an exotoxin. The exotoxin has a multiplicity of effects and is neurotoxic, cytotoxic, and enterotoxic. (**Ref. 4,** p. 558)

506. (**D**) Virulence-associated factors that have been identified for *Yersinia pestis* include (1) Ca^{2+} dependency, (2) V and W antigens, (3) outer membrane proteins (Yops), (4) F-1 envelope antigen, (5) pesticin, coagulase, and fibrinolysin products, and (6) pigment absorption. The importance of each of these factors has been difficult to assess separately. (**Ref. 4,** p. 585)

507. (**D**) In primary genital herpes, patients will have systemic symptoms, including fever, malaise, myalgias, headache, and regional adenopathy. (**Ref. 4,** p. 956)

508. **(C)** Secretory IgA antibodies in respiratory tract are probably critical for successful protection against influenza. However, the current inactivated influenza vaccines induce only low levels of IgA antibodies in the respiratory tract. Antibodies begin to decrease in about 3 months after immunization and immunity is often lost within 6 months. (**Ref. 3**, p. 1003)

509. **(D)** Fluid loss in severe cases of cholera approaches 15–20 L/day. The voided fluid is watery without traces of odor or enteric organisms. Hypovolemic shock and metabolic acidosis are consequences of the fluid loss, so the eyes and cheeks are sunken, skin turgor is diminished, and the hands have the appearance of a washerwoman's. (**Ref. 4**, p. 569)

510. **(B)** Spirochetes are best seen in the living state by dark-field illumination since they are too slender and may be below the resolution of light microscopy. When examined by dark-field illumination, spirochetes have a characteristic motility, including apparent rotation around their long axis, flexion, and a boring corkscrew motion. Species differ somewhat in motility which may be useful in differential diagnosis. (**Ref. 3**, pp. 673–674)

511. **(C)** Infectious hepatitis A is predominantly spread by ingestion. In epidemics, the source of virus can usually be traced to water and food contaminated by human carriers. (**Ref. 3**, p. 1099)

512. **(A)** The incidence of echinococcosis is high in humans in grazing countries, including southern Europe, where association with dogs is intimate. Infection often begins in childhood when children have unhygienic habits and transmission occurs by ingestion of eggs from infected dogs. The hydatid cysts are primarily located in the right lobe of the liver, mostly toward the inferior surface, so that they extend downward into the abdominal cavity. Clinical diagnosis is based upon the slowly growing cystic tumor, history of residence in an endemic area, and close association with dogs. (**Ref. 5**, pp. 203–205)

513. **(E)** Spores are formed within certain Gram-positive cells under conditions of inadequate nutrition. The spores have no metabolic activity; hence, they are "cryptobiotic." They are much more resistant to the lethal effect of heat, drying, freezing, toxic chemicals, and radiation than the parental vegetative cells. The surrounding mother cell is known as a sporangium. (**Ref. 3,** p. 45)

514. (D) *Rhodococcus equi* is a Gram-positive organism that exhibits a rod-coccus morphogenetic cycle. It causes several zoonoses, primarily a bronchopneumonia in horses. However, human infections have been reported in immunocompromised patients with severly impaired cell-mediated immunity and with histories of exposure to animals. It produces a necrotizing pneumonia, resembling mycobacterial infection. (**Ref. 4,** p. 495)

515. (D) The source of *Microsporidium* spp. is fecal contamination. The oocysts are taken in by mouth and reside in the small intestine. *Microsporidium* is responsible for diarrhea and malabsorption seen in immunosuppressed individuals, mainly AIDS patients. (**Ref. 5,** p. 11)

516. (D) Pili or fimbriae are fine filamentous appendages which are present in several hundred per cell. Most fimbriae function as adhesins, mediating adhesion to specific surfaces. Hence, they play an important role in pathogenesis. This has been established for the gonococcus and the pathogenic strains of *E. coli*. (**Ref. 3,** p. 24)

517. (D) About 0.1 to 1% of the adult population are asymptomatic carriers, and approximately 5% of the recognized cases of acute HBV infection become carriers of HBV. Most persist as carriers beyond 6 months, and patients more likely to be long-term carriers are: (1) nonwhites; (2) males; (3) infants; and (4) those who are immunosuppressed. (**Ref. 4,** p. 1043)

518. (D) Flagella occur most commonly among bacilli, and they are attached either at or near the poles of the cell or distributed over the rest of the cell surface. Those having tufts of flagella along the cylinder of the cells are designated peritrichous. (**Ref. 3,** p. 24)

519. (D) The portal of entry for *Babesia microti* is by the bite of the vector, *Ixodes* tick, through the exposed human skin. (**Ref. 5,** p. 102)

520. (A) Infection of the cervicofacial area by *Actinomyces* is the most common site. Lesions in the submandibular region and the angle of the jaw give the face a swollen appearance. The diagnostic sulfur granules in the pus, when crushed between two slides and stained, will give a Gram-positive center with individual branching rods at the periphery. (**Ref. 6,** pp. 464–465)

521. (B) Thayer–Martin medium is a variant of chocolate agar medium selective for the pathogenic *Neisseria, N. gonorrhoeae* and *N. meningitidis.* Growth of most other bacteria and fungi in the genital or respiratory flora is inhibited by the addition of vancomycin, colistin, trimethoprim, and anisomycin. (**Ref. 6,** p. 271)

522. (C) *Pseudomonas aeruginosa* is the pathogenic organism most consistently resistant to antimicrobics. The resistance is largely due to the structure of the outer membrane porins that restrict the entry of antimicrobics to the periplasmic space. *P. aeruginosa* strains are resistant to penicillin, ampicillin, cephalothin, tetracycline, chloramphenicol, sulfonamides, and the earlier aminoglycosides, such as streptomycin and kanamycin. The newer aminoglycosides are still active against most strains, as are carbenicillin and ticarcillin. A primary feature of the third-generation cephalosporins is their activity against *Pseudomonas.* (**Ref. 6,** p. 397)

523. (A) *Bacteroides fragilis* constitutes less than 10% of *Bacteroides* species in the normal colon but it predominates among Gram-negative infections in the abdominal cavity. Its polysaccharide capsule confers resistance to phagocytosis. It is almost always resistant to penicillin and many other β-lactams partly because of chromosomally encoded β-lactamase. (**Ref. 6,** p. 338)

524. (B) Skin infections caused by *Candida albicans* is an occupational disease of dishwashers and laundry workers. The initial lesions are erythematous papules or confluent areas associated with tenderness, erythema, and fissures of the skin. When exudate and epithelial scrapings are examined in potassium hydroxide, yeast cells are abundant, and if pseudohyphae are present, the infection can be assumed to be caused by *C. albicans.* (**Ref. 6,** pp. 654, 656)

525. (B) The enzyme catalase catalyzes the conversion of hydrogen peroxide to water and oxygen. The liberation of oxygen is seen as gas bubbles. This test is very useful in differentiating staphylococci, which produce catalase, from streptococci, which do not. (**Ref. 6,** p. 272)

526. (C) Streptomycin binds irreversibly to the 30S ribosomal subunit at the initiation of protein synthesis, thereby interrupting the ribosome cycle. Although it does not inhibit the formation of the initiation complex, it inhibits the initiation of the peptide chains on the complex. (**Ref. 4,** p. 170)

527. (A) Erythromycin is the most important of the macrolides. The 50S ribosomal subunit is the target site of erythromycin. In intact bacteria, erythromycin blocks the translocation step by specifically interfering with the release of the charged tRNA bound to the donor site of the ribosome after peptide bond formation. (**Ref. 4,** p. 175)

528. (C) *Legionella pneumophila* is a Gram-negative rod that attacks the lung and associated structures. The pneumonia it causes is necrotizing and multifocal with a tendency for coalescence of the lesions. The inflammatory exudate contains abundant fibrin and a mixture of neutrophils and macrophages. (**Ref. 6,** p. 423)

529. (E) *Mycoplasma pneumoniae* accounts for approximately 20% of all cases of pneumonia in general. It causes pneumonia that has been described as primary atypical pneumonia or walking pneumonia as it is less severe than the common bacterial pneumonia. X-ray reveals a lobar pneumonia, usually of the lower lobes. Small pleural effusions are seen in about 25% of the cases. (**Ref. 6,** pp. 415, 417)

530. (C) HBeAg is a low-molecular-weight glycoprotein. It is associated with the core antigen. It is present when HBsAg is also present but disappears from serum with the development of antibodies, anti-HBe and anti-HBs. (**Ref. 6,** pp. 551, 553)

531. (D) The development of anti-HBs against HBsAg is associated with the elimination or resolution of infection and, hence, also with protection against reinfection. (**Ref. 6,** pp. 553, 554)

532. (E) *Coxiella burnetii* is a strict intracellular parasite that is taken into the host cell by a phagocytic process to cause Q fever. Q fever is primarily a zoonosis and is transmitted from animals to humans by inhalation. The disease occurs in those who work with infected animals or their products, such as workers in abattoirs where slaughtering of infected animals produce aerosols for massive contamination. It also occurs in textile workers who break open bales of wool. **(Ref. 6,** pp. 486, 498)

533. (D) *Chlamydia psittaci* is an obligate intracellular bacteria that causes human psittacosis. It is a zoonosis that is contracted through inhalation of dust from droppings of infected birds. It is an occupational hazard of poultry workers, especially those who process turkey carcasses, as well as owners of pet psittacine birds. **(Ref. 6,** pp. 469, 472)

534. (C) Erythrogenic toxin, which is elaborated only by lysogenic streptococci, causes the rash in scarlet fever. Only strains elaborating this toxin can cause scarlet fever. Strains devoid of the temperate phage genome do not produce this toxin. **(Ref. 2,** p. 203)

535. (D) Streptolysin S is the enzyme responsible for the hemolytic zones around streptococcal colonies on the surface of blood agar plates. Complete disruption of erythrocytes with release of hemoglobin is classified as β hemolysis, while incomplete lysis of erythrocytes with the formation of green pigment is classified as α hemolysis. **(Ref. 2,** p. 203)

536. (E) After the resolution of chickenpox in childhood, the varicella-zoster virus may persist for decades. Reactivation of the latent virus results in a unilateral vesicular eruption, involving one to three dermatomes. This is clinically diagnosed as herpes zoster or shingles. It is seen in all ages but its frequency is increased with advancing age. **(Ref. 6,** pp. 566–567)

537. (A) One to three days after the onset of measles, pinpoint gray-white spots surrounded by erythema appear on the mucous membranes of the mouth. This sign is called Koplik's spots. The spots are most noticeable over the buccal mucosa opposite the molars and persist for 1 to 2 days. **(Ref. 6,** p. 520)

538. (C) The trypomastigotes of *T. cruzi* appear in stained blood smears in a U- or S-shape. It has a free flagellum about one third of the body length, a deeply staining central nucleus, and a large terminal kinetoplast. (**Ref. 5,** p. 66)

539. (B) The mature schizont of *P. malariae* contains 8 to 10 merozoites. The compact mass of greenish-black pigment is located in the center surrounded by the merozoites. Hence, the mature schizont resembles a "rosette" or "daisy." (**Ref. 5,** p. 82)

540. (B) Group B streptococci are a leading cause of pneumonia, sepsis, and meningitis during the first 2 months of life. Most cases result from contamination of the infant with the group B streptococci from the mother's genital tract. The morbidity in this age group is 1 to 3 cases per 1000 births and the mortality is between 30 to 60% of infected cases. (**Ref. 6,** p. 305)

541. (A) Some group A strains of streptococci form erythrogenic toxin, which has no clear role in the pathogenesis of invasive streptococcal disease. However, it is responsible for the rash seen in scarlet fever. The rash is probably caused by a combination of the direct effect of the erythrogenic toxin on the skin and delayed-type hypersensitivity to toxin. (**Ref. 6,** p. 298)

542. (B) Pneumocystosis is the most common opportunistic infection seen in AIDS patients. Approximately 50% of patients develop *Pneumocystis carinii* pneumonia. (**Ref. 6,** p. 931)

543. (D) Candidiasis in the form of oral thrush and esophagitis is a commonly encountered opportunistic infection in AIDS patients. (**Ref. 6,** p. 931)

544. (E) Gene transfer from one bacterial cell to another by the uptake of naked DNA is known as transformation. Transformation has been observed in a wide variety of both Gram-positive and Gram-negative bacteria. Three mechanisms of transformation have been described. The pneumococcus, for example, binds double-stranded DNA nonspecifically and the molecules are cut by an endonuclease in the membrane and only one strand enters. In the Gram-negative *Haemophilus,* uptake depends on a specific sequence of about 10 nucleotides. DNA enters as a double strand.

With enteric bacteria, transformation occurs only after artificial modification of the cell envelope. (**Ref. 3,** pp. 128, 130–131)

545. (C) When gene transfer from one bacterium to another is accomplished through infection by a nonlethal virus, it is known as transduction. Transduction of bacterial genes by a bacteriophage introduces only a small fraction of a bacterial chromosome. There are two mechanisms; in generalized transduction the phage may transfer any genes, while in specialized transduction the phage DNA that has been integrated into the host chromosome is excised and transferred by the phage. (**Ref. 3,** pp. 128, 131)

546. (A) Most cases (75%) of sporotrichosis (*S. schenckii*) are lymphocutaneous with lesions first appearing in the cutaneous or subcutaneous tissue and progressively involving the draining lymphatics. The subcutaneous nodule becomes discolored and the overlying skin eventually blackens. This necrotic lesion subsequently erupts to form an ulcer, which heals in a few weeks. (**Ref. 4,** p. 1115)

547. (F) Sputum, tissue, or scrapings of mucocutaneous lesions will reveal multiple budding yeast cells that are pathognomonic for *P. brasiliensis*. When *P. brasiliensis* is grown on a rich medium at 35°C to 37°C, the yeast forms will show multiple buds. (**Ref. 4,** pp. 1108–1109)

548. (A) Recent studies of Lyme disease have implicated the hard tick, *Ixodes dammini,* as the most probable vector in the Northeast and Midwest and another hard tick *I. pacificus,* in the western United States, and *I. ricinus* in Europe. *Ambylomma americanum,* the Lone Star tick is also a known vector. (**Ref. 4,** p. 670)

549. (E) Rocky Mountain spotted fever is directly related to the life cycle of four species of hard ticks that are indigenous to the United States: *Dermacentor andersoni, D. variabilis, Amblyomma americanum,* and *Haemaphysalis leporispalustris. D. andersoni,* the wood tick, is the major vector in the Rocky Mountain region; *D. variabilis,* the American dog tick, is the major vector in the eastern and southeastern United States. (**Ref. 4,** p. 705)

550. **(C)** Ketoconazole is one of the antifungal agents that is active against dermatophytes, dimorphic fungi, and yeasts, as well as bacteria and protozoa. It is efficacious when administered orally and when administered parenterally causes few adverse reactions. It interferes with ergosterol synthesis by the fungus cell. (**Ref. 4,** p. 166)

551. **(D)** Metronidazole, a nitroimidazole, was first used against trichomoniasis. It has been found to be effective against giardiasis, amebiasis, and a variety of infections produced by anaerobic bacteria. It reduces the 5-nitro group of the imidazole to produce intermediate products responsible for the death of the protozoal and bacterials cell, possibly by alkylation of DNA. (**Ref. 5,** p. 697)

552. **(E)** *T. trichiura* egg must undergo extrinsic development under ideal environmental conditions, such as moist shaded soil, humidity, and warm temperature, for about 3 weeks. The embryonated egg is now infective for humans. (**Ref. 5,** p. 120)

553. **(A)** *N. americanus* egg undergoes development to a rhabditiform larva in 1 to 2 days in the environment under favorable conditions and optimal terperature (23° to 33°C). It develops into the filariform larva in a few days. The active filariform larva, which projects from the soil surface, has a strong thigmotaxis that facilitates access to the skin. The filariform larva enters the exposed human skin to initiate the infection. (**Ref. 5,** p. 129)

554. **(B)** *Microsporum audouinii* is a typical dermatophyte; it causes epidemic tinea capitis, dermatophytosis of the scalp and hair. It does not invade the nails. (**Ref. 4,** pp. 1129–1130)

555. **(D)** *Histoplasma capsulatum* is a fungus that causes a systemic infection, primarily a pulmonary mycosis in humans. Histoplasmosis is the most prevalent mycosis of humans and animals. It is initiated by inhalation of the fungus, which occurs worldwide. (**Ref. 4,** p. 1097)

556. **(C)** Amantadine specifically inhibits all influenza viruses by blocking viral penetration of the host cell or by blocking viral uncoating. It is not prophylactically effective against influenza B. (**Ref. 2,** p. 401)

557. (F) Acyclovir strongly inhibits herpes simplex virus but has little effect on other DNA viruses. Parenteral administration of acyclovir has prevented the reactivation of latent herpesvirus infections. **(Ref. 2,** p. 399)

558. (E) Azidothymidine (AZT) inhibits the replication of human immunodeficiency virus (HIV) by blocking the synthesis of proviral DNA. The reverse transcriptase of the virus is 100 times more sensitive than the cellular DNA polymerase to inhibition by this drug. **(Ref. 2,** p. 398)

559. (A) Methisazone inhibits poxvirus replication by blocking a late stage in viral replication, resulting in the formation of immature, noninfectious viral particles. It is no longer used, since smallpox has been eradicated. **(Ref. 2,** p. 401)

560. (D) Ribavirin is believed to interfere with synthesis (capping) of viral mRNA. It has been approved for aerosol treatment of respiratory syncytial virus infections in infants. **(Ref. 2,** p. 401)

561. (B) Purified polysaccharide meningococcal vaccines have been shown to prevent group A and C disease in military and civilian populations. Quadrivalent vaccine containing A, C, Y, and W-135 polysaccharides has now been licensed for use in the United States. The lack of an effective serogroup B vaccine is still a problem. **(Ref. 6,** p. 348)

562. (H) The live attenuated yellow fever virus vaccine (17-D strain) is used to protect rural populations exposed to sylvatic cycle in certain countries and for international travelers to these endemic areas. Countries, such as those in tropical Africa, Asia, and South America, require proof of yellow fever vaccination. The vaccine correlates well with protective immunity. **(Ref. 6,** pp. 591–592)

563. (D) The pneumococcal vaccine is a purified multivalent polysaccharide prepared from the 23 types of *S. pneumoniae* most commonly encountered. It is protective against these 23 types and is recommended for patients susceptible to pneumococcal infection due to age, underlying disease, or immune status. **(Ref. 6,** p. 311)

564. (F) The rabies vaccine employs an attenuated rabies virus grown in human diploid cell culture and inactivated with β-propiolactone. Preexposure prophylaxis consists of two subcutaneous injections of the vaccine 1 month apart, followed by a booster dose several months later. Postexposure prophylaxis is based on immediate washing of the wound with soap and water, passive immunization with hyperimmune globulin of which at least half the dose should be around the wound site, and active immunization in 6 doses on days 1, 3, 7, 14, an 90. (**Ref. 6,** pp. 599–601)

565. (C) The mumps vaccine is an attenuated vaccine that has proven to be safe and highly effective. It is prepared by propagating the virus in chick embryo cell tissue cultures. It is recommended for infants after the first year of life and for seronegative susceptible adult men to prevent orchitis. (**Ref. 6,** p. 519)

566. (E) Granuloma inguinale is a very uncommon disease caused by *Calymmatobacterium granulomatis,* a Gram-negative bacillus morphologically and antigenically similar to *Klebsiella.* It is characterized by chronic, persistent genital papules or ulcers, which may extend into the inguinal region. (**Ref. 6,** p. 905)

567. (D) *Haemophilus ducreyi* is a Gram-negative bacillus that tends to be coccobacillary like other *Haemophilus.* It causes chancroid, a rare venereal disease in North America. It is characterized by a painful genital chancroid ulcer. Involvement of the inguinal lymph nodes is rapid and may develop into an abscess within a node (bubo), which can rupture. (**Ref. 6,** pp. 408, 904)

568. (A) The most common manifestation of gonococcal infection in men is urethritis which persists for several weeks, with unilateral epididymitis developing in 5 to 10% of cases. Gonorrhea is manifested in women by discharge and pain associated with infection of the cervix, as well as endometritis and salpingitis with upward spread. Gram stain of infected material reveals typical Gram-negative intracellular diplococci, *N. gonorrhoeae.* (**Ref. 6,** pp. 896–897)

569. (I) *T. vaginalis* is the etiologic agent of a persistent vaginitis in females. It is transmitted primarily by sexual intercourse, especially by asymptomatic infected male. However, transmission by contaminated fomites, such as toilet articles and toilet seats, is possible. Newborns can become infected while passing through the birth canal of an infected mother. In males there may be urethritis. (**Ref. 5,** p. 43)

570. **(B)** *C. trachomatis* causes the venereal disease lymphogranuloma venereum. The clinical spectrum is similar to that caused by *Neisseria gonorrhoeae*. Like gonorrhea, it is most prevalent in young adults of lower socioeconomic groups who have multiple sex partners. Lymphogranuloma verereum is a distinct venereal disease caused by 3 serotypes of *C. trachomatis* that is not associated with other chlamydial infections. (**Ref. 6,** p. 475)

571. **(B)** The narrow, barrel-shaped, whipworm egg (20 × 40 μm) is evacuated in the stool in an unembryonated condition. It has a golden brown color (due to bile) and a transparent prominence at each end referred to as "polar plugs." It is easily identified in the stool due to these characteristic features. (**Ref. 4,** p. 1190)

572. **(E)** The egg of *N. americanus* is thin-shelled, transparent, and broadly ovoidal and measures 60 × 40 μm. In freshly passed stool, it ranges in development from four-celled to a morula stage. The eggs may develop and hatch in 1 to 2 days, releasing the rhabditiform larvae which must be differentiated from those of *S. stercoralis.* (**Ref. 4,** p. 1197)

573. **(A)** *Taenia* eggs are characterized by broad radial striations in the shell. Eggs of *T. saginata* are indistinguishable from those of *T. solium.* The egg measures 35 μm in diameter. (**Ref. 4,** p. 1208)

574. **(C)** At the time of oviposition, the fertilized egg of *A. lumbricoides* is broadly ovoidal and measures 45 to 70 × 35 to 50 μm. The various layers account for the thick shell, which is characteristic. The outer layer is coarsely mammillated. (**Ref. 4,** p. 1194)

575. **(D)** The egg of *E. vermicularis* discharged in the perianal skin is essentially mature and within a few hours contains a fully developed, infective-stage larva. The egg measures 50 to 60 × 20 to 30 μm and has a double shell. The eggs are asymmetrical, being flattened on one side. (**Ref. 4,** p. 1190)

References

1. Braude AI, Davis CE, Fierer J (eds): *Infectious Diseases and Medical Microbiology,* 2nd Ed. WB Saunders, Philadelphia, 1986.
2. Brooks GF, Butel JS, Ornston LN, Jawetz E, Melnick JL, Adelberg EA: Jawetz, Melnick & Adelberg's *Medical Microbiology,* 19th Ed. Appleton & Lange, Norwalk, CT, 1991.
3. Davis BD, Dulbecco R, Eisen HN, Ginsberg HS: *Microbiology,* 4th Ed. JB Lippincott, Philadelphia, 1990.
4. Joklik WK, Willett HP, Amos DB, Wilfert CM (eds): *Zinsser Microbiology,* 20th Ed. Appleton & Lange, Norwalk, CT, 1992.
5. Neva FA, Brown HW: *Basic Clinical Parasitology,* 6th Ed. Appleton & Lange, Norwalk, CT, 1994.
6. Sherris JC (ed): *Medical Microbiology: An Introduction to Infectious Diseases,* 2nd Ed. Elsevier, New York, 1990.
7. Stites DP, Terr AI: *Basic and Clinical Immunology,* 7th Ed. Appleton & Lange, Norwalk, CT, 1991.

4

Pathology
Alfred Olusegun Fayemi

DIRECTIONS (Questions 576 through 614): This section of the test consists of cases, each followed by a series of questions. Study each case and select the ONE best answer to each question following it.

CASE 1 (Questions 576 through 578): Figures 4–1A and B show histologic sections from an hemithyroidectomy specimen from a 40-year-old woman with a diffusely enlarged thyroid gland.

576. The histologic features most strongly suggest
- **A.** follicular carcinoma
- **B.** tuberculous thyroiditis
- **C.** chronic lymphocytic thyroiditis
- **D.** medullary carcinoma
- **E.** malignant lymphoma

577. Most likely to be encountered in this patient is
- **A.** exophthalmos
- **B.** elevated thyroid-stimulating hormone (TSH)
- **C.** bilateral cervical lymphadenopathy
- **D.** positive tuberculin test
- **E.** C-cell hyperplasia

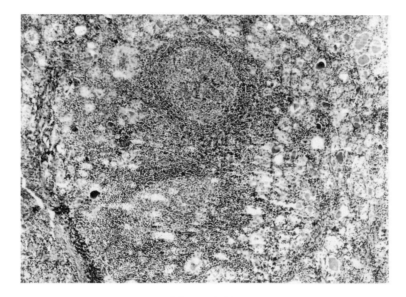

Figure 4.1A

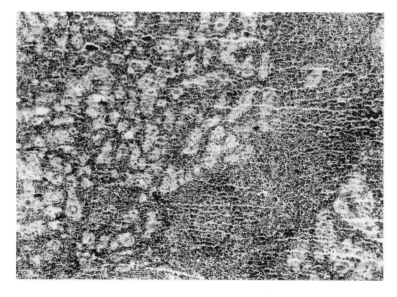

Figure 4.1B

578. Which of the following is most closely associated with the etiopathogenesis of this disease?
   A. ionizing radiation
   B. autoimmunity
   C. *Mycobacterium tuberculosis*
   D. iodine deficiency
   E. none of the above

CASE 2 (Questions 579 through 581): A 47-year-old white HIV-positive man was admitted to the hospital for the investigation of fever, headaches, vomiting, intermittent confusion, and an episode of generalized convulsion. Physical examination revealed right hemiparesis and variable sensory loss in the right lower extremity. The CSF showed mildly elevated protein, normal glucose, and few lymphocytes. CT scan of the brain showed two well circumscribed masses in the left cerebral cortex. A craniotomy was performed and one of the lesions was resected. Sections show areas of necrosis with scattered enlarged cells (arrow—Fig. 4.2).

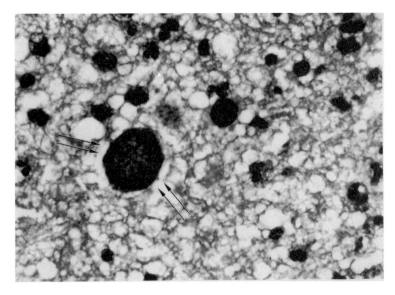

Figure 4.2

579. The most probable diagnosis is
  A. North American blastomycosis
  B. cryptococcosis
  C. histoplasmosis
  D. toxoplasmosis
  E. herpes encephalitis

580. Which organ is most frequently involved in toxoplasma infection in immunocompetent adults?
  A. lymph nodes
  B. brain
  C. liver
  D. spleen
  E. myocardium

581. Which of the following most accurately characterizes the tissue response to toxoplasma infection?
  A. hemorrhagic necrosis with minimal inflammatory response
  B. necrotizing granulomatous inflammation
  C. tissue necrosis and vasculitis with thrombosis
  D. intense acute inflammation with abscess formation
  E. granulation tissue and nonspecific chronic inflammation with exuberant repair

CASE 3 (Questions 582 through 585): Light microscopic features of a kidney biopsy from a 68-year-old man with a 20-year history of diabetes mellitus and azotemia.

582. Figure 4.3 best illustrates which of the following renal lesions?
   A. chronic glomerulonephritis (chronic GN)
   B. diffuse glomerulosclerosis (diffuse GS)
   C. nodular glomerulosclerosis (nodular GS)
   D. membranous nephropathy
   E. focal segmental glomerulosclerosis

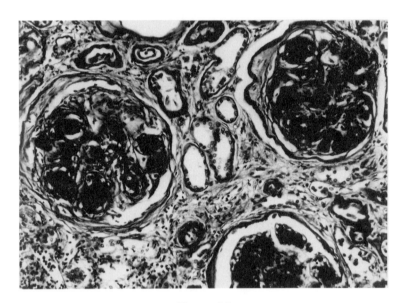

Figure 4.3

583. Which of these is LEAST likely to be found in the late stages of diabetic nephropathy?
- **A.** hypertension
- **B.** hematuria
- **C.** widespread microangiopathy
- **D.** severely depressed glomerular filtration rate (GFR)
- **E.** massive proteinuria

584. Electron microscopy of advanced diabetic glomerulosclerosis will most likely show
- **A.** loss of foot processes
- **B.** dense subendothelial deposits
- **C.** dense subepithelial deposits
- **D.** massive increase in mesangial matrix
- **E.** splitting of basement membrane

585. Which of the following is NOT true concerning the pathogenesis of diabetic glomerulosclerosis?
- **A.** the development of diabetic GS has been linked to a separate genetic defect
- **B.** diabetic GS is intimately linked with that of generalized microangiopathy
- **C.** hemodynamic changes, specifically glomerular vasodilation, increased intraglomerular plasma flow and filtration pressure have been implicated
- **D.** increased synthesis of collagen type IV
- **E.** nonenzymatic glycosylation of proteins

CASE 4 (Questions 586 and 587): An 11-year-old boy presented with mild fever, nausea, vomiting, and abdominal pain. Physical examination showed right lower quadrant tenderness. Temperature: 101°F; pulse: 92/min. Laboratory investigation revealed WBC 16,000 with a predominance of neutrophils, Hb 15.2 G/100 mL, normal electrolytes and BUN. After observation for 12 hours, he underwent an appendectomy. Figure 4.4 shows a cross section of the resected appendix.

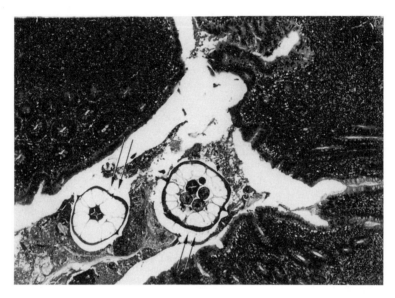

Figure 4.4

586. The objects indicated in the lumen of the appendix (arrows) most likely are
   A. nonspecific debris
   B. enterobius vermicularis
   C. fecal matter
   D. vegetable matter
   E. trichuris trichiura

587. Symptomatology attributable to this condition includes
- **A.** acute appendicitis
- **B.** constipation
- **C.** perianal pruritus
- **D.** recurrent abdominal pain
- **E.** none of the above

CASE 5 (Questions 588 and 589): Histologic findings in the lungs of a 50-year-old man with interstitial pulmonary fibrosis.

588. The structure indicated with the arrows (Fig. 4.5) represents
- **A.** Charcot–Leyden crystals
- **B.** Curschmann's spirals
- **C.** asteroid bodies
- **D.** asbestos bodies
- **E.** Mallory bodies

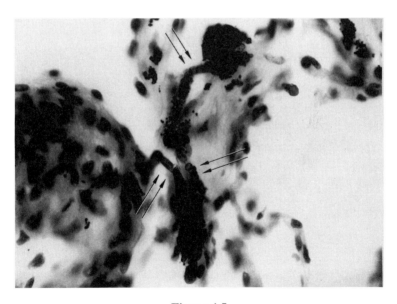

Figure 4.5

589. The disease most commonly associated with this structure is
   A. pulmonary emphysema
   B. chronic bronchitis
   C. bronchioloalveolar carcinoma
   D. non-caseating epithelioid granuloma
   E. mesothelioma

CASE 6 (Questions 590 through 592): Figure 4.6 shows representative section from the lung of a 50-year-old man with a history of dyspnea on exertion and dry cough. Physical examination revealed fine crackling inspiratory and expiratory rales and accentuated second heart sound in the pulmonic area. Roentgenogram of the chest revealed bilateral reticulonodular densities, most prominent at the lung bases. Blood chemistry and CBC were normal.

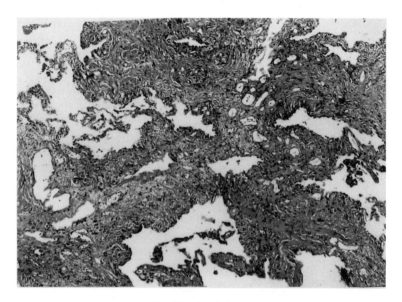

Figure 4.6

590. The etiology most commonly associated with this condition is
   A. tuberculosis
   B. viral infection
   C. asbestosis
   D. collagen vascular disease
   E. sarcoidosis

591. Typical morphologic changes in this disease include all of the following EXCEPT
   A. honeycomb lung
   B. hyperplasia of type II pneumocytes
   C. destruction and dilatation of bronchi
   D. thickening of pulmonary interstitium with edema and fibroblasts
   E. right ventricular hypertrophy

592. Which of the following has not been implicated in the pathogenesis of this lesion?
   A. direct toxicity of free radicals and chemicals to endothelial cells
   B. release of neutrophil chemotactic factor
   C. cell mediated (type IV) immune reaction
   D. type I hypersensitivity reaction
   E. immune complex (type III) reaction

CASE 7 (Questions 593 and 594): A 70-year-old man was admitted with frequency, urinary retention, and intermittent dysuria. For a few years he had noticed a decrease in the force of urinary stream. Physical examination showed moderate enlargement of the prostate. Urinalysis: 50 WBC/high power field, 10 RBC/HPF. A transurethral prostatectomy was performed. The specimen, which weighed 32 gm, was composed of fragments of rubbery, pinkish-gray tissue. The microscopic sections in Figures 4.7A and B are representative of the lesion.

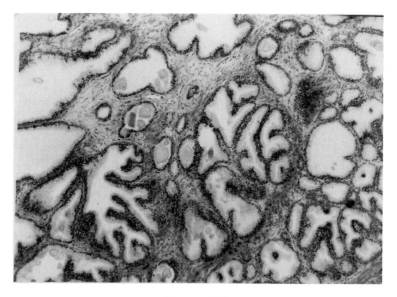

Figure 4.7A

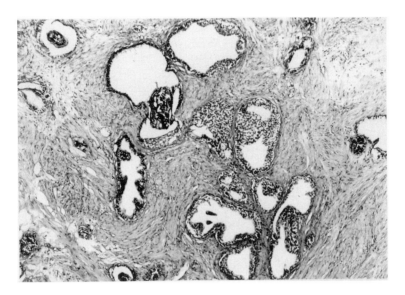

Figure 4.7B

593. The most appropriate diagnosis is
    A. benign prostatic hyperplasia
    B. nonspecific chronic prostatitis
    C. granulomatous prostatitis
    D. well differentiated prostatic adenocarcinoma
    E. prostatic adenoid cystic carcinoma

594. Which of the following is not true concerning this disease?
    A. although common in men over 60 years, surgical treatment is required only in about 10%
    B. the disease develops only in the presence of intact testes
    C. the lesion is surrounded by a pseudocapsule
    D. the disease occurs with the same frequency in both blacks and whites of the same age
    E. squamous metaplasia may occur in this lesion

CASE 8 (Questions 595 and 596):   Sections from a brain tumor in a 51-year-old white woman (Figs. 4.8A, B, and C).

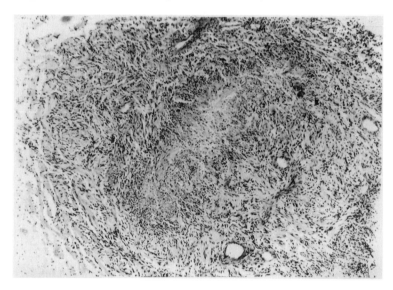

Figure 4.8A

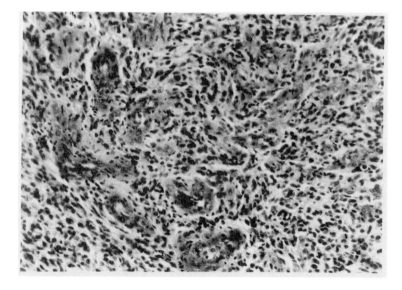

Figure 4.8B

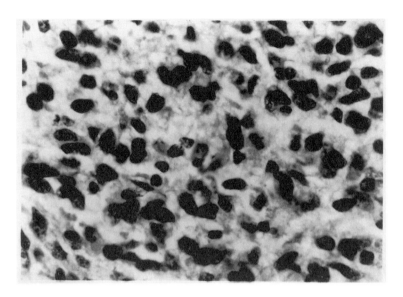

Figure 4.8C

595. The morphologic features strongly suggest
    A. primary malignant lymphoma of the brain
    B. glioblastome multiforme
    C. oligodendroglioma
    D. ependymoma
    E. meningioma

596. This tumor will be least expected to arise from
    A. cerebral hemispheres
    B. spinal cord
    C. pons
    D. cerebellum
    E. medulla oblongata

CASE 9 (Questions 597 and 598):

597. The clinical setting and finding most likely to be associated with the renal lesion (arrows) in Figure 4.9 is
- **A.** acute pyelonephritis
- **B.** a blood pressure of 180/135
- **C.** massive proteinuria
- **D.** amyloidosis
- **E.** minimal change disease (lipoid nephrosis)

598. The pathogenesis of this lesion has been associated with all of the following EXCEPT
- **A.** high levels of renin
- **B.** elevated serum levels of angiotensin
- **C.** intravascular coagulation
- **D.** microangiopathic hemolytic anemia
- **E.** excessive production of prostaglandins and kinins

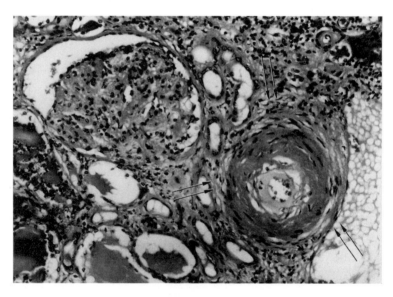

Figure 4.9

CASE 10 (Questions 599 and 600): Liver biopsy from a 35-year-old black man (Fig. 4.10).

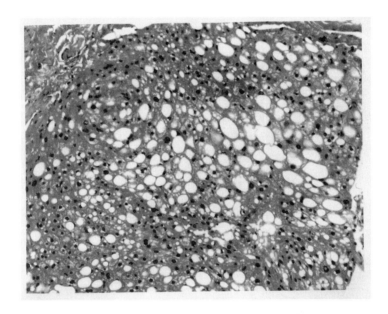

Figure 4.10

599. All of the following may cause this disease EXCEPT
  A. carbon tetrachloride poisoning
  B. protein–calorie malnutrition
  C. alcohol consumption
  D. acute viral hepatitis
  E. obesity

600. Which of the following is NOT true regarding this lesion?
  A. it may progress to liver cirrhosis
  B. the involved liver is usually enlarged and greasy
  C. it may be confirmed histochemically by Sudan IV stain
  D. it may be caused by decreased apoprotein synthesis
  E. patients manifest no abnormal serum biochemical parameters

CASE 11 (Questions 601 through 603): Section of the biopsy of an enlarged prostate in a 75-year-old man (Fig. 4.11).

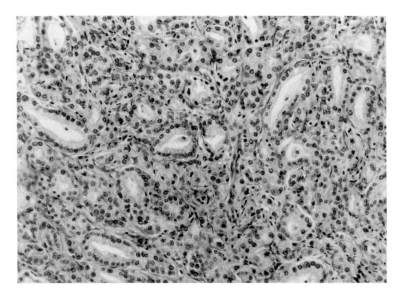

Figure 4.11

601. This lesion should be treated
   A. by observation and annual follow-up physical examination
   B. periodic laboratory testing following measurement of prostatic specific antigen
   C. transurethral prostatectomy followed by orchiectomy and estrogen administration
   D. medical treatment to diminish the size of the prostate
   E. pelvic lymphadenectomy followed by radiation

602. This lesion is least prevalent among
   A. the Japanese
   B. American whites
   C. American blacks
   D. Europeans
   E. Scandinavians

603. From which part of the prostate is the lesion most likely to have arisen?

    A. submucosa of the proximal urethra

    B. peripheral and lateral

    C. central and posterior

    D. peripheral and posterior

    E. central and lateral

CASE 12 (Questions 604 through 606): Figure 4.12 on page 202 shows a biopsy of a pigmented skin lesion in the upper arm of a 35-year-old white woman. The lesion, which recently became itchy, was slightly elevated. It was dark brownish, had irregular external borders, and was not ulcerated.

604. The clinical and histopathologic findings are most consistent with

    A. epithelioid nevus (Spitz nevus)

    B. malignant melanoma

    C. dysplastic nevus

    D. seborrheic keratosis

    E. dermatofibroma (fibrous histiocytoma)

605. A large pigmented skin lesion with numerous hairs which, histologically, shows intraepidermal and dermal melanocytes which extend into the subcutaneous tissue and around skin adnexa is most probably a

    A. lentigo maligna

    B. acral lentiginous melanoma

    C. dermal nevus

    D. congenital nevus

    E. blue nevus

606. Which of the following statements concerning malignant melanoma is inaccurate?

    A. lightly pigmented persons are at a greater risk than darkly pigmented individuals

    B. the tumor may occur in the leptomeninges

    C. it does not metastasize during its radial growth phase

    D. mitotic rate is a reliable prognostic indicator

    E. the rarest clinical subtype in blacks is acral lentiginous melanoma

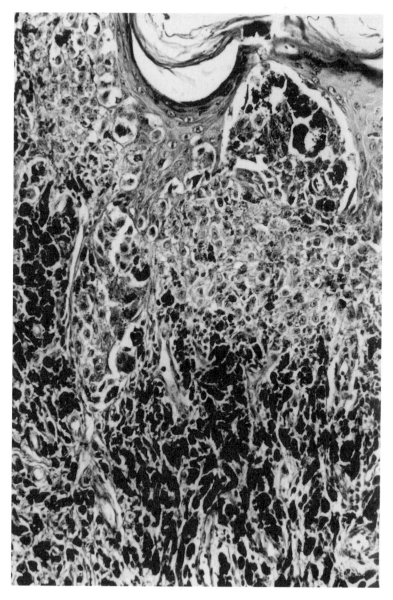

Figure 4.12

CASE 13 (Questions 607 through 609): A 34-year-old white man presented with diarrhea, abdominal cramps, and periumbilical pain. He had lost about 5 lb body weight in the previous few days. The diarrhea was accompanied by rectal bleeding. Physical examination showed a tired-looking man in obvious distress. Temperature: 100°F; Hb 10.5 Gm/100 mL. A proctosigmoidoscopy was performed and a colonic biopsy was obtained (Figs. 4.13A and B).

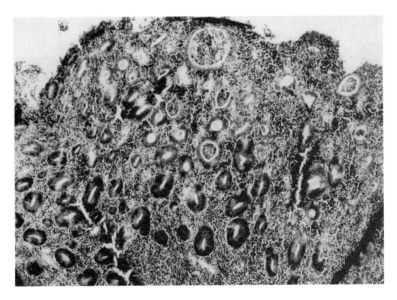

Figure 4.13A

607. The clinical and histologic findings strongly suggest
   A. amebic colitis
   B. ulcerative colitis
   C. Crohn's colitis
   D. *Shigella* colitis
   E. pseudomembranous colitis

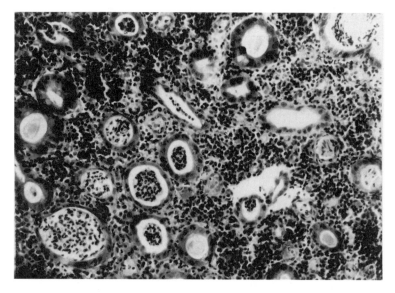

Figure 4.13B

608. This disease is characterized by all of these EXCEPT
  A. pseudopolyps
  B. iron deficiency anemia
  C. "skip" lesions
  D. crypt abscesses
  E. predominant involvement of left colon

609. Toxic megacolon is typically observed in
  A. Hirschsprung disease
  B. bacillary dysentery
  C. acute colitis of toxigenic strains of *E. coli*
  D. acute colitis caused by *Campylobacter* spp
  E. acute ulcerative colitis

CASE 14 (Questions 610 through 614): Section from the my-ocardium of a 65-year-old woman who was admitted for substernal chest pain with radiation to the neck and left arm. In spite of intensive treatment she expired after a few days of hospitalization. Figure 4.14 represents a section from the heart.

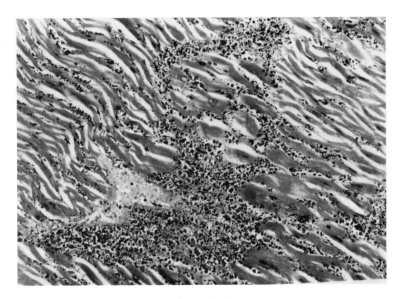

Figure 4.14

610. At the cellular level, the early changes of this lesion is character-ized by all of these EXCEPT
   A. $\downarrow$ ATP
   B. $\downarrow$ intracellular Ca^{++}
   C. $\uparrow$ intracellular Na^+
   D. $\uparrow$ intracellular H^+
   E. $\uparrow$ proteases

611. The earliest histologic lesion of irreversible cell death in this lesion is
  A. coagulative necrosis
  B. outpouring of polymorphonuclear leukocytes
  C. myocytolysis
  D. wavy myocardial fibers
  E. fatty change

612. Alterations in serum enzymes are sensitive and reliable indicators of acute myocardial infarction. Which of the following rises in 2 to 4 hours, peaks within 12 hours, and returns to normal within 48 to 96 hours?
  A. CK-MB
  B. LDH-1
  C. CK-MM
  D. SGOT
  E. SGPT

613. An acutely ill 38-year-old man was admitted with a fever of 105°F, shaking chills, moderate respiratory distress, and severe right-sided chest pain aggravated by coughing and deep breathing. His cough occurred in paroxysms and was productive of rusty sputum. Except for a bout of nasopharyngitis a few days previously, he had enjoyed good health. Examination of the chest revealed right-sided respiratory lag, dullness and tenderness on percussion, bronchial breath sounds, increased tactile fremitus and pleural friction rub. Moderate leukocytosis with "shift to the left" was present. Chest x-ray showed consolidation of the right middle and lower lobes. The most likely causative organism is
  A. group A streptococcus
  B. *Haemophilus influenzae*
  C. *Streptococcus pneumoniae*
  D. *Klebsiella pneumoniae*
  E. Mycoplasma pneumoniae

614. Macroscopic examination of the lungs would reveal which characteristic morphology?
  A. heavy, boggy, red, and subcrepitant lobe
  B. frothy, blood-tinged fluid can be squeezed from lung parenchyma

C. fleshy, brownish-pink lobe with leathery tough areas and pleural adhesions

D. red–gray consolidation of lobe with extensive abscess formation

E. red, firm, and airless lobe with liverlike consistency

DIRECTIONS (Questions 615 through 700): Each of the numbered items or incomplete statements in this section is followed by answers or completions of the statement. Select the ONE lettered answer or completion that is best in each case.

---

615. The descriptive term "cleaved" or "non-cleaved," when applied to a non-Hodgkin lymphoma refers to which cell component?
    A. cell membrane
    B. nucleolus
    C. nucleus
    D. nuclear chromatin
    E. cytoplasmic organelles

616. The most common organism encountered in the infective endocarditis of the intravenous drug abuser is
    A. *Streptococcus viridans*
    B. *Staphylococcus aureus*
    C. *E. coli*
    D. *Candida albicans*
    E. *Aspergillus fumigatus*

617. Barett esophagus is characterized by all of the following EXCEPT
    A. columnar metaplasia of esophageal squamous epithelium
    B. association with smoking and alcohol
    C. presence of longitudinal mucosal tears and ulceration
    D. chronic gastroesophageal reflux
    E. serious risk of malignant transformation

618. Most of transfusion-related hepatitis is caused by
  A. hepatitis A (HAV) and hepatitis B (HBV)
  B. HBV and hepatitis D (HDV)
  C. hepatitis C (HCV) and HBV
  D. hepatitis E (HEV) and HBV
  E. HAV and HEV

619. Which of the following cancers of the lung is LEAST associated with a history of cigarette smoking?
  A. squamous cell
  B. small cell, oat cell type
  C. small cell, intermediate cell type
  D. adenocarcinoma
  E. bronchioloalveolar

620. Which of these is not typical of anemia due to intravascular hemolysis?
  A. reticulocytosis in peripheral blood
  B. erythroid hyperplasia of bone marrow
  C. indirect bilirubinemia
  D. hemosiderinuria
  E. elevated serum haptoglobin

621. The following are true of toxoplasmosis EXCEPT
  A. the infection occurs in tissue cells as bradyzoites or tachyzoites
  B. adults can be infected by transfusion of contaminated blood
  C. toxoplasma lymphadenitis is the most common manifestation in immunocompetent adults
  D. maternal infection during pregnancy may result in stillbirth
  E. toxoplasmosis should be considered in an AIDS patient with protean neurologic symptoms and signs

622. "Feathery degeneration" is most likely to be found in which of the following liver diseases?
  A. chronic passive congestion
  B. Gilbert syndrome
  C. hepatitis A infection
  D. choledocholithiasis
  E. hemochromatosis

623. The most common complication of acute myocardial infarct is
   A. cardiogenic shock
   B. congestive heart failure
   C. rupture of the free wall of the left ventricle
   D. mural thrombosis and embolism
   E. cardiac arrhythmias

624. Richter syndrome may be expected to occur with
   A. hairy cell leukemia
   B. chronic myelogenous leukemia
   C. chronic lymphocytic leukemia
   D. acute lymphoblastic leukemia
   E. none of the above

625. Chronic cor pulmonale is least likely to be caused by
   A. recurrent pulmonary emboli
   B. bronchial asthma
   C. cystic fibrosis
   D. Hamman–Rich syndrome
   E. kyphoscoliosis

626. All of these have similar morphology EXCEPT
   A. Cushing ulcer
   B. duodenal ulcer
   C. ulcer at gastroenterostomy stoma
   D. Barett ulcer
   E. jejunal ulcer associated with Zollinger–Ellison syndrome

627. A 55-year-old man with a blood pressure of 160/100 for 20 years is being treated with low salt diet and chlorothiazides. Which of the following lesions is most likely to be present in this patient?
   A. "flea-bitten" kidneys
   B. hyaline arteriolosclerosis
   C. papilledema
   D. necrotizing glomerulitis
   E. dilated left ventricle

628. Which of the following pathologic changes is LEAST likely to be found in chronic congestive heart failure?
   A. "brown induration" of the lung
   B. ventricular dilatation
   C. "nutmeg" liver
   D. splenic infarcts
   E. pleural effusion

629. The risk of atherosclerotic ischemic heart disease bears an inverse relationship to serum levels of
   A. triglycerides (TG)
   B. very low-density lipoprotein (VLDL)
   C. intermediate-density lipoprotein (IDL)
   D. high-density lipoprotein (HDL)
   E. low-density lipoprotein (LDL)

630. A lung neoplasm located in the subpleural parenchyma and showing pleural puckering and pigmentation on cut section is most likely to be
   A. small cell carcinoma
   B. squamous cell carcinoma
   C. malignant melanoma
   D. adenocarcinoma
   E. mesothelioma

631. Which of the following is NOT typical of polycythemia vera?
   A. bone marrow panhyperplasia
   B. hepatosplenomegaly
   C. low leukocyte alkaline phosphatase
   D. risk of progression to acute myelogenous leukemia
   E. diminished bone marrow iron stores

632. Which of these will be expected to be MOST severely involved by atherosclerosis?
   A. abdominal aorta
   B. coronary arteries
   C. internal carotid arteries
   D. cerebral arteries
   E. thoracic aorta

633. Which antibody will be expected to occur MOST frequently in patients with Sjörgren syndrome?
   A. anti-nuclear antibodies (ANA)
   B. SS-B (La)—antibody against ribonucleoprotein antigens
   C. rheumatoid factor
   D. anti-histone antibody
   E. anti-ribonucleoprotein (Smith antigen)

634. Which of the following MOST accurately describes AIDS lymphadenopathy?
   A. histiocytic necrotizing lymphadenitis
   B. angiofollicular hyperplasia, plasma cell type
   C. angioimmunoblastic lymphadenopathy
   D. follicular involution with generalized lymphocytic depletion
   E. viral lymphadenitis with Warthin–Finkeldey cells and granulomas

635. The currently accepted pathogenesis of pulmonary emphysema stipulates
   A. progression from chronic bronchitis in susceptible patients
   B. intrinsic skeletal weakness, particularly of the chest wall permitting progressive expansion of the lung
   C. destruction of alveolar wall from derangement of protease–antiprotease mechanism
   D. insidious recurrent inflammation of bronchi and bronchioles
   E. immunological mechanism involving cytotoxic antibodies

636. In which histologic type of Hodgkin disease would "lacunar" Reed–Sternberg cells be most commonly found?
   A. lymphocytic predominant
   B. mixed cellularity
   C. lymphocyte depleted, reticular type
   D. lymphocyte depleted, diffuse fibrosis
   E. nodular sclerosis

637. All of these are true of immune complex disease EXCEPT
  A. very large complexes formed in antibody excess are most injurious to tissues
  B. IgA-containing complexes can activate complement through the alternate pathway
  C. immune complex vasculitis is characterized by fibrinoid necrosis of small blood vessels
  D. by immunofluorescence, immune complexes can be recognized as granular deposits
  E. the Arthus reaction is a prototype of local immune complex disease

638. Disorganization and haphazard arrangement of myocardial fibers with mild interstitial fibrosis will be most typically observed in
  A. dilated cardiomyopathy
  B. hypertrophic cardiomyopathy
  C. restrictive cardiomyopathy
  D. endomyocardial fibrosis
  E. endocardial fibroelastosis

639. Which of the following have been unequivocally associated with the pathogenesis of atherosclerosis?
  A. platelets, lymphocytes, macrophages
  B. plasma cells, smooth muscle cells, lymphocytes
  C. endothelial cells, smooth muscle cells, neutrophils
  D. smooth muscle cells, endothelial cells, macrophages
  E. macrophages, plasma cells, endothelial cells

640. Degranulation of mast cells with the release of preformed and secondarily generated mediators is the pathogenetic mechanism in which of the following diseases?
  A. systemic lupus erythematosus
  B. allergic rhinitis (hay fever)
  C. pulmonary tuberculosis
  D. poststreptococcus glomerulonephritis
  E. rheumatoid arthritis

641. A lung disease characterized by diffuse alveolar damage, interstitial and intraalveolar edema, fibrin deposition, hyaline membranes, and patchy atelectasis is typically found in all of these EXCEPT

    A. oxygen toxicity
    B. septic shock
    C. paraquat poisoning
    D. radiation
    E. Goodpasture syndrome

642. Significant clinical and the most common manifestations of reactive systemic amyloidosis is most likely to be encountered in

    A. gastrointestinal tract
    B. respiratory tract
    C. liver
    D. kidney
    E. spleen

643. All of the following are well recognized causes of osteoporosis EXCEPT

    A. hyperadrenocortism
    B. hypogonadism in young men
    C. acromegaly
    D. rheumatoid arthritis
    E. thyrotoxicosis

644. Comedocarcinoma is a subtype of which histologic type of breast carcinoma?

    A. lobular
    B. medullary
    C. intraductal
    D. colloid
    E. Paget disease

645. All of the following are typical of the renal disease associated with HIV-positive patients EXCEPT

    A. rapid progression to end-stage renal failure
    B. focal segmental glomerular sclerosis
    C. electron dense immune complex deposits in the mesangium
    D. nonspecific interstitial inflammation
    E. linear deposits by immunofluorescence

646. Which of the following is INCORRECT regarding hepatitis A?
- **A.** the large majority of infections are asymptomatic and anicteric
- **B.** hepatitis A virus (HAV) is a single-stranded RNA virus
- **C.** the disease may be transmitted by eating inadequately cooked shellfish
- **D.** the infection rate is higher among male homosexuals
- **E.** chronic infection manifests morphologically as chronic active hepatitis

647. The adverse reaction resulting from the transfusion of a BRh+ blood to a recipient with ORh+ blood group is most likely caused by
- **A.** complement-dependent hypersensitivity lysis
- **B.** systemic anaphylactic reaction
- **C.** antibody-dependent cell-mediated cytotoxic reaction
- **D.** immune complex reaction
- **E.** T cell-mediated cytotoxicity

648. Demonstrated risk factors for esophageal cancer include all of the following EXCEPT
- **A.** Barett esophagus
- **B.** Plummer–Vinson syndrome
- **C.** achalasia
- **D.** reflux esophagitis
- **E.** cigarette smoking

649. The immune deposit in IgA nephropathy is predominantly
- **A.** subendothelial
- **B.** mesangial
- **C.** subepithelial
- **D.** intramembranous
- **E.** along the Bowman's capsule

650. The antigen-binding site of an immunoglobulin molecule resides specifically in
- **A.** F_c fragment
- **B.** F_{ab} fragment
- **C.** V regions of H and L chains
- **D.** C regions of H and L chains
- **E.** the entire L chain

651. The best prognosis would be expected in which type of non-Hodgkin malignant lymphoma?
  A. small, non-cleaved cell
  B. diffuse, large cell
  C. follicular, predominantly large cell
  D. diffuse, small cleaved cell
  E. follicular, predominantly mixed, small cleaved, and large cell

652. A diarrheal illness following the intake of broad spectrum antibiotics such as cephalosporins will most likely be caused by
  A. enterotoxigenic *E. coli*
  B. *Staphylococcus aureus*
  C. *Clostridium difficile*
  D. *Salmonella typhimurium*
  E. *Shigella sonnei*

653. Natural killer (NK) cells are so called because they
  A. are activated macrophages that readily engulf particulate matter
  B. are a subset of B lymphocytes that participate in type 1 hypersensitivity reaction
  C. are immune cells that indiscriminately kill both virus-infected and normal human cells
  D. monocytoid cells that eliminate foreign cells through the activation of the complement system
  E. are lymphocytes that possess the ability to kill tumor cells and virus-infected cells

654. A 23-year-old man presented at the emergency room with abrupt onset of hematuria, nausea, and vomiting. Physical examination showed mild periorbital edema. Blood pressure: 180/100; urinalysis: many WBC, RBC with scattered RBC casts; protein 3+. Serum BUN: 40 mg/dL. Which of the following is the LEAST likely cause of this disease?
  A. poststreptococcal glomerulonephritis
  B. IgA nephropathy
  C. Goodpasture syndrome
  D. membranous nephropathy
  E. rapidly progressive glomerulonephritis

655. A skin lesion showing acantholysis with suprabasal blister formation, positive Nikolsky's sign, demonstration of IgG and/or complement in the intercellular spaces of keratinocytes, is most likely to be

A. bullous pemphigoid

B. dermatitis herpetiformis

C. psoriasis

D. pemphigus vulgaris

E. Stevens–Johnson syndrome

656. An intracranial tumor characterized by cellular pleomorphism, hypercellularity, anaplasia, necrosis with pseudopalisading of cells and striking endothelial proliferation is most likely to be

A. ependymoma

B. angioblastic meningioma

C. glioblastoma multiforme

D. ganglioglioma

E. oligodendroglioma

657. Vitamin B_{12} deficiency (pernicious anemia) is not characterized by

A. increased excretion of formiminoglutamic acid after histidine loading

B. hypersegmented neutrophils

C. atrophic gastritis

D. subacute combined degeneration of the spinal cord

E. parietal canalicular antibody

658. Which of the following is INCORRECT regarding T lymphocytes?

A. they constitute 10 to 20% of peripheral blood lymphocyte population

B. CD3 is demonstrable on all peripheral T lymphocytes

C. CD4 to CD8 ratio is about 2

D. they may be found in periarteriolar sheaths of the spleen

E. they participate in cell-mediated immunity

659. In which of the following genetic disorders are sex chromosomes predominantly involved?

A. Edward syndrome

B. Down syndrome

C. Patau syndrome
D. Turner syndrome
E. cri-du-chat syndrome

660. In the description of malignant nodular melanoma, the term level III indicates the tumor
  A. is confined to the epidermis
  B. invades but does not fill up the papillary dermis
  C. invades through the papillary dermis to the border of the reticular dermis
  D. invades into the reticular dermis
  E. invades into the subcutaneous tissues

661. Which type of emphysema is associated with α_1-antitrypsin deficiency?
  A. panacinar
  B. centriacinar
  C. paraseptal
  D. localized
  E. irregular

662. The presence of e antigen (HB_eAg) in the serum of a patient with hepatitis B infection (HBV)
  A. is best demonstrated during the "window period"
  B. implies active viral replication and maximal infectivity
  C. heralds the beginning of convalescence
  D. indicates co-infection with hepatitis E
  E. has been implicated in the pathogenesis of immune-complex glomerulonephritis associated with hepatitis infection

663. The brain of a patient with Down syndrome who lives longer than 35 years may be expected to show morphologic changes similar to those observed in
  A. Alzheimer's disease
  B. Creutzfelt–Jakob disease
  C. subacute sclerosing panencephalitis (SSPE)
  D. progressive multifocal leukoencephalopathy
  E. subcortical leukoencephalopathy

664. Epstein–Barr virus (EBV) has been unequivocally implicated as contributing to the pathogenesis of
  A. nasopharyngeal carcinoma
  B. Hodgkin disease
  C. Burkitt lymphoma
  D. B and C
  E. A and C

665. Typical features of dilated cardiomyopathy include all of the following EXCEPT
  A. may be caused by chronic alcoholism
  B. macroscopic dilatation of both cardiac ventricles and atria
  C. specific diagnostic electron microscopic changes
  D. normal cardiac valves and coronary arteries
  E. association with heart failure occurring one month before or after childbirth

666. Which of the following amyloid protein is most likely to be found in a patient with multiple myeloma?
  A. AA fibril protein
  B. β_2-microglobulin
  C. β_2-amyloid protein
  D. AL fibril protein
  E. transthyretin

667. A 50-year-old woman who had been on broad spectrum antibiotics for the previous ten days for the treatment of a chronic sinus infection presented at the emergency room with sudden onset of diarrhea, fever, and abdominal cramps. Peripheral blood showed leukocytosis. Which of the following is true of this illness?
  A. patients such as this usually carry class 1 histocompatibility antigen HLA-B8
  B. the small bowel mucosa of this patient will most probably show villous atrophy and chronic inflammation of the lamina propria
  C. this gastrointestinal disease may herald the onset of malabsorption syndrome

D. this disease is most probably caused by the toxin of *Clostridium difficile*

E. a chronic form of this disease shows morphologic features similar to those of ulcerative colitis

668. Autosplenectomy is typically observed in

A. idiopathic thrombocytopenia purpura (ITP)

B. thrombotic thrombocytopenia purpura (TTP)

C. recurrent *Plasmodium falciparum* malaria infection

D. sickle cell disease

E. acute myelogenous leukemia

669. There is unequivocal association of congenital heart disease with all of the following EXCEPT

A. Down syndrome

B. Turner syndrome

C. trisomy 18

D. Klinefelter syndrome

E. maternal infection with rubella virus

670. Biochemical and clinical pathologic sequelae of chronic pancreatitis include all of the following EXCEPT

A. steatorrhea

B. diabetes mellitus

C. pancreatic pseudocyst

D. hypoalbuminemia

E. elevated serum lipase

671. Shock characterized by arteriolar dilatation, reduction in systemic vascular resistance, endothelial cell injury and disseminated intravascular coagulation is most likely due to which of the following?

A. cardiac tamponade

B. massive gastrointestinal bleeding

C. extensive third degree burns

D. gram-negative septicemia

E. acute myocardial infarction

672. Which combination of immunological and clinical chemistry parameters most closely suggests primary biliary cirrhosis?

A. ↑ AMA, ↑ AP, ↓ ASA, ↓ C_4
B. ↓ AMA, ↑ AP, ↓ ASA, ↑ C_4
C. ↑ AMA, ↓ AP, ↑ ASA, ↑ C_4
D. ↑ AP, ↑ AMA, ↓ C_4 ↑ ASA
E. ↓ AMA, ↓ ASA, ↑ AP, ↓ C_4

AMA: antimitochondrial antibody; AP: alkaline phosphatase; ASA: antismooth muscle antibody; C_4: complement

673. A previously healthy 8-year-old boy with a 10-day history of upper respiratory infection develops sudden cardiac failure and decompensation accompanied by ST-T wave changes on the ECG. At autopsy the heart would be expected to

A. reveal extensive ischemic changes
B. show concentric myocardial hypertrophy
C. be dilated, pale, and flabby
D. reveal glycogen-filled myocardial fibers
E. show no significant histopathologic changes

674. Which of the following is directly involved in angiogenesis during chronic inflammation and repair?

A. epidermal growth factor(EGF)
B. platelet dermal growth factor (PDGF)
C. fibroblast growth factor (FGF)
D. interleukin-1 (IL-1)
E. transforming growth factor (TGF$_\alpha$ and TGF$_\beta$)

675. The cardiac lesions of carcinoid syndrome are located mainly in the right ventricle because of

A. inactivation of serotonin in the lung
B. lower oxygen in the right ventricle
C. different microscopic composition of the endocardium of the right ventricle when compared with that of the left
D. slower velocity of the circulation in the right ventricle
E. the difference in the thickness of the right and left ventricular myocardium

676. Which of the following is true of the pathogenesis of hereditary spherocytosis?
  A. deficiency of glutathione reductase
  B. deletion of two alpha globulin genes
  C. deficiency of spectrin
  D. substitution of glutamic acid by valine on β hemoglobin chain
  E. deficiency of glucose-6-pyruvate dehydrogenase

677. The reduction of the oncotic pressure of the plasma is the pathogenetic mechanism of the following EXCEPT
  A. nephrotic syndrome
  B. kwashiorkor
  C. congestive heart failure
  D. liver cirrhosis
  E. malabsorption syndrome

678. The complement system plays an important role in the acute inflammatory process. Which of the following is not partly or wholly mediated by components of the complement system?
  A. vascular permeability
  B. vasoconstriction
  C. chemotaxis
  D. opsonization
  E. cell lysis

679. All of the following are typical of gonococcal infection EXCEPT
  A. in the male, severe gonococcal infection often progresses from acute urethritis to bilateral orchitis
  B. intracellular organisms can be demonstrated in Gram stain of smear from gonococcal discharge
  C. a petechial rash may occur during the bacteremic phase of the infection
  D. it is the most common sexually transmitted disease in the United States
  E. gonococcal proctitis, arthritis, and pharyngitis are known to occur

680. Pathophysiologic changes in congestive heart failure include all of the following EXCEPT
   A. increased serum catecholamines
   B. decreased glomerular filtration rate
   C. increased renin secretion
   D. decreased aldosterone secretion
   E. increased vasopressin secretion

681. Which of the following statements is NOT true regarding the human leukocyte antigen (HLA) complex?
   A. HLA complex is the major histocompatibility complex
   B. blood group antigens are linked to HLA
   C. four closely linked HLA foci have been recognized on chromosome 6
   D. HLA-A, -B, -C antigens can evoke the synthesis of complement-fixing antibodies
   E. platelets are rich in cell-surface HLA antigens

682. A liver biopsy shows portal tracts densely infiltrated by lymphocytes, plasma cells and histiocytes which penetrate the limiting plate and which is associated with piecemeal necrosis and focal lobular necrosis. Which of the following hepatitis virus should be suspected as etiologic agents?
   A. A and D
   B. A and B
   C. B and C
   D. C and A
   E. D and E

683. In the diagnosis and evaluation of colorectal lesions, carcinoembryonic antigen (CEA) is of greatest use in
   A. monitoring postoperative recurrence of colonic carcinoma
   B. the initial diagnosis of colonic carcinoma
   C. assessing the size of tubulovillous adenomas
   D. determining if a villous adenoma has undergone malignant change
   E. monitoring the emergence of malignancy in inflammatory bowel disease

684. Which of the following will typically manifest rapidly progressive crescentic glomerulonephritis with linear immunofluorescence deposit?
- **A.** Henoch–Schönlein syndrome
- **B.** poststreptococcal glomerulonephritis
- **C.** systemic lupus erythematosus
- **D.** Goodpasture syndrome
- **E.** membranoproliferative glomerulonephritis

685. The histologic diagnosis of the early lesions of esophagitis depends on the demonstration of
- **A.** metaplastic epithelium
- **B.** submucosal lymphocytes and plasma cells
- **C.** submucosal edema and congestion
- **D.** intraepithelial eosinophils
- **E.** superimposed *Candida* organisms

686. All of the following are true of alcoholic liver disease EXCEPT
- **A.** alcohol metabolism in the liver occurs primarily by cytosolic NAD-dependent alcohol dehydrogenase
- **B.** alcoholic fatty liver is characterized by enlarged mitochondria and increased activity of cytochrome P_{450}-dependent enzymes
- **C.** alcoholic liver injury usually results from associated poor nutrition
- **D.** alcoholic hepatitis may progress to liver cirrhosis but alcoholic fatty liver does not
- **E.** alcoholic cirrhosis is micronodular

687. Which of the following is not true concerning glucose-6-phosphatase dehydrogenase (G6PD) deficiency?
- **A.** this red blood cell deficiency protects against *Plasmodium falciparum* malaria infection
- **B.** it is inherited as an autosomal recessive trait
- **C.** oxidant drugs such as primaquine may trigger hemolytic episodes
- **D.** peripheral red blood cells reveal Heinz bodies
- **E.** G6PD Mediterranean variant is clinically more severe than G6PD A- variant

688. Which of the following statements concerning radiation injury is false?
   A. lymphoid tissue is more radiosensitive than connective tissue
   B. the biologic effect of radiation is induced almost exclusively by excitation of atoms and/or molecules
   C. the biologic effect of radiation is dependent on the total dosage and the rate of delivery and absorption of radiation
   D. the gastrointestinal syndrome occurs with absorbed radiation of greater than 300 rads
   E. radiation injury may cause cellular pleomorphism, giant cell formation, and endothelial proliferation

689. Genital chlamydial infection is characterized by all of the following EXCEPT that
   A. it morphologically reveals epithelial intranuclear inclusions
   B. the treatment of choice is third-generation penicillins
   C. the diagnosis may be made by culturing the organism in living cell culture media
   D. the disease can be transmitted to sex partners
   E. in women, the disease may progress to pelvic inflammatory disease

690. A carcinoma that is confined to the colon wall but has extended to the muscularis propria, with no lymph node metastases belongs to which Duke type?
   A. A
   B. B1
   C. B2
   D. C
   E. D

691. Lung infection by *legionella pneumophila* (legionnaire's disease) can be expected to show
   A. interstitial inflammation
   B. confluent fibrinopurulent bronchopneumonia
   C. granulomatous inflammation (pneumonia alba)
   D. lobar pneumonia with lesions at same stage of development
   E. hemorrhagic and necrotizing lobar pneumonia

692. Which of the following is not a cytokine?
   A.   colony-stimulating factor (CSF)
   B.   prostaglandin E_2 (PGE_2)
   C.   interferon α (IFNα)
   D.   interleukin-1 (IL-1)
   E.   tumor necrosis factor alpha (TNFα)

693. The most accurate definition of aspergilloma is
   A.   colonizing aspergillosis
   B.   invasive aspergillosis
   C.   allergic aspergillosis
   D.   aspergillus flavus pulmonary lesions
   E.   none of the above

694. The most significant characteristic parameter defining chronic bronchitis is
   A.   squamous metaplasia of bronchial epithelium
   B.   hypertrophy of submucosal smooth muscle
   C.   recurrent viral and bacterial infections
   D.   hypertrophy of submucosal mucous glands
   E.   lymphocytic and plasma cell infiltration of bronchial walls

695. Progressive worsening of the prognosis of Hodgkin disease may be represented by which of the following sequence?
   A.   lymphocyte predominant (LP), nodular sclerosis (NS), mixed cellularity (MC), lymphocyte depletion (LD)
   B.   NS, MC, LD, LP
   C.   MC, NS, LP, LD
   D.   LD, LP, MC, NS
   E.   NS, LP, LD, MC

696. Progressive massive fibrosis is typically associated with
   A.   anthracosis
   B.   tuberculosis
   C.   silicosis
   D.   asbestosis
   E.   berylliosis

697. A 54-year-old patient with nephrotic syndrome presents with an enlarged kidney. The gross and microscopic morphology of the kidney required histochemical stains. Light microscopy showed pinkish deposits which, under polarized light revealed green birefringence. The substance thus demonstrated is most likely
   A. immune complexes
   B. fibrinous deposits
   C. lipid droplets
   D. amyloid deposits
   E. collagen fibers

698. The demonstration of terminal deoxynucleotidyl transferase (Tdt) is very useful in the diagnosis of which leukemia
   A. chronic lymphocytic (CLL)
   B. chronic myelogenous (CML)
   C. acute monocytic (AMML)
   D. acute lymphoblastic (ALL)
   E. acute myeloblastic

699. Chronic constrictive pericarditis is most likely to be associated with
   A. healed rheumatic pericarditis
   B. restrictive cardiomyopathy
   C. systemic lupus erythematosus
   D. metastatic carcinoma
   E. tuberculosis

700. Which of the following is not characteristic of acute rheumatic fever?
   A. immune pathogenesis
   B. erythema marginatum
   C. McCullum plaques
   D. destructive vegetative valvulitis
   E. acute arthritis which resolve without sequelae

DIRECTIONS (Questions 701 through 725): For each numbered word, phrase, or statement, select the ONE lettered heading that is most closely associated with it. Each lettered heading may be used once, more than once, or not at all.

Questions 701 and 702

		A	B	C	D	E
A.	random plasma osmolality	↓	↑	↓	↑	N
B.	random urine osmolality					
C.	urine osmolality during hypertonic saline administration	↓	↓	↑	↓	N
D.	urine osmolality following intravenous vasopressin	↑	NC	↑	NC	NC
E.	plasma vasopressin	↑	↑	NC	NC	↑
F.	NC: no change; L: low; N: normal	L	L	N	N/↑	L

701. Neurogenic diabetes insipidus

702. Nephrogenic diabetes insipidus

Questions 703 and 704

A. cholangiocarcinoma
B. veno-occlusive disease
C. primary biliary cirrhosis
D. hepatocellular carcinoma
E. micronodular cirrhosis
F. macronodular cirrhosis
G. angiosarcoma

703. Aflatoxin

704. Thorotrast

Questions 705 through 707

A. alpha-fetoprotein
B. calcitonin
C. neuron specific enolase
D. synaptophysin
E. CA-125
F. acid phosphatase
G. immunoglobulins
H. CD 45
I. none of the above

705. Medullary carcinoma of thyroid

706. Choriocarcinoma

707. Hepatocellular carcinoma

Questions 708 through 711

A. homogentisic oxidase
B. hexosaminidase A
C. sphingomyelinase
D. α-L-iduronidase
E. debranching enzyme
F. muscle phosphorylase
G. arylsulfatase A
H. α-1, 4 glucosidase
I. acid lipase
J. heparin N-sulfatase

708. Hurler syndrome

709. Niemann Pick disease

710. Pompe disease

711. Tay–Sacks disease

Questions 712 and 713

   A. autosomal recessive trait; defective adhesion of platelets to subendothelial collagen

   B. defective platelet aggregation due to deficiency of glycoprotein, GPIIb, and GPIIIa

   C. transient neurologic deficit, hemolytic anemia, renal failure

   D. chronic ineffective megakaryopoiesis

   E. improvement or cure by splenectomy; platelet-associated IgG detected in serum

712. Idiopathic thrombocytopenic purpura (ITP)

713. Thrombotic thrombocytopenic purpura (TTP)

Questions 714 and 715

   A. crosses the placenta, constitutes about 75% of total serum immunoglobulins; capable of fixing serum complement

   B. predominant immunoglobulin in the mucosal immune system; important antiviral defense mechanism; 7S globulin

   C. present in the serum only in trace amounts; function not entirely certain but probably related to activity toward certain antigens such as insulin, milk proteins, diphtheria toxoid; not known to fix complement

   D. 0.004% of total serum immunoglobulins; reaginic activity; binds with high affinity to mast cells; exists in monomeric form; found in high levels in patients with helminthic infection

   E. 19S globulin; prominent antibody in early immune responses to most antigens; most efficient complement-fixing immunoglobulin

714. IgM

715. IgE

Questions 716 and 717

    A. Crokhite–Canada syndrome

    B. Gardner syndrome

    C. familial adenomatous polyposis

    D. Peutz–Jeghers syndrome

    E. Turcot syndrome

716. Hamartomatous gastrointestinal polyps; melanin pigmentation of the buccal mucosa, lips, and digits

717. Diffuse pedunculated colonic polyposis and sigmoid carcinoma in a 35-year-old man

Questions 718 and 719

    A. type I hypersensitivity reaction (anaphylactic reaction)

    B. type II hypersensitivity reaction (cytotoxic)

    C. type III hypersensitivity reaction (immune complex)

    D. type IV hypersensitivity reaction (cell mediated)

    E. none of the above

718. Arthus reaction

719. Erythroblastosis fetalis

Questions 720 and 721

    A. monocytoid B cell lymphoma

    B. follicular small cleaved cell lymphoma

    C. anaplastic large cell lymphoma (Ki-1 lymphoma)

    D. Burkitt lymphoma

    E. Waldenstrom macroglobulinemia

    F. lymphoblastic lymphoma

    G. adult T cell lymphoma

    H. Hodgkin disease, nodular sclerosis type

    I. mycosis fungoides

    J. none of the above

720. Most frequently associated with HTLV-1

721. Predominantly extranodal. 80% show translocation of c-myc protooncogene on chromosome 8 to chromosome 14, 2, or 22

Questions 722 and 723
A. coagulative necrosis
B. gummatous necrosis
C. fat necrosis
D. caseous necrosis
E. gangrenous necrosis
F. fibrinoid necrosis
G. liquefactive necrosis
H. none of the above

722. Acute tubular necrosis

723. Encephalomalacia

Questions 724 and 725
A. pneumonia most commonly associated with chronic alcoholism. Mucoid feel to the cut surface of the lung; may be complicated by bronchopleural fistula
B. often seen in patients with burns; necrotizing bronchopneumonia associated with vasculitis in which large quantities of bacteria are demonstrable
C. pneumonia which typically undergoes the states of congestion, red hepatization, gray hepatization, and resolution.
D. confluent bronchopneumonia; alveoli contain fibrin, neutrophils, and macrophages, many showing leukocytoclasis; abundant organisms which may be visualized with the Dieterle silver stain
E. interstitial pneumonia with insidious onset; little or no leukocytosis; alveoli may contain hyaline membranes; elevated cold agglutinins

724. *Streptococcus pneumoniae*

725. *Klebsiella pneumoniae*

Pathology

Answers and Comments

576. (C), **577.** (B), **578.** (B) Also called Hashimoto's thyroiditis or struma lymphomatosa, chronic lymphocytic thyroiditis is the prototype autoimmune disease. It occurs predominantly in women in their fourth and fifth decades. The female:male ratio is 10:1. The evidence for autoimmune pathogenesis of this disease derives from clinical and laboratory observations. To illustrate, the sera of patients with chronic lymphocytic thyroiditis contain many antibodies to a variety of thyroid antigens. 90% of patients have antibody to thyroid microsomal antigen while 60% have antibody to thyroglobulin. Other evidence supporting this thesis comes from the incidence of other autoimmune diseases such as Sjörgren's syndrome, rheumatoid arthritis, systemic lupus erythematosus, pernicious anemia and Graves disease in patients with chronic lymphocytic thyroiditis. The pathogenesis of the disease is unknown but certain mechanisms have been proposed, among them, antibody-dependent complement-mediated cytotoxicity, direct T-cell killing, antibody-dependent cell-mediated toxicity and immune complex deposition.

The laboratory findings in chronic lymphocytic thyroiditis vary according to the stage of the disease. Early on, patients are metabolically normal. Later, free serum T_4 index is reduced and TSH is elevated. As hypothyroidism becomes established, serum T_4 and T_3 levels decline.

Macroscopic pathology: the gland is symmetrically enlarged and rubbery or it may reveal intense fibrosis. Histological sections typically show extensive infiltration of the gland by an infiltrate of lymphocytes and plasma cells. Lymphoid aggregates with germinal centers may be seen as is observed in the case presented here. The follicular epithelium is transformed into oncocytes or Hurthle cells. Definitive diagnosis may be made by needle biopsy or from surgical specimens. (**Ref. 1**, p. 1126; **Ref. 4**, p. 1952)

579. (D), 580. (A), 581. (C) Figure 4.2 shows a cyst containing many bradyzoites surrounded by an area of necrosis with inflammatory cells. Acquired toxoplasma infection has recently become more common, particularly in HIV positive patients. Caused by *Toxoplasma gondii* (*T gondii*), a protozoan, the disease is transmitted to humans through accidental ingestion of cysts or oocysts from cat feces or by the consumption of inadequately cooked meat. Congenital infection occurs through transplacental infection of the fetus from an infected mother. The organism occurs in human tissues in two forms, the bow-shaped tachyzoites and cystically dilated cells containing numerous small bradyzoites.

In normal immunocompetent adults the organisms usually do not cause clinical symptoms and signs. In a small number of people, however, there may be symmetrical lymph node enlargement, most commonly posterior cervical. Microscopically such lymph nodes reveal characteristic follicular hyperplasia with irregular clusters of epithelioid cells. In immunodeficient patients (AIDS, malignant lymphoma, posttransplantation) disseminated organ involvement is the rule. Mass lesions of the brain is common; other clinical manifestations include myocarditis, hepatosplenomegaly, myositis, pneumonitis, and meningoencephalitis. Neonatal (congenital) toxoplasmosis also affects numerous organs, notably the brain—microcephaly, seizures, and cerebral calcifications. Other signs and symptoms include fever, lymphadenopathy, pneumonitis, hepatosplenomegaly, and retinochoriditis. Infection of the mother early in pregnancy may be the cause of spontaneous abortion, stillbirth, or prematurity. (**Ref. 4**, pp. 903–908; **Ref. 1**, pp. 311, 1325)

582. (C), 583. (B), 584. (D), 585. (A) The consequences of diabetes mellitus are borne by multiple organ systems but most prominently by the kidney. End-stage diabetic renal disease is much more common in type 1 (insulin-dependent) diabetes. The natural history of diabetic glomerulopathy runs through three stages: occult, intermediate, and advanced. In early stages there is an elevation of glomerular filtration rate to be followed in late stages by progressive decline in GFR. The intermediate stage is marked by increasing proteinuria, declining GFR, hypertension, and the development of edema but hypoproteinemia is lacking. In the advanced stage which ensues after about a 20- to 25-year history of diabetes, azotemia supervenes; this is characterized by the retention of urea, creatinine, and other nitrogenous compounds. The proteinuria is now accompanied by hypoproteinemia and frank nephrotic syndrome. At the same time there is widespread microangiopathy with particular devastating effects on the retina and peripheral nerves.

The classic characteristic renal lesion in diabetes are diffuse and nodular GS. The latter, almost pathognomonic for diabetes, is also called intercapillary GS or Kimmelstiel–Wilson disease. Two other glomerular lesions in diabetes are the fibrin cap and capsular drop. Diabetic patients are also susceptible to pyelonephritis and papillary necrosis.

The clinical course of diabetic nephropathy, though variable, is progressive and relentless. Diabetic GS is more severe and more progressive in type 1 disease and is characterized by proteinuria and hypertension. In the vast majority of patients, end-stage diabetic nephropathy supervenes, ending in treatment with maintenance hemodialysis. (**Ref. 1**, pp. 909–922; **Ref. 4**, p. 1995)

586. (B), 587. (C) The lumen of the appendix contains a cross section of a round worm with thick external cuticle, internal to which are sections of its internal organs. The helminth found most commonly in the appendix is *Enterobius vermicularis* (pinworm). Measuring about 1.0 cm in length, the adult female worm resides in the cecum and appendix from where it migrates to the anal skin for laying eggs causing anal, perianal, and perineal itching. The diagnosis is made by the inspection of the anus for worms or by sticking a piece of Scotch tape to the anus and examining it under the microscope for the presence of eggs. Although suspected of causing acute appendicitis, the worm is too small to obstruct the appendiceal lumen and trigger an inflammatory reaction. The disease is common worldwide but particularly so in the temperate countries. It is estimated that more than 200 million are infected, most commonly young children. (**Ref. 3**, p. 608; **Ref. 2**, p. 441)

588. (D), 589. (E) The photomicrograph illustrates a high-power view of asbestos bodies with typical beading and knobbed ends. They are found in the walls of bronchioles or within alveolar macrophages. In routine histologic sections, they appear golden brown, coated by complexes of hemosiderin and glycoprotein. Asbestos occurs naturally in many forms: slender serpentine (chrysotile) of which two types are known—crocidolite and amosite. Together they account for about 90% of commercially used asbestos. The other type, amphiboles, is brittle and straight. Although all asbestos fibers excite fibrous tissue formation, crocidolite is the most carcinogenic. These fibers cause asbestosis, most often in people who work with asbestos and its products, among them those who work in roofing, insulation sewers, water conduits, and shipyards. Additional to pulmonary fibrosis, asbestos may also lead to the development of pleural plaques, pleural effusion, and mesothelioma. Bronchogenic carcinoma, predominantly adenocarcinoma, and relatively fewer squamous cell carcinoma is a dreaded complication of asbestosis. The relationship between asbestos and exposure and malignant mesothelioma is irrefutable. (**Ref. 1**, p. 710; **Ref. 2**, p. 596)

590. (E) The photomicrograph shows alveolar septa severely thickened by fibrocollagenous tissue containing scattered inflammatory cells. The alveolar spaces are empty and reduced in size. The findings are those of chronic interstitial lung disease (interstitial fibrosis, fibrosing alveolitis). These diseases can be divided broadly into two categories—those with known causes and those whose etiology is not known (idiopathic interstitial lung disease). The former can be further subdivided into various groups of etiologies; among them, those due to occupational and environmental inhalants, constituting about 24% of cases (organic and inorganic dusts, gases, fumes, and aerosols), drugs and toxins, infections (viral, bacterial, fungal, parasitic). Sarcoidosis is responsible for about 20% of chronic interstitial lung disease while collagen vascular disease is diagnosed in another 8%. In 15% no antecedent disease or etiology is identifiable. There is a myriad of rare causes such as idiopathic pulmonary hemosiderosis, histiocytosis X, and alveolar proteinosis. (**Ref. 1**, p. 704; **Ref. 4**, p. 1206)

591. (C) The macroscopic and microscopic morphology of chronic interstitial lung disease are distinctive. Injury to the alveolar wall by a multitude of factors leads to interstitial edema and interstitial inflammation. Subsequently there is proliferation of fibroblasts with progressive fibrosis and collagenization. Simultaneously there is destruction of alveolar pneumocytes type I which are replaced by alveolar pneumocytes type II. Continuation of these processes finally produces a lung that is solid with air spaces lined by cuboidal epithelium separated by thick fibrous tissue, the typical appearance of honeycomb lung. (**Ref. 1**, p. 705)

592. (D) The pathogenesis of chronic interstitial lung disease involves direct toxicity of chemicals, participation of lymphocytes, macrophages, and neutrophils, or immunological reactions. Neutrophil recruitment is caused by activation of complement and release of chemotactic factors. Macrophages elaborate several factors that cause tissue destruction and promote fibroblast proliferation and collagen deposition. Immune complexes are demonstrable as granular deposits of IgG in alveolar septa; cell-mediated reactions have also been implicated in sarcoidosis. (**Ref. 1**, p. 704)

593. (A), 594. (D) Benign prostatic hyperplasia (BPH, nodular hyperplasia, benign prostatic hypertrophy) occurs in 20% and 70% of men of about 40 and 60 years, respectively. By age 70 and above, 90% of men would have developed enlarged prostates. However, clinically significant disease necessitating surgical resections observed only in 10 to 15% of men.

Two factors are known to be associated with the development of BPH: aging and intact testes. The pathogenesis of BPH is closely related with hormonal factors; specifically, androgens and estrogens. Much of the knowledge in this area is derived in dogs, the only animal species which develops BPH. Dihydrotestosterone is thought to be the ultimate mediator of prostatic growth.

BPH affects predominantly the inner prostatic mass of the middle and lateral lobes. The nodules are grossly visible both externally and on cut section. Some show microcyst formation which may exude milky white prostatic fluid. Microscopically there may be glandular proliferation, smooth muscle and stromal hyperplasia, and hypertrophy. An important diagnostic point is the double layering of the proliferating glands—an inner columnar and an outer cuboidal or flattened epithelium.

The consequences of BPH are multiple: urethral compression with attendant difficulty of urnination and urinary retention which subsequently may cause distention and hypertrophy of the urinary bladder. Urinary tract infection is also common. (**Ref. 1,** p. 1025)

595. (B), 596. (D) The photomicrographs illustrate the salient features of glioblastoma multiforme. So called because of its variegated appearances, the tumor shows gray-white firm areas, yellowish necrotic foci, focal hemorrhage, and cyst formation. Microscopically the tumor shows necrosis often with features of palisading (Fig. 4.8A), prominent endothelial proliferation (Fig. 4.8B), and pleomorphic anaplastic cells (Fig. 4.8C). Glioblastoma multiforme, combined with the less malignant lower grade astrocytomas together constitute about 80% of adult primary tumors of the brain. Recently, however, there has been an increase in the incidence of primary malignant lymphoma of the brain in AIDS patients. Nearly all the tumors arise in the cerebral hemispheres; the remainder arise from the brain stem and the spinal cord.

The symptoms and signs of the tumors reflect their site of origin, the effect of increased intracranial pressure, and cerebral edema. These tumors rarely metastasize outside the cranium but may spread along cerebrospinal fluid pathways. The prognosis is very poor with fewer than 10% of patients surviving above two years after the diagnosis. (**Ref. 1,** p. 1342)

597. (B), 598. (E) The photomicrograph shows arteriolar intimal thickening by proliferating concentrically arranged smooth muscle cells causing considerable narrowing of the lumen. The changes are those of hyperplastic arteriolosclerosis, typical of malignant hypertension. Similar changes may be observed in the interlobular arteries. In malignant hypertension, arterioles may also undergo fibrinoid necrosis, which, when accompanied by inflammatory cells leads to necrotizing arteriolitis. Focal necrosis may also be observed in the glomeruli. The macroscopic appearance of the kidney reflects the underlying renal disease and the duration of hypertension. In addition, the cortical surface shows petechial hemorrhages owing to ruptured arterioles or glomeruli—the "flea-bitten kidney."

Malignant hypertension often occurs as a complication of pre-existing benign essential hypertension or a chronic renal disease. Less commonly, it may arise in normotensive individuals. Clinically, patients manifest persistent elevated diastolic pressure in excess of 130 mm Hg. This is often accompanied by papilledema, increased intracranial pressure, headaches, vomiting, convulsion, visual symptoms, and loss of consciousness. The syndrome is a true medical emergency requiring the institution of aggressive medical treatment.

The triggering mechanism for the development of malignant hypertension and associated vascular lesion has been related to high levels of renin, angiotensin, and aldosterone. Severely elevated blood pressure causes endothelial injury, platelet thrombosis, and intravascular coagulation. Associated with them are arteriolar and arterial narrowing causing severe ischemic changes. (**Ref. 1,** p. 977)

599. (D), 600. (A) The photomicrograph shows fatty liver (hepatic steatosis). The cytoplasm of most hepatocytes contain fat, sometimes in minute quantities but in other cases, large enough to distend the cells. The nuclei of these cells are compressed and pushed to one side of the cell. Inflammation or fibrous tissue is not present.

Fatty liver occurs under many clinically unrelated conditions. Probably the most common cause in the western world is chronic alcoholism. Other causes include obesity, corticosteroid administration, protein–calorie malnutrition (kwashiorkor), uncontrolled diabetes mellitus, certain hepatotoxins, and prolonged chronic illnesses.

Several possible mechanisms have been propounded in the pathogenesis of fatty liver—excess entry of free fatty acids to the liver (starvation, corticosteroids), enhanced fatty acid synthesis, decreased fatty acid oxidation, increased esterification of fatty acids to triglyceride (alcohol), decreased apoprotein synthesis (carbon tetrachloride, phosphorus poisoning), and impaired lipoprotein secretion from the liver (alcohol, orotic acid). (**Ref. 1,** pp. 25, 857)

601. (C), 602. (A), 603. (D) Figure 4.11 shows well to moderately differentiated prostatic adenocarcinoma characterized by small- to medium-sized glands lined by one layer of uniform cuboidal epithelial cells. The cytoplasm of the tumor cells is pale and the nuclei are round to oval and vesicular. Nucleoli, often times large and conspicuous, are seen in many cells. The glands are closely packed with almost no fibrous stromal between them—the so-called "back-to-back" pattern. This is only one of the histologic types of prostatic adenocarcinoma. The spectrum of histologic variation has led to several grading systems; currently, the most widely used is the Gleason's grading system which is based on the degree of glandular differentiation and growth pattern of tumor in relation to the stroma. The system recognizes five histologic patterns. The Gleason's score is the sum of the grade of the most and least prominent patterns. The best and most poorly differentiated tumors have a score of 1 and 5 respectively. Thus, Gleason's score varies from 2 to 10.

Prostatic carcinoma is the most common cancer diagnosed in American men and is the third leading cause of cancer deaths. Wide variation exists in the geographical distribution of age-related death rates. The tumor is rare in Asians and among the Japanese the prevalence is 3 to 4/100,000 compared with 50 to 60 among white Americans. The highest incidence in the world is found among American blacks whose rate is twice that of American whites. Low rates are also found in Mexico and Greece.

The grading and staging are important in the choice of treatment and establishing a prognosis. The staging usually does not include lymph node involvement; for this reason several techniques such as lymphangiography, CT scan, and fine-needle aspiration are employed to assess lymph node involvement. The range of therapeutic options vary from clinical follow-up (stage A1) through surgery or radiation (stage B) to surgery, lymphadenectomy, hormonal manipulation, and radiation. (**Ref. 1,** pp. 1026–1030; **Ref. 2,** p. 899)

604. (B) The photomicrograph shows a malignant neoplasm composed of highly atypical polygonal cells (melanocytes) infiltrating the epidermis reaching to the stratum corneum. The malignant cells are readily identified by the pericellular halo probably due to tissue retraction during processing. The tumor cells, particularly those in the reticular dermis, contain large amounts of melanin. Malignant melanomas present two types of growth: radial (superficial usually within the epidermis and superficial dermis) and vertical (downward into the deep dermis and subcutaneous tissue). It is the latter type of growth that determines the possibility for metastases. (**Ref. 1,** p. 1180)

605. (**D**) Nevi are composed of aggregates of round, uniform melanocytes which lack atypical features or conspicuous nucleoli. When such cells occur in the dermo-epidermal junction, a junctional nevus results; when they occur in the dermis in addition to that site, the lesion is called compound nevus. Older lesions may lose their epidermal component and a dermal nevus results. In congenital nevi, there is infiltration of the deep dermis and subcutaneous tissue as well as of neuromuscular and adnexal structures. Other types of nevi are compound nevus of Spitz, halo nevus, and blue nevus. (**Ref. 1,** p. 1176)

606. (**E**) Clinically, malignant melanoma manifests as an asymmetrical irregular lesion with papules and nodules. The borders of the tumor are irregular with notching and pigment spilling out of the edges. The color is variegated with hues of brown, black, blue, and red. Usually the lesion is larger than 6 mm. Several clinical forms are recognized: lentigo malignant melanoma, superficial spreading melanoma, nodular melanoma, and acral lentiginous melanoma. The last mentioned is one of the most common types in blacks. (**Ref. 1,** p. 1178; **Ref. 2,** p. 1226)

607. (**B**) The figures show the salient histomorphology of acute ulcerative colitis—focal denudation of colonic surface epithelium, severe inflammation of the lamina propria (lymphocytes, histiocytes, and copious polymorphonuclear leukocytes), inflammation of glands with crypt abscess formation, distortion of glandular architecture and diminution of goblet cells. Clinical symptoms and signs of ulcerative colitis may be mild, moderate, or severe. Severe disease, which occurs in about 15% of patients, manifests severe constitutional symptoms, high fever, profuse diarrhea, rectal bleeding, and profound weakness. (**Ref. 1,** p. 804; **Ref. 4,** p. 1407)

608. (**C**) The gross pathologic features of ulcerative colitis are sometimes distinct but at times overlap with those of other colitides, especially Crohn's disease. In 75% of patients the disease involves the left colon, in others the entire colon is involved, and in yet another 10% or so, there is involvement of the terminal ileum (backwash ileitis). The mucosa is patchily involved areas of disease alternating with normal mucosa. Over time the inflammatory disease leads to fibrosis and thickening of bowel wall resulting in shortening of the bowel. Long-term disease may be complicated by the development of adenocarcinoma; the incidence is about 1% in diseases of less that 10 years' duration, gradually rising to about 30% at 30 years' duration. (**Ref. 1,** pp. 804–805)

609. (E)   Toxic megacolon is a dreaded complication of ulcerative colitis. It may occur spontaneously or may be secondary to barium enema examination, potassium depletion, or anticholinergic or narcotic medication. The patients manifest fever, abdominal tenderness, and distention with loss of bowel sounds. There may be tachycardia, dehydration, marked leukocytosis, anemia, and hypoalbuminemia. Mortality may be as high as 10 to 20%. (**Ref. 4,** p. 1412; **Ref. 1,** p. 805)

610. (B)   The photomicrograph shows necrosis of myocardial fibers accompanied by profound leukocytic infiltrate typical of acute myocardial infarction. Myocardial ischemia leads to a variety of biochemical alterations at the cellular level ultimately resulting in cell death. These changes are heralded by decreased oxygen supply to the myocardium. The metabolism shifts from aerobic to anaerobic with a dramatic fall in intracellular ATP with attendant impaired ATPase ion pump. These changes result in the elevation of intracellular Na^+ and Ca^+ and extracellular K^+. The last mentioned causes alterations of membrane potential and development of arrhythmias. The changes in Ca^{++} is probably the common pathway to all necrosis. (**Ref. 5,** p. 116; **Ref. 1,** p. 531)

611. (D)   Edema of the myocardium, one of the earliest changes in acute myocardial infarction, occurs within 4 to 12 hours. However, wavy myocardial fibers and contraction bands may be observed earlier. Wavy myofibers are due to the tugging effect of the contracting healthy myocardium in the vicinity of the acute infarct. Within the first half of myocardial infarct enzymatic changes occur, demonstrable by histochemical techniques; they include decreased dehydrogenases, oxidases, phosphorylases, and glycogen. (**Ref. 5,** p. 116; **Ref. 1,** p. 533)

612. **(A)** Currently the preferred enzymatic diagnosis of acute myocardial infarction relies on the temporal sequences of the rise and fall of creatine kinase (CK) and lactic dehydrogenase (LDH) isoenzymes. CK-MB, one of the three common isoenzymes of CK, becomes elevated within 2 to 4 hours, reaches a peak at about 12 hours, and returns to normal within 48 to 96 hours. CK-MB is usually greater than 5 to 6% of total serum CK. The other clinically useful enzyme assay is that of LD_1 and LD_2 isoenzymes. The former is specific for the heart and an LD_1/LD_2 ratio greater than 1.0 is indicative of acute myocardial infarct. (**Ref. 5,** p. 121; **Ref. 4,** p. 1066)

613. **(C)** Bacterial pneumonia occurring in a healthy individual usually is due to *Streptococcus pneumoniae* and it is responsible for most cases of lobar pneumonia and many cases of bronchopneumonia. *Klebsiella pneumoniae* accounts for approximately 1 to 2% of cases of lobar pneumonia and tends to affect older men (fifth to seventh decades), alcoholics, diabetics, and debilitated individuals. The pulmonary lesions produced by *Mycoplasma pneumoniae* show no obvious consolidation and pleuritis is uncommon. *Haemophilus influenzae,* a frequent cause of primary pneumonia in children, rarely causes pneumonia in adults but may do so as a complication of influenza or primary atypical pneumonia. (**Ref. 1,** p. 697)

614. **(E)** Four stages of inflammatory reaction account for the distinguishing pathologic features of lobar pneumonia. These features, however, are modified by effective antibiotic therapy and the natural sequence is frequently interrupted today. The four phases are: (1) Stage of congestion and edema representing the initial phase of bacterial infection and characterized by serous exudation with accompanying vascular congestion. Many bacteria are present in the edema fluid and large numbers also are observed in smears made from the cut surface of the lung. Understandably, the sputum is slightly turbid and watery. (2) Stage of red hepatization occurs 2 to 4 days after the onset of illness and is characterized by fibrinocellular exudation resulting in consolidation (dullness on percussion, increased tactile fremitus, bronchial breath sounds) and fibrinopurulent pleuritis (pleural friction rub, chest pain aggravated by deep breathing and coughing). Bacteria are engulfed by neutrophils. The sputum is typically rusty. (3) Stage of gray

hepatization, a more advanced stage of consolidation, characterized by continuing accumulation of fibrin with progressive red
blood cell and neutrophilic disintegration giving a grayish-brown,
dry appearance of the cut surface of the lung. Microorganisms are
no longer present. (4) Stage of resolution characterized by progressive enzymatic digestion producing granular and semifluid intraalveolar debris which is either resolved or engulfed by
macrophages. Grossly, the lung is moist and mottled gray, red,
and dirty brown and large amounts of yellowish fluid can be
squeezed from the lung parenchyma. In general, resolution in
pneumococcal pneumonia is complete. Rarely does organization
occur leading to fibrosis. (**Ref. 1,** p. 697)

615. **(C)**   In its development in the germinal center of lymph nodes,
four distinctive morphologic stages can be identified: small
cleaved cells which become transformed to large cleaved cells
and which subsequently become small and large non-cleaved
cells. Outside of the germinal center, these cells are transformed
into the large immunoblast which may proliferate to plasma cells
or revert to dormant resting B lymphocytes. Lukes and Collins
classified non-Hodgkin lymphomas on the basis of their cell of
origin and thus these tumors as small or large, cleaved or non-
cleaved, and immunoblastic. (**Ref. 1,** p. 635)

616. **(B)**   Infective endocarditis may be acute or chronic. Implicated
as the leading cause of acute infective endocarditis in intravenous
drug abusers, *S. aureus* has the ability to implant on normal cardiac valves in contrast to *Streptococcus viridans* which, though
overall is the commonest organism encountered in infective endocarditis (65%), affects previously damaged cardiac valves. In
drug addicts, right-sided valve lesions are common; implicated
organisms include *Candida* and *Aspergillus*. (**Ref. 1,** p. 551)

617. **(C)**   Three types of metaplastic epithelium are recognized in
Barett esophagus: cardiac type, composed of mucus glands without parietal or chief cells, a fundic type with short glands containing Paneth and chief cells and an intestinal type with villi and
goblet cells. The epithelium may show inflammatory changes and
ulceration which subsequently may cause esophageal stricture.
Malignant transformation occurs predominantly in the intestinal
type of epithelium. Most primary adenocarcinomas of the lower

esophagus probably arise from Barett epithelium. (**Ref. 2**, p. 624; **Ref. 3**, p. 563)

618. (C) In spite of screening donor blood for HB$_s$Ag, post-transfusion hepatitis abated only somewhat until recently. Those cases of hepatitis were thought to be caused by nonA nonB virus, now known to be mostly hepatitis C. HCV contains a single-stranded DNA with 5000 to 10,000 nucleotides. Today, blood in the United States is now screened not only for HB$_s$Ag but also for HCV. Blood transfusion, however, accounts for only a small proportion of HCV infection. The clinical course of HCV is similar to that of HBV infection; however, chronic hepatitis supervenes on HCV more frequently than with HBV. In fact, about 50% of patients with hepatitis C would progress to chronic active hepatitis or chronic persistent hepatitis with 20% of the former eventually ending up with liver cirrhosis. (**Ref. 2**, p. 726)

619. (E) Constituting 1.1 to 9% of lung carcinomas, these tumors arise in the peripheral parts of the lung. They are derived from Clara cells, mucus-secreting bronchiolar cells or rarely from type II alveolar pneumocytes. The tumor occurs in patients of all ages, without any sex predilection from the third decade on. They may occur as solitary masses or involve the lung diffusely mimicking pneumonic consolidation. The tumors have no relationship to tobacco smoking. The lesions may resemble the infectious disease of the South African sheep called jagziekte. (**Ref. 1**, p. 725; **Ref. 2**, p. 611)

620. (E) The hemoglobin released during intravascular hemolysis becomes bound by haptoglobin into a complex, which, in turn, is taken up by the reticuloendothelial system. When the capacity of haptoglobin is exhausted, hemoglobin is oxidized to methemoglobin which is excreted with unbound hemoglobin in the urine (hemoglobinuria and methemoglobinuria). During the passage through the kidney, hemoglobin may be taken up by renal tubular cells and may be degraded in those cells to hemosiderin. Upon desquamation into the urine, such cells may be identified with iron stain and a diagnosis of hemosiderinuria made. (**Ref. 1**, p. 587; **Ref. 3**, p. 390)

621. (B) Toxoplasmosis is caused by *Toxoplasma gondii*, a coccidian protozoan. Humans are infected by the ingestion of incompletely cooked meat that harbors *T. gondii* cysts or the ingestion of food contaminated by cat feces containing toxoplasma oocysts. In normal immunocompetent adults toxoplasmosis manifests mainly as lymphadenopathy, seen histologically as follicular hyperplasia with scattered accumulation of epithelioid histiocytes. In immunocompromised hosts (AIDS, post-transplantation), *T. gondii* produces a necrotizing encephalitis in which organisms exist as bradyzoites and tachyzoites. Transplacental transmission of *T. gondii* causes congenital toxoplasmosis, a devastating multisystem disease which is particularly severe in central nervous system and the eyes. (**Ref. 2**, p. 425; **Ref. 1**, p. 358)

622. (D) In "feathery degeneration" which occurs in long-standing cholestasis, groups of hepatocytes show hydropic degeneration, intracellular bile accumulation, and reticulated cytoplasm. Continued cholestasis leads to necrosis of such cells, extravasation of bile pigment and cellular debris, a condition known as bile infarct. The lesion is found in the peripheral areas of the liver lobule and may be encountered in diverse clinical conditions that have in common intra- and/or extrahepatic cholestasis such as hepatocellular injury, drugs, pregnancy, primary biliary cirrhosis, sclerosing cholangitis, or obstruction of extrahepatic bile ducts. (**Ref. 2**, p. 714)

623. (E) Cardiac arrhythmias may occur in as many as 95% of acute MI patients. The rhythm disorders include heart blocks, premature ventricular beats, sinus bradycardia, paroxysmal atrial tachycardia, ventricular tachycardia, and ventricular fibrillation. The last mentioned is usually serious and may be the cause of sudden death. Continuous monitoring in cardiac intensive care units have significantly reduced the mortality resulting from these arrhythmias. The cause of the arrhythmias is unknown but cellular electrolyte shifts and increased catecholamines have been implicated. (**Ref. 1**, p. 537; **Ref. 2**, p. 529)

624. (C) The majority (>95%) of chronic lymphocytic leukemia (CLL) are B cell neoplasms; the remainder originate from T lymphocytes. One complication of B-CLL is the development of a second neoplasm, frequently pulmonary neoplasms, malignant melanoma, or plasma cell tumors. Richter syndrome comprises the superimposition of a large cell immunoblastic lymphoma on B-CLL. The disease is heralded by progressive lymphadenopathy and constitutional symptoms such as fever and weight loss. The disease is fulminant and aggressive with death ensuing in about two months. (**Ref. 2**, p. 1067)

625. **(B)** Cor pulmonale is characterized by right ventricular hypertrophy secondary to pulmonary hypertension. The latter may be caused by diseases of lung parenchyma, pulmonary vessels, or disorders affecting chest movement, and diseases inducing pulmonary arteriolar constriction. Chronic cor pulmonale occurs in 10 to 30% of patients with congestive heart failure, the high prevalence being a reflection of how common chronic pulmonary diseases are. The most common causes of cor pulmonale are chronic bronchitis and emphysema. Other causes include primary pulmonary hypertension, Pickwickian syndrome, intravenous drug abuse, and neuromuscular diseases. In bronchial asthma, intervals of freedom alternate with periods of respiratory difficulty. There are only minimal parenchymal or vascular changes, although in more severe form, superimposed infection may lead to chronic bronchitis or bronchiectasis. (**Ref. 1**, p. 542; **Ref. 2**, p. 533)

626. **(A)** Cushing's ulcer, which occurs in patients with intracranial lesions, is a prototype of acute stress ulcer in contradistinction to the more chronic peptic ulcer. Acute ulcers are superficial gastric mucosal defects which may occur singly or multiple. The ulcer occurs randomly in the stomach, less commonly in the duodenum; by contrast, gastric ulcer has a predilection for the gastric antrum or lesser curvature. Acute ulcers are small (1 cm or less) and lack the induration, scarring, and thickening of blood vessels so typical of peptic ulcers. Acute ulcers may be caused by alcohol, cigarette smoking, and drugs (aspirin, steroids). (**Ref. 1**, p. 777)

627. **(B)** The patient has benign, probably essential, hypertension. "Flea-bitten" kidneys are associated with the malignant phase of hypertension and are due to necrotic ruptured glomerular capillaries or arterioles. Other lesions found in malignant hypertension include hyperplastic arteriolosclerosis (malignant nephrosclero-

sis). Usually in these cases the diastolic pressure rises above 130 mm Hg. Benign nephrosclerosis occurs in benign hypertension and is characterized by hyaline arteriolosclerosis, focal ischemic atrophy, glomerular obsolescence, and interstitial fibrosis. The heart shows concentric hypertrophy; dilatation occurs only in decompensated cases and is a sign of heart failure. (**Ref. 1**, p. 976)

628. **(D)** Most organ systems in the body suffer the effects of congestive heart failure (CHF). Left-sided failure affects predominantly the lungs, kidneys, and brain. Heart failure leads to an increase in left atrial and pulmonary venous pressures, which, in turn, leads to pulmonary congestion and edema. Late in the course of the failure, there is interstitial pulmonary fibrosis with intraalveolar hemosiderin-laden macrophages imparting a brown color to the lungs—"brown induration." The brunt of right-sided failure is borne by the liver, spleen, and subcutaneous tissues. The liver and spleen are both enlarged and show chronic passive congestion. In the liver there is centrolobular congestion accentuating the central areas which are surrounded by paler periportal areas—the "nutmeg" liver. The spleen shows dilatation of sinuses, fibrosis, recent and old hemorrhage with many hemosiderin-laden macrophages. (**Ref. 1**, pp. 522–523; **Ref. 2**, p. 510)

629. **(D)** Ultracentrifuge of serum yields five types of lipoproteins: chylomicrons, VLDL, IDL, LDL, and HDL. Cholesterol is transported mainly by LDL and HDL; the former contains about 70% of total plasma cholesterol. LDL and cholesterol levels correlate directly with the severity of atherosclerosis whereas HDL levels bear an inverse relationship to the development of atherosclerosis. Low LDL levels are associated with cigarette smoking, diabetes mellitus, and physical inactivity. Levels of HDL below 35 mg/dL may be associated with increased risk for atherosclerosis even in the presence of "normal" levels of plasma cholesterol. (**Ref. 1**, p. 475; **Ref. 3**, p. 319; **Ref. 6**, p. 206)

630. **(D)** Most pulmonary adenocarcinomas arise in the periphery of the lung. Less than 10% are associated with areas of scarring (old tuberculosis, healed infarcts, trauma). Sometimes, however, the scar represents a desmoplastic reaction to the tumor rather than preexisting scarring. Two histologic types of adenocarcinoma are known: the usual adenocarcinoma with its usual morphologic at-

tributes and bronchioloalveolar type. The tumor occurs with equal frequency in males and females and is associated with cigarette smoking. (**Ref. 2,** p. 610; **Ref. 1,** p. 723)

631. **(C)** Polycythemia vera is one of four chronic myeloproliferative syndromes. The others are agnogenic myeloid metaplasia (idiopathic myelofibrosis), chronic myelogenous leukemia, and idiopathic thrombocythemia. They all arise from the proliferation of multipotential stem cells which may differentiate along predominant cell lines. In polycythemia vera, erythroid proliferation predominates; however, there is also an increase in other bone marrow elements, thus the panhyperplasia. The clinical course of the disease is marked by specific phases: the proliferative, spent, post-polycythemia myelofibrosis with myeloid metaplasia and acute myelogenous leukemia, the last complication occurring in 5 to 10% of cases. (**Ref. 2,** p. 1051)

632. **(A)** Generally atherosclerosis involves the abdominal aorta much more severely than thoracic aorta. The orifices of major branches of the aorta usually show severe involvement. Arteries of the upper extremities show minimal involvement as do mesenteric and renal arteries. (**Ref. 1,** p. 476)

633. **(B)** Immunological injury in Sjörgren's syndrome may be mediated through cytotoxic T lymphocytes, specifically CD4+ or by autoantibodies. Many of the latter are found in these patients. By far the most common, detectable in 90% of patients, are two antibodies directed against ribonucleoprotein antigens—SS-A (Ro) and SS-B (La), of which the latter is more specific. Other autoantibodies which have been detected include ANA (50 to 80%) and antibodies to salivary duct cells, smooth muscle mitochondria, and thyroid antigens. Salivary and lacrimal glands are the major targets; they show enlargement and lymphocytic (predominantly T cell) infiltrate. The affected patients manifest dry eyes (keratoconjunctivitis sicca) and dry mouth (xerostomia). (**Ref. 1,** p. 201)

634. **(D)** Early on in the course of AIDS there is generalized lymphadenopathy. Histologically there is marked ("explosive") follicular hyperplasia with loss of mantle zone lymphocytes. The medulla shows prominent plasmacytosis. The interfollicular areas show hemorrhage ("follicular lysis") accompanied by focal perisinusoidal cell hyperplasia. Additionally there are varying degrees of vascular proliferation. Later generalized lymphocyte depletion and involution of follicles and interfollicular areas occur. Terminally the lymph nodes may be the site of an array of opportunistic infections, malignant lymphomas or Kaposi's sarcoma. (**Ref. 2,** p. 1040; **Ref. 1,** p. 230)

635. (**C**) Although cigarette smoking is the major cause of emphysema, the pathogenesis of the lesion is still unsettled. The most widely accepted hypothesis is the proteolysis–antiproteolysis theory. It has been proposed that there is a disturbance of the balance between proteases (mainly elastase) and antiproteases in the lung. Decrease of antielastase and/or increase in the elastase will cause destruction of the elastin of lung tissue leading to emphysema. The principal antielastase activity resides in α_1-antitrypsin while the principal antielastase activity is found in neutrophils. Cigarette smoking causes recruitment of neutrophils and macrophages, stimulating and enhancing the release of elastase from these inflammatory cells. Additionally oxidants in cigarette smoke inhibit α_1-antitrypsin, thus reducing antielastase activity. (**Ref. 1,** p. 683; **Ref. 2,** p. 587)

636. (**E**) The lacunar RS cell is large and has a single-to-multiple hyperlobated nucleus with multiple small nucleoli. The cytoplasm is abundant and pale-staining; the cytoplasmic membrane is distinct. In formalin-fixed tissue the cytoplasm of the cells retract from the adjacent tissue giving rise to a pericellular halo or "lacuna." This type of RS cell may occasionally be encountered in mixed cellularity type Hodgkin disease. The classic RS cell presents a binucleated or bilobed cell with prominent nucleoli and each nucleus appearing as a mirror image of the other—the "owl eye" feature. Many variants of RS cell are described: mononuclear, pleomorphic, lymphocytic, and histiocytic variant. (**Ref. 2,** p. 1087; **Ref. 1,** p. 645)

637. (**A**) Central to the pathogenesis of immune complex type hypersensitivity reaction (type III) is the formation of antigen–antibody complexes. The complexes formed in moderate antigen excess are most effective for activating complement. Those complexes formed in antibody excess are usually rapidly removed from the circulation by reticuloendothelial cells. The soluble antigen–

antibody complexes are deposited in the basement membrane of glomeruli and the internal elastic laminae of blood vessels. The complexes may also activate complement; while complexes formed with IgG and IgM activate complement through the classic pathway, IgA can do a similar thing through the alternate pathway. Activation of complement leads to neutrophil aggregation, release of vasoactive amines, and tissue necrosis. (**Ref. 1,** pp. 184–187; **Ref. 8,** p. 135)

638. **(B)** Hypertrophic cardiomyopathy is characterized by cardiac enlargement with myocardial hypertrophy of ventricular muscle. In some cases the hypertrophy may affect the septum disproportionately (asymmetrical septal hypertrophy) or the apical portion of the left ventricle or the basal septum may be more severely involved. Obstructive hypertrophic cardiomyopathy results when the submitral valve myocardial is involved. The intramyocardial arteries show markedly thickened walls. Clinically, patients may be asymptomatic for years while others may manifest intractable heart failure or die suddenly. (**Ref. 1,** p. 560; **Ref. 3,** p. 369)

639. **(D)** The pathogenesis of atherosclerosis is complex and many hypotheses have been propounded. Most of these hypotheses invoke injury to arterial endothelium, smooth muscle proliferation, and the participation of platelets and monocytes. Endothelial injury may be initiated by hemodynamic forces, hypertension, chronic hyperlipidemia, cigarette smoking, or in experimental animals, by immune complex deposits or chemicals. Smooth muscle proliferation may be caused by mitogens; among them, platelet growth factor, fibroblast growth factor, epidermal growth factor, and transforming growth factor alpha. (**Ref. 1,** p. 477)

640. **(B)** The F_c portion of IgE molecule is uniquely structured for attachment to mast cells. During re-exposure to the specific antigen (allergen) that stimulated the IgE, a series of reactions occurs which lead to the degranulation and release of vasoactive amines and other mediators from basophils and mast cells. The process of degranulation involves active influx of Ca^{++}, transient elevation of cyclic AMP, activation of CAMP-dependent kinases, and phosphorylation of perigranular protein. Degranulation leads to the release of primary (preformed) and secondary (newly synthesized) mediators. Some of the latter include histamine, eosinophil chemotactic factors of anaphylaxis, and granule-matrix-derived mediators; among the latter are arachidonic acid derivatives (leukotrienes and prostaglandins) and platelet-activating factor. (**Ref. 1,** p. 179; **Ref. 8,** p. 368)

641. (E) Diffuse alveolar damages, also known as adult respiratory distress syndrome (ARDS), is a clinicopathologic syndrome characterized by distinctive morphologic changes and clinically by acute and rapid onset of severe respiratory insufficiency, decreased lung compliance, severe arterial hypoxemia refractory to oxygen therapy and associated with extensive radiologic opacities in both lungs. The lesion is the final common pathway for a variety of insults among them, shock due to any cause, fat embolism, diffuse viral pulmonary infections, septicemia, oxygen toxicity, inhalation of irritant gases, narcotic overdose, and aspiration pneumonitis. The pathogenesis invokes capillary endothelial and alveolar epithelial cell injury through the generation of oxygen-derived free radical or through the liberation of mediators that involve leukocyte aggregation in the lung. These in turn, secrete oxygen-derived free radicals, lysosomal enzymes, and products of arachidonic acid metabolism which then injure the endothelium and epithelium. (**Ref. 2,** p. 576; **Ref. 1,** p. 704)

642. (D) Clinical manifestations of renal amyloidosis include proteinuria with or without hypoalbuminemia, nephrotic syndrome, renal failure, and uremia. The kidneys may be normal in size or may be enlarged, firm, brownish, and waxy. In late stages of the disease, they may be contracted and small due to ischemic changes caused by vascular involvement. Amyloid involvement of the heart may cause congestive heart failure, cardiomegaly, and arrhythmias. In the gastrointestinal tract, amyloidosis is known to cause constipation, diarrhea, or malabsorption syndrome. (**Ref. 1,** pp. 234, 236; **Ref. 2,** p. 1173)

643. (D) Most cases of osteoporosis are idiopathic. In a small number of cases, however, some underlying condition may be evident, such as hypopituitarism, malnutrition, malabsorption, and prolonged glucocorticoid administration. Joint disease is the hallmark of rheumatoid arthritis characterized morphologically by diffuse proliferative synovitis. (**Ref. 1,** p. 1219)

644. (C) Comedocarcinoma is a variant of intraductal breast carcinoma (ductal carcinoma-in-situ). In DCIS the tumor cells are confined within the basement membrane of the duct. The disease is frequently multifocal and is bilateral in 15 to 20% of cases. Histologically the ducts are distended by tumor cells which may be arranged in papillary, cribriform, or solid patterns. Some show central necrosis which may be extruded when pressure is applied, thus the designation, "comedocarcinoma." **(Ref. 1, p. 1102; Ref. 3, p. 825)**

645. (E) About 50% of AIDS patients develop some degree of proteinuria; in about 10%, full-blown nephrotic syndrome may occur. A variety of glomerular and tubular alterations have been observed in these patients. By light microscopy one sees focal segmental sclerosis and a nonspecific interstitial chronic inflammation. By electron microscopy tubuloreticular inclusions may be found in the endothelial cells of the kidney and some other organs. Although not diagnostic, these inclusions are useful in distinguishing AIDS-associated focal glomerulosclerosis from the idiopathic form. The tubules show focal necrosis, atrophy, and cystic dilatation. **(Ref. 2, p. 818; Ref. 1, p. 954)**

646. (E) HAV is a picornavirus that is transmitted by the fecal–oral route. HAV never pursues a chronic protracted clinical course and does not cause chronic hepatitis; neither do patients become chronic carriers. Fatal fulminant hepatitis rarely occurs (about 0/1%). The disease is endemic in developing countries and it is common in children in daycare centers and those housed in institutions for the mentally retarded. Following infection with HAV, detectable IgM-antiHAV appear in the serum during the acute illness, begins to fall a few weeks later, and is then replaced by IgG-antiHAV which persists for life. **(Ref. 2, p. 720)**

647. (A) Hemolytic transfusion reaction is a prototype type II hypersensitivity disorder in which antibodies are directed towards antigens present on the surface of cells. The case in question represents the transfusion of cells from an incompatible donor to a patient with autochthonous antibodies. The disease, often heralded by fever and chills, may progress to hypotension, dyspnea, shock, and renal failure. Transfusion of ABO incompatible blood may be fatal in up to 10% of cases. Other complement-dependent type II hypersensitivity reactions include erythroblastosis fetalis and autoimmune hemolytic anemia. (**Ref. 1,** p. 183; **Ref. 8,** p. 288)

648. (**D**)   Esophageal cancers constitute 7 to 10% of malignant neoplasms of the GIT. The great majority are squamous cell carcinomas. Very wide variations exist in the prevalence of these tumors even in adjacent geographic locations. Relatively high incidence is found in northern China, Iran, Russia, and South Africa. Many risk factors have been identified which include excessive consumption of alcohol, particularly hard liquor, cigarette smoking, diets deficient in certain vitamins and trace metals, the presence of chronic esophagitis (not reflux esophagitis), food contaminated by fungi such as *Aspergillus* and primary esophageal diseases (achalasia, Plummer–Vinson syndrome and esophageal stricture). (**Ref. 1,** p. 764; **Ref. 2,** p. 628)

649. (**B**)   IgA nephropathy (Berger disease) is a disease of young adults affecting females twice as frequently as males. It is a common cause of gross hematuria and has been regarded by some as a monosymptomatic form of Henoch–Schönlein purpura. Kidney biopsies reveal focal and segmental proliferation. Crescents may be observed in rare cases. By immunofluorescence, immune deposits are found mainly in the mesangium and less commonly in the subepithelial or subendothelial regions. In addition to IgA, C3 is demonstrable in 60% and IgG in 30% of cases. (**Ref. 1,** p. 957; **Ref. 4,** p. 1305)

650. (**C**)   Each of the four polypeptide chains of the immunoglobulin molecule contains an amino-terminal V (variable) and a carboxy-terminal C (constant) portions. Digestion of the IgG molecule by papain yields two F_{ab} (antigen binding) and one F_c (crystallizable) fragments. The antigen-binding property resides in the F_{ab}, but specifically in a small number of amino acids in the V portion of the molecule of both the H and L chains. (**Ref. 8,** p. 110)

651. (**E**)   In the last three decades, a number of classifications of non-Hodgkin lymphoma (NHL) have emerged, each employing morphologic, immunologic, and clinical aspects of these tumors. While the Rappaport, Lukes–Collins, and the Kiel classification have their adherents, the most widely used classification is the

Working Formulation which employs clinical criteria to classify the NHLs. Based on five-year survival statistics, three major groups are identified: low-grade, intermediate, and high-grade NHLs, which have survival rates of 50 to 75%, 35 to 45%, and 23 to 32%, respectively. The Working Formulation also recognizes a fourth category of miscellaneous NHLs which include histiocytic tumors, HTLV-1-induced T lymphoma and other T cell lymphomas. (**Ref. 1,** p. 638)

652. (**C**)   *C. difficile* colitis (pseudomembranous colitis) occurs in severely ill patients receiving broad spectrum antibiotics for long periods of time. The antibiotics destroy the normal bowel flora permitting proliferation of *C. difficile,* which, in turn, produce toxins that destroy the bowel mucosa. Pathologically the "pseudomembrane" composed of necrotic debris, fibrin, and acute inflammatory cells adhere to the mucosa but can be easily wiped off to reveal superficial mucosal erosions. The lesions may be punctate, patchy, or confluent and may be diagnosed by screening fecal extracts for *C. difficile* toxins or by culture. (**Ref. 1,** p. 795; **Ref. 2,** p. 379)

653. (**E**)   NK cells are a subset of lymphocytes that recognize and kill certain tumor cells and virus-infected cells without previous recognition of these antigens. Hence, they function as the first line of defense against viral infection. The rare patient who has no NK cells show susceptibility to viral infections such as cytomegalovirus and varicella. NK cells are larger than small lymphocytes, have a granular cytoplasm, and are therfore called large granular lymphocytes. Antigens expressed on the surface of NK cells and which may serve as markers for them include CD2, $CD11_a$, $CD11_b$, CD38, CD45. (**Ref. 1,** p. 173; **Ref. 8,** p. 69)

654. (**D**)   The symptoms, signs, and laboratory findings are characteristic of acute nephritic syndrome of which hematuria is the cardinal symptom. Patients with this syndrome also manifest edema usually in non-dependent parts of the body such as eyelids, face, and hands. Impaired renal function is seen as mild or severe diminished glomerular filtration rate (oliguria or anuria). Membranous nephropathy is the classic example of renal disease which manifests nephrotic syndrome. (**Ref. 2,** p. 813; **Ref. 4,** p. 1295)

655. (D) The location of the blister forms an important basis for differentiating various bullous disorders of the skin. Three sites most commonly described are subcorneal, suprabasal, and subepidermal regions of the skin. Other lesions that may form vesicles include impetigo contagiosa, eczematous dermatitis, and viral infections of the skin such as chickenpox and herpes zoster. (**Ref. 1,** p. 1201)

656. (C) Occurring most frequently in the cerebral cortex and almost never in the cerebellum, glioblastoma multiforme is an anaplastic glial tumor that usually develops in preexisting astrocytomas. The name "multiforme" derives from the variegated gross appearance of the tumor—solid and cystic areas, foci of necrosis and hemorrhage are often present. (**Ref. 1,** p. 1342)

657. (A) Excretion of formiminoglutamic acid after the administration of histidine is typical of folic acid deficiency. Vitamin B_{12} is involved in the isomerization of methylomalonyl coenzyme A to succinyl coenzyme A and its deficiency leads to increased levels of methylmalonate (as methylmalonic acid) in the urine. Pernicious anemia is regarded by some as an autoimmune disease. Three types of autoantibodies are known to occur: blocking antibodies against vitamin B_{12}-intrinsic factor binding, binding antibodies against intrinsic factor, and intrinsic factor-B_{12} complex and antibodies against gastric parietal cells which can be demonstrated in the serum of 95% of patients. (**Ref. 1,** pp. 605–608; **Ref. 3,** p. 383)

658. (A) T lymphocytes comprise 65 to 75% of peripheral blood lymphocytes, >95% of thymic lymphocytes, and 70 to 80% of lymphocytes in the lymph node. In the spleen, however, they account for only 20 to 30% of lymphocytes while B lymphocytes predominate. T, B, and NK lymphocytes are distinguished by their antigen receptors and characteristic surface markers called cluster differentiation (CD). For example, T cells recognize antigens by a receptor complex called CD3/TCR. T lymphocytes not only participate in cell-mediated immunity but also secrete potent cytokines including gamma interferon and interleukins. (**Ref. 8,** p. 61)

659. (D) 95% of patients with Down syndrome, the most common chromosomal disorder, reveal trisomy 21, the extra chromosome being derived from the mother in 80% and the father in 20% of cases. 95% of Edward syndrome occur as trisomy 18, a disease which is observed in one of every 8,000 births. It is characterized by mental retardation and a multitude of somatic anomalies. In over 80% of Patau syndrome the chromosomal abnormality is trisomy 13; patients manifest microcephaly and mental retardation in addition to numerous severe malformations. The major chromosomal abnormality in cri-du-chat syndrome is the deletion of the short arm of chromosome 5. Turner syndrome (gonadal dysgenesis), which occurs in one of every 3,000 female births results from nondisjunction of the X chromosome leading to the absence of one X chromosome (45, XO). The patients present with short stature, poor breast development, webbed neck, primary amenorrhea, and infertility. (**Ref. 1**, pp. 156–161; **Ref. 3**, pp. 235–237)

660. (C) There are three principal variants of malignant melanoma: superficial spreading melanoma, lentigo maligna melanoma, and nodular melanoma. The last behaves most aggressively and has the worst prognosis. Both the superficial spreading and lentigo maligna melanoma pass through an initial phase of lateral spread during which the neoplasm seems to have no potential for distant metastases. By contrast, dermal invasion occurs early in nodular melanoma which does not pass through an initial lateral spread phase. Clearly the prognosis depends on the level of invasion of the deeper tissues. (**Ref. 1**, p. 1179)

661. (A) α_1-antitrypsin, a glycoprotein produced by the liver, inhibits a variety of proteases, among them elastase, trypsin, and chymotrypsin. In the lung, α_1-antitrypsin inhibits neutrophil elastase which is responsible for digestion of elastin in alveolar walls, a mechanism that has been proposed for the pathogenesis of emphysema. A deficiency of α_1-antitrypsin disturbs the protease–antiprotease balance with resulting destructive effects on lung tissue. Homozygous patients with α_1-antitrypsin deficiency have a marked tendency for developing emphysema occurring predominantly as panacinar emphysema. Panacinar emphysema affects the entire acinus and tends to occur more commonly in the lower zones and anterior margins of the lung. (**Ref. 1**, p. 685; **Ref. 2**, p. 587)

662. (B) The next marker after HB_sAg to appear in the serum of patients infected with hepatitis B virus is HB_eAg. It is usually seen before the onset of symptoms and, with HBV-DNA and DNA polymerase constitute evidence of active viral replication. HB_eAg peaks during the acute illness and disappears before HB_sAg has cleared from the serum. In chronic carriers with HB_eAg, sustained high serum levels of HB_eAg persists. (**Ref. 2**, p. 724; **Ref. 1**, p. 845)

663. (A) Improved medical care has contributed to increasing the survival of patients with Down syndrome; many now survive to 30 years, and a few more till age 50. Nearly all Down syndrome patients who survive beyond 35 years show brain morphologic changes similar to those of Alzheimer patients. Many of these patients also manifest symptoms of the disease. (**Ref. 1**, p. 156)

664. (E) A DNA virus, EBV has been implicated in the pathogenesis of Burkitt lymphoma and nasopharyngeal carcinoma (poorly differentiated squamous cell carcinoma). Cells from 98% of African Burkitt lymphoma and 15 to 20% on non-African Burkitt lymphoma contain EBV genome and EBV nuclear antigen (EBNA). It has been suggested that other risk factors such as malaria may be involved in the genesis of Burkitt lymphoma. 100% of nasopharyngeal carcinoma contain EBV DNA and EBNA. Additionally, titers to EBV viral antigens are elevated in both African Burkitt tumor and nasopharyngeal carcinoma. (**Ref. 1**, p. 348; **Ref. 2**, p. 169)

665. (C) The gross and microscopic changes in dilated cardiomyopathy (CMP) are nonspecific: cardiac hypertrophy with four-chamber dilatation, histologic changes varying from normal to focal interstitial necrosis, and myofiber alterations such as atrophy or hypertrophy. Electron microscopy or histochemistry reveal nonspecific changes. Among pathogenetic considerations are alcohol or its metabolites, peripartum (pre- or postpartum), genetic influences, and postviral myocarditis. (**Ref. 1**, p. 558)

666. (D) AL (amyloid light chain) fibril protein is derived from plasma cells and contains predominantly complete immunoglobulin kappa or lamda light chains, NH_2-terminal fragments of light chains, or both. AL protein occurs in primary amyloidosis or amyloidosis associated with plasma cell dyscrasia such as multiple myeloma. AA fibril protein is found in the amyloidosis associated with chronic inflammation, neoplasia, or hereditary diseases, the most prominent being familial Mediterranean fever. The amyloidosis seen in patients on long-term hemodialysis is due to deposition of β_2 macroglobulin while β_2 amyloid protein is found in the cerebral plaques of Alzheimer patients. (**Ref. 1,** p. 233)

667. (D) The most likely diagnosis is pseudomembranous colitis, usually caused by the toxin of *Clostridium difficile*. It is an acute colitis characterized by patchy areas of mucosal inflammation to which are attached gray-yellowish plaques; sometimes these lesions coalesce to form extensive pseudomembrane. Microscopically, the lesion is composed of an admixture of fibrin, mucus, disintegrated epithelial cells, and leukocytes. Typically, the lesions occur as "volcanic eruptions" from crypt abscesses in the colonic mucosa. The lesions are found not only in association with antibiotic therapy but may also be encountered in other enteric infections by *Staphylococcus, Shigella,* and *Candida.* (**Ref. 2,** p. 673; **Ref. 1,** p. 795)

668. (D) In early childhood the spleen of the sickle cell patient is slightly to moderately enlarged (about 500 gm) owing to marked congestion of the red pulp and reticuloendothelial hyperplasia. Late in the course of the disease, however, repeated thrombosis and infarction leads to fibrosis with or without iron deposits (Gamna–Gandy bodies) and decrease in splenic size. Subsequently only a small nodule of tissue remains—autosplenectomy. This condition predisposes to bacteremia and osteomyelitis, in particular, *Salmonella* organisms. Such patients are also prone to *Streptococcus pneumoniae* and *H. influenzae* infections. (**Ref. 1,** p. 594; **Ref. 3,** p. 396)

669. (D) The cause of congenital heart diseases is unknown in the great majority of cases (90%). In the remainder, multifactorial genetic factors and environmental influences are suspected. Among the chromosomal abnormalities associated with increased congenital heart disease are trisomies 18, 13, 22, 9 (mosaic) and +14q-. Maternal infection with rubella in the first trimester is a cause of multiple congenital anomalies, among them, patent ductus arteriosus, tetralogy of Fallot, and ventricular septal defect. Klinefelter syndrome is characterized by male hypogonadism (testicular atrophy and azoospermia), 47XXY or 46XY/47XXY karyotypes, eunuchoid body habitus and slightly decreased IQ. (**Ref. 1,** pp. 154–157, 571; **Ref. 2,** p. 511)

670. (**E**) The most common type of chronic pancreatitis is chronic calcifying pancreatitis, often seen in alcoholics. This is characterized by atrophy of pancreatic acini, marked interstitial and interlobular fibrosis, chronic inflammation, and dilatation of pancreatic ducts. Focal calcification and pancreatic calculi are typical. The islets are spared and appear normal. The second type of pancreatitis is the chronic obstructive form in which there is stenosis of the sphincter of Oddi. (**Ref. 1,** pp. 902–904; **Ref. 2,** p. 792)

671. (**D**) The features are those found in septic shock which in early stages shows normal or increased cardiac output and warm and dry skin. In late stages, however, the peripheral pooling of blood results in the reduction of effective circulating blood volume, hypotension, diminished cardiac output, and poor tissue perfusion. The pathogenesis of septic shock is poorly understood. Usually caused by gram-negative bacteria, it is probably due to release into the circulation of bacterial endotoxic liposaccharides. Sometimes septic shock may be caused by gram-positive organisms such as streptococcus and pneumococcus. (**Ref. 1,** pp. 114–121)

672. (**D**) Primary biliary cirrhosis (PBC), defined as nonsuppurative destructive cholangitis and most common in middle-aged women, constitutes about 2% of deaths from cirrhosis. The serum of patients with PBC usually shows elevated IgM and a variety of autoantibodies, among them, antinuclear, antithyroid, and antiplatelet antibodies. Three major pathologic states of the disease are recognized: the duct lesion (chronic destructive cholangitis), the stage of scarring (disappearance of bile ducts, proliferation of bile ductules) and the stage of cirrhosis (finely nodular dark-green, bile-stained liver). (**Ref. 2,** p. 740; **Ref. 1,** p. 868)

673. (**C**) The features are those found in acute myocarditis. The dilatation affects all cardiac chambers; focal petechial hemorrhages may also be observed. The valves and endocardium are unaffected. Microscopically there is edema, hyperemia, myocytolysis, and diffuse inflammatory infiltrate composed of lymphocytes, macrophages, and plasma cells. Eosinophils are found in those cases where immune pathogenesis or parasitic infection (eg, trichinosis) is involved. Giant cells are found in idiopathic giant cell (?Fiedler's) myocarditis. The disease may be asymptomatic but may also be heralded by sudden onset of congestive heart failure. (**Ref. 1**, pp. 562–564; **Ref. 2**, p. 368)

674. (**B**)   Although TGF_{α}, TGF_{β}, and tumor necrosis factor may be involved indirectly in angiogenesis, of the factors mentioned, only fibroblast growth factor is directly involved in the four phases of angiogenesis—degradation of basement membrane of pre-existing parent blood vessel, migration of endothelial cells, proliferation of endothelial cells, and organization into capillaries. PDGF, derived from α granules of platelets, activated macrophages, endothelium, and smooth muscle cells, causes proliferation and migration of fibroblasts, smooth muscle, and monocytes. (**Ref. 1**, pp. 79–80)

675. (**A**)   Carcinoid heart disease is characterized by a peculiar plaque-like fibrous thickening of the endocardium of the right ventricular outflow tract which may result in pulmonic and tricuspid valvular stenosis. The pathogenesis of this lesion is uncertain but it has been suggested that it may be related to serotonin, bradykinin, and tachykinins P and K; elevated serum levels of the latter peptides tend to correlate with carcinoid heart syndrome. The lesion predominates on the right because there is inactivation of bradykinin and serotonin in the blood during passage through the lungs by monoamine oxidase. If these substances are not totally inactivated, lesions of the left heart may ensue. (**Ref. 1**, p. 555)

676. (**C**)   Hereditary spherocytosis, an autosomal dominant disease, results probably from a fundamental defect in the skeletal framework of the erythrocyte. The membrane skeleton is composed of a complex arrangement of proteins dominated by spectrin; other proteins include ankryin, actin, and glycophorin-3. The most common abnormality in the disease is a deficiency of spectrin. Other abnormalities are abnormal polymerization of spectrin and defective membrane autophosphorylation. (**Ref. 1**, p. 559; **Ref. 3**, p. 390)

677. **(C)** Edema is the accumulation of excessive fluid in the interstitial (intercellular) tissue space or body cavities. Caused by a derangement of Starling forces, edema may result from decreased intravascular osmotic pressure or increased hydrostatic pressure. The latter may be caused by impaired venous return (congestive heart failure, liver cirrhosis), constrictive pericarditis, or arteriolar dilatation. Clinical antecedents of the former include nephrotic syndrome, malnutrition, protein-losing gastroenteropathies, and hypoproteinemia. Edema may also be caused by sodium retention and lymphatic obstruction. (**Ref. 1,** pp. 93–97)

678. **(B)** During acute inflammation, the complement system is activated either through the classic pathway, which itself is initiated by antigen–antibody complexes, or through the alternate pathway by stimuli such as bacterial endotoxins, aggregated globulins, and complex polysaccharides. C3a and C5a increase vascular permeability mainly by liberating histamine from mast cells and platelets. C5a is strongly chemotactic for neutrophils, eosinophils, basophils, and monocytes. C3b and C3bi are opsonins, facilitating the process of phagocytosis. C5b-9, also called membrane attack complex, is responsible for cell lysis. (**Ref. 1,** pp. 66–68)

679. **(A)** In the male the anterior urethra is the site of early infection and is characterized by suppurative inflammation with production of copious pus. Untreated, the infection progresses to involve the epididymis, seminal vesicles, and prostate; the testis is remarkably resistant to this infection. In late stages, the acute inflammation leads to fibrosis and sometimes sterility. In women, the urethra, Bartholin glands, Skene glands, and fallopian tubes are involved and the infection may progress to pyosalpinx and tuboovarian abscess. (**Ref. 1,** p. 343; **Ref. 3,** p. 802)

680. **(D)** The central cause of heart failure is decreased contractility of the myocardium; this sets in motion a sequence of events starting with decreased cardiac output leading to decreased effective arterial blood volume. This then triggers increased sympathetic discharge and serum catecholamines with attendant widespread vasoconstriction. The stimulation of the renin–angiotensin system causes increased aldosterone production, increased tubular reabsorption of Na^+ and water, and edema. The stimulation of the sympathetic nervous outflow also causes renal vasoconstriction, decreased glomerular filtration rate, diminished urinary excretion of Na^+ and water, and subsequent edema. (**Ref. 9**, p. 584; **Ref. 1**, pp. 520–522)

681. **(B)** The major histocompatibility complex (MHC) gene products can be classified into three categories—class I comprising HLA-A, HLA-B, HLA-C; class II antigens coded for in HLA-D region, and class III proteins with components of the complement system. The HLA complex in man is regarded as the major histocompatibility complex; the cell-surface antigens coded for this region are capable of invoking strong transplantation reactions. The ABO blood group antigen system, however, is an exception. These antigens are not linked to HLA. As is true of other haplotypes (sets of closely linked genes on one chromosome which tend to be inherited en bloc) the HLA complex includes one gene each from HLA-A, HLA-B, HLA-C, and HLA-D loci. (**Ref. 1**, pp. 175–177; **Ref. 3**, p. 118)

682. **(C)** The histologic features aptly describe chronic active hepatitis. Piecemeal necrosis, an irregular appearance of the periportal zone, although most often seen in chronic active hepatitis, has also been described in other acute and chronic liver diseases. In addition to the features enumerated, chronic active hepatitis, may also reveal bridging necrosis and progressive fibrosis extending from the portal tracts into the lobular parenchyma. (**Ref. 2**, p. 732; **Ref. 1**, p. 852)

683. **(A)** Serum levels of CEA are directly related to the size of colonic carcinoma and the extent of the disease. Thus, the serum levels are elevated in 5% and 25% of patients with Duke A and Duke B tumors respectively. The test is therefore not useful in early lesions. CEA is also not specific for colonic carcinoma; it may be elevated in tumors of the lung, ovary, breast, urinary bladder, and in nonneoplastic lesions such as alcoholic cirrhosis, pancreatitis, and ulcerative colitis. Measurement of serum levels of CEA is therefore of greatest use to assess possible recurrence of colonic carcinoma following resection. (**Ref. 1**, p. 300; **Ref. 2**, p. 694)

684. **(D)** Rapidly progressive glomerulonephritis refers to a group of renal diseases characterized by rapid decline of renal function as-

sociated with widespread (>50%) glomerular crescent formation. Crescents result from proliferation of epithelial cells which fill the Bowman's space, often compressing the glomerular tuft. Fibrin can be demonstrated in these lesions, a finding that has been used to ascribe a pathogenetic role to leakage of fibrin from severely damaged glomeruli. RPGN may be caused by antiglomerular membrane disease-mediated diseases such as Goodpasture syndrome, idiopathic antiglomerular basement membrane nephritis, or immune complex disease such as poststreptococcal glomerulonephritis, IgA nephropathy, bacterial endocarditis, membranoproliferative glomerulonephritis, Henoch–Schönlein purpura, or renal lesions without glomerular immune deposits (polyarteritis nodosa, Wegener's granulomatosis). (**Ref. 2,** p. 839; **Ref. 4,** p. 1297)

685. (D) Reflux esophagitis is caused by reflux of gastric contents owing to incompetence of lower esophageal sphincter or disordered esophageal motility. The histologic changes include basal cell hyperplasia and infiltration of the mucosa by eosinophils. The presence of intraepithelial neutrophils marks the presence of esophageal ulceration. Continued gastroesophageal reflux may lead to Barett esophagus. (**Ref. 1,** p. 761)

686. (C) There is convincing evidence in experiments in both humans and baboons that alcohol is a direct hepatotoxin. Alcohol affects the oxidative capacity of hepatocytes and causes impaired formation of ATP. Mitochondria are enlarged and the smooth endoplasmic reticulum become hyperplastic; the latter is reflected by increased activity of cytochrome P_{450}-dependent mixed function oxidases. (**Ref. 2,** p. 737)

687. (B) G6PD deficiency is inherited as a sex-linked trait, hence, all red blood cells of affected males manifest the deficiency whereas in females, only mild enzyme deficiency is observed. The disease is the most common erythrocyte enzyme deficiency affecting millions of people all over the world, and about 10% of American blacks. Dozens of variants are known to occur of which only two are clinically significant—G6PD A- and G6PD Mediterranean. Many oxidant drugs such as antimalarials, sulfonamides, and nitrofuratoin may trigger hemolysis. (**Ref. 1,** pp. 591–592; **Ref. 3,** p. 393)

688. (B) Two hypotheses have been proposed to explain the biologic effects of radiation. The "target" theory proposes that radiation energy acts by direct hits on target molecules within the cell. In this, the linkage bonds of the DNA are disrupted, a process that may lead to mutations, inhibition of cell division, or cell death. The other hypothesis, the "indirect action" theory proposes the damages is caused by the production of active free radicals resulting from radiolysis of water molecules. Such free radicals include H_2O^+, H_2O^-, which in turn, form free radical H• and OH• and the reactive radicals H_2O_2•. These radicals then react with vital cell components such as cell membranes, enzymes, and nucleic acids producing cell injury. (**Ref. 1,** pp. 402–408)

689. (B) Genital chlamydial infection is caused by *Chlamydia trachomatis,* an obligate intracellular organism which though possessing DNA, RNA, and a cell wall, lacks the ability to produce ATP. Two forms are recognized in its life cycle—the elementary body, metabolically inactive and the reticulate body which takes over the host cells metabolism and replicates repeatedly forming numerous daughter elementary bodies. In tissue the organism is recognized as intracytoplasmic inclusions. *Chlamydial* infection incites a neutrophilic and lymphocytic response. The disease responds to tetracycline but not penicillin administration. (**Ref. 2,** p. 394; **Ref. 1,** p. 307)

690. (B) The prognosis of colon cancer depends largely on the extent of the disease and the involvement of regional lymph nodes and the presence of distant metastases and to a lesser extent, the histologic differentiation of the tumor and the part of the colon (left or right) involved. Several staging classifications exist but by far the most well known and used is the Duke classification or any of its modifications. In essence the Asteler and Coller modification of Dukes classification recognized the following stages:

A: tumor confined to the mucosa
B1: tumor invading muscularis propria but not penetrating the serosa
B2: tumor invading the serosa
C1: B1 tumor with metastasis to regional lymph nodes
C2: B2 tumor with metastasis to regional lymph nodes
D: tumor with distant metastasis

Another classification by the American Joint Committee for Cancer Staging and End Result Reporting employs the TNM system. (**Ref. 1**, p. 817; **Ref. 2**, p. 692)

691. **(B)** The lung infection caused by legionella pneumophili is necrotizing bronchopneumonia, sometimes confluent, rarely lobar, with or without microabscesses. The alveoli and bronchioles contain an inflammatory exudate consisting of fibrin, neutrophils, and macrophages with a predominance of the latter. Some macrophages are enlarged with myriad of organisms which are difficult to visualize in routine stains; however, they can be demonstrated with the Diederle silver impregnation stain. Secondary inflammation of vessel walls may lead to thrombosis and more tissue necrosis. (**Ref. 1**, p. 353; **Ref. 2**, p. 374)

692. **(B)** Prostaglandins are derivatives of arachidonic acid metabolism through the cyclooxygenase pathway. Intermediate metabolites include PGG_2 and PGH_2; the latter is converted enzymatically into thromboxane A_2, prostaglandin I_2, $PGF_{2\alpha}$ and PGD_2, which are involved in the vascular components of acute inflammation—vasodilation and edema formation. Cytokines, by contrast, are peptide or glycoprotein mediators of immunologic, inflammatory, and reparative reactions to injury. When produced by lymphocytes and macrophages, they are called lymphokines or monokines, respectively. At least eight interleukins (IL-1–IL-8) and three interferons (IFN-α, IFN-β, and IFN-gamma) have been described. (**Ref. 1**, pp. 41, 174; **Ref. 8**, p. 78)

693. **(A)** Aspergillus infection may take one of three forms: allergic, colonizing, and invasive. The growth of spores of aspergillus in the warm atmosphere of pre-existing pulmonary cavities (eg, tuberculous or bronchiectatic cavities) with minimal or no invasion of surrounding tissue, results in an aspergilloma also called a fungus ball. Inflammatory reaction to the aspergilloma is usually minimal. Invasive aspergillosis occurs in immunocompromised patients and may be widely disseminated in many organs. Allergic aspergillosis may manifest as allergic alveolitis, allergic bronchopulmonary aspergillosis, or bronchial asthma. (**Ref. 1**, p. 356; **Ref. 2**, p. 410)

694. (D) Secretion and production of mucus is the clinical hallmark of chronic bronchitis. Thus, the definition of the disease—persistent cough with sputum production for at least three months in at least two consecutive years. The major cause of this mucus production is hyperplasia and hypertrophy of mucous-secreting cells. There is also a marked increase in the goblet cells of small airways (small bronchi and bronchioles) which may contribute in part to the obstruction associated with chronic bronchitis. The increased mucous gland enlargement is quantitated in the Reid index—the ratio of the thickness of the mucous glands to the thickness of the bronchial wall between the basement membrane of the surface epithelium to the perichondrium of the bronchial cartilage. The Reid index is normally less than 0.4; in chronic bronchitis it is usually greater than 0.5. (**Ref. 1,** p. 689; **Ref. 2,** p. 584)

695. (A) The cure rate of LP, NS, MC, and LD types of Hodgkin's disease are >90%, 80 to 85%, 75%, and 40 to 50%, respectively. Advances with chemotherapy has significantly improved the survival rates of patients with Hodgkin disease. Overall there is a 70% cure rate. The prognosis depends not only on the histologic type but also on the age of the patient, clinical stage, and whether the patient is symptomatic. In general, patients with the less favorable histologic types tend to present with disease at a higher stage—III or IV. (**Ref. 2,** p. 1091; **Ref. 1,** pp. 644–648)

696. (C) Silicosis is a pneumoconiosis caused by the inhalation of silicon dioxide (silica). It is encountered in a variety of occupations—mining gold, tin, copper, and coal, in sandblasting, quarrying, ceramic manufacturing, and cleaning of boilers. The most common form of the disease, simple nodular silicosis begins insidiously and evolves slowly over a span of decades. The severity depends on the type of silica, the duration and intensity of inhalation, and individual susceptibility. Pathologically the lung reveals silicotic nodules—characteristic whorled nodule with concentric rings of collagen fibers within which silica fragments are visible by polarized light. Progressive massive fibrosis typically shows large coalescent nodules that may measure 5 to 10 cm in diameter. The lesions may cavitate. Clinically, patients manifest severe, sometimes fatal, respiratory failure. Silicosis may also be accompanied by tuberculosis or the development of Caplan syndrome. (**Ref. 1,** p. 708; **Ref. 2,** p. 595)

697. (D) The histochemical stain with the features enumerated in the question are typical of Congo Red staining of amyloid. With hematoxylin and eosin amyloid appears amorphous extracellular eosinophilic hyaline deposits. Amyloid also stains metachromatically with crystal violet or methyl violet. With thioflavin T or thioflavin S, amyloid demonstrates secondary fluorescence when viewed with ultraviolet light. Congo Red, by far, is the most widely used stain for amyloid and the reaction is shared by all forms of amyloid. On electron microscopy amyloid appears as non-branching fibrils of varying lengths and about 75 to 10 nm wide. (**Ref. 1,** p. 236; **Ref. 2,** p. 1166)

698. (D) While the diagnosis of acute leukemias can be made on Wright-Giemsa stained preparation of bone marrow and peripheral blood smears, a more accurate classification can be achieved with the use of cytochemistry. For example, whereas ALL cells contain PAS-positive material, myeloblasts are usually positive for myeloperoxidase. Tdt, a DNA polymerase, is demonstrable in 95% of ALL and in less than 5% of AML. In all ALL cases, the enzyme is specifically present in the subtype L1 and L2 and is usually absent in the L3 subtype. (**Ref. 1,** p. 650; **Ref. 2,** p. 1072)

699. (E) In chronic constrictive pericarditis the heart is encased in a greatly thickened fibrotic or fibrocalcific pericardium and the pericardial cavity is obliterated. The disease most commonly follows pyogenic or tuberculous pericarditis. The fibrous pericardium restricts right atrial filling and constricts the cardiac chambers, which, in turn, leads to reduced minute volume output, reduced pulse pressure, and elevated jugular venous pressure. (**Ref. 1,** p. 568; **Ref. 3,** p. 372)

700. (D) The vegetations of acute rheumatic carditis are usually small (1 to 2 mm) and are found along the lines of closure of valve leaflets. They may extend into the chordae tendinae. The verrucae heal with minimal sequelae and do not cause destruction of valve leaflets as may be observed in infective endocarditis. Sometimes, however, the verrucae may cause fibrosis and in recurrent acute rheumatic infections, may contribute to the valvular deformity characteristic of chronic rheumatic heart disease. (**Ref. 1,** p. 547)

701. (B), 702. (D) Diabetes insipidus (DI), characterized by polyuria, polydypsia, and thirst, is due to inadequate antidiuretic hormone (ADH) secretion (central or neurogenic), or the inability of the renal tubules to respond to the hormone (nephrogenic). The former may be caused by trauma to the neurohypophysis, or primary or secondary intracranial tumor, less frequently by granulomatous lesions of the central nervous system, encephalomyelitis, or vascular lesions. Nephrogenic DI may result from renal parenchymal disease or may be associated with hypokalemia, hypercalcemia, or lithium therapy.

The laboratory findings in DI are distinctive: persistent hyposthenuria (specific gravity 1.005 or <) and urine osmolality of <200 mOsm/kg. The diagnosis of DI and the differentiation between neurogenic and nephrogenic types is achieved by water deprivation tests or less commonly measurement of antidiuretic response to infusion of hypertonic saline. The results of such tests for both conditions are seen in responses B and D. These two groups of patients must be distinguished from those suffering from primary polydypsia and psychogenic polydypsia. (**Ref. 7,** p. 314; **Ref. 6,** p. 312; **Ref. 4,** p. 1925)

703. (D) Mycotoxins from *Aspergillus flavus,* particularly aflatoxin B$_1$, have been shown to cause hepatocellular carcinoma (HCC) in experimental animals. HCC exists in high prevalence in areas of the world (mostly developing countries) where aflatoxin-contaminated food is consumed. Hepatitis B is also endemic in many of these countries and has been linked to the prevalence of HCC. The role of the aflatoxin in the pathogenesis of HCC under these circumstances remains intriguing but difficult to assess. (**Ref. 2,** p. 772; **Ref. 1,** p. 880)

704. (G) Hepatic angiosarcoma (hemangiosarcoma) is rare and has been associated with exposure to thorotrast (thorium dioxide), vinyl chloride, or inorganic arsenic. It is an extremely aggressive tumor with poor prognosis. The latent period between exposure and the development of tumor ranges up to several decades. (**Ref. 1,** p. 879; **Ref. 2,** p. 774)

705. (B) Medullary carcinoma originates from parafollicular (C) cells of the thyroid. About 80 to 90% of medullary carcinomas secrete calcitonin which may be measured in the serum by radioimmunoassay. Calcitonin may also be demonstrated in the tumor cells by immunoperoxidase. The tumor cells may also produce other secretions such as somatostatin, histaminase, prostaglandins, and vasoactive intestinal peptide. Patients may manifest diarrhea and less commonly hypocalcemia. (**Ref. 1**, p. 1140; **Ref. 3**, p. 854)

706. **(I)** Choriocarcinoma produces β-HCG and serum levels may be elevated; its measurement may be used to follow the effectiveness of therapy and the clinical course of the patient. Elevated HCG may also be found in other trophoblastic tumors such as hydatidiform mole and invasive mole and occasionally in non-trophoblastic tumors such as lung carcinoma. (**Ref. 1**, p. 1084)

707. **(A)** Serum alpha-fetoprotein (AFP) is elevated in about 80% of patients with hepatocellular carcinoma. Carcinoembryonic antigen (CEA) is also elevated but only in about 30% of patients. Serum AFP may be normal when the liver tumor is small. Elevated levels have also been found in chronic hepatitis, liver cirrhosis, germ cell tumors, normal pregnancy, and during fetal distress. (**Ref. 1**, p. 881; **Ref. 3**, p. 658)

708. **(D)** An autosomal recessive disease, Hurler syndrome, is one of seven recognized diseases characterized by deficiencies of specific lysosomal enzymes involved in the breakdown of mucopolysaccharides resulting in the accumulation of one or more of the following: dermatan sulfate, heparan sulfate, keratan sulfate, and chondroitin sulfate. In Hurler syndrome there is accumulation of heparan and dermatan sulfates. Patients manifest symptoms and signs in the second half of the first year of life—dwarfism, grotesque facies (gargoylism), hepatosplenomegaly, and progressive mental retardation. (**Ref. 1**, p. 140)

709. **(G)** Niemann Pick disease is characterized by a deficiency of sphingomyelinase, an enzyme involved in the cleavage of sphingomyelin resulting in the accumulation of sphingomyelin and cholesterol in the reticuloendothelial and parenchymal cells. Two variants are recognized, types A and B. Type B, comprising about 20% of all cases, shows normal levels of sphingomyelinase while in type A there is a deficiency of the enzyme. Clinically, there is severe neurologic disease, progressive wasting, and death in the

first three years of life. The cells of the brain, liver, spleen, lymph nodes, and bone marrow are engorged with lipid accumulation. (**Ref. 1,** p. 141)

710. **(I)**   Deficiency of enzymes in the glycogen metabolism produces a variety of glycogen storage diseases (glycogenosis). The organs involved and the severity of the corresponding clinical disease depends on the distribution of the enzyme in question. Thus, some of the disorders may be systemic while others are limited to specific organs. Three clinicopathologic categories are recognized: hepatic (von Gierke disease—type I), myopathic (McArdle syndrome—type V), and generalized (Pompe disease—type II). Although Pompe disease is systemic, involvement of the heart is the most prominent and most patients die from cardiac failure. (**Ref. 1,** p. 146)

711. **(B)**   One of the lysosomal storage diseases, Tay–Sachs, is an autosomal recessive disease, prevalent among Jews in which there is a deficiency of hexosaminidase A resulting in the accumulation of G_{M2}-ganglioside. At about the age of six months affected infants begin to manifest motor and mental symptoms which progressively deteriorate. Lipid deposition in the macula of the retina produces the characteristic "cherry red spot." Death usually ensues at two or three years of age. (**Ref. 1,** p. 140)

712. **(E)**   ITP may occur as either an acute or chronic disease. Acute ITP is a disease of children usually following viral infections such as measles, rubella, or viral hepatitis. It is self-limiting and is probably due to immune complexes (viral antigen–antiviral antibodies) bound to the surface of platelets making them vulnerable to phagocytosis by the reticuloendothelial system. In contrast, chronic ITP is a disease of adults and is generally believed to be mediated by immunologic mechanisms involving humoral antibodies or immune complexes. Females are affected more than males (3:1). The serum contains platelet-associated immunoglobulins (PAIgG), detectable in up to 90% of patients. The bone marrow shows megakaryocytic hyperplasia. The spleen is the major site of platelet destruction and production of autoantibodies, hence splenectomy leads to recovery in 75 to 80% of patients. (**Ref. 1,** p. 618; **Ref. 3,** p. 423)

713. **(C)** TTP is characterized by thrombocytopenia, microangiopathic hemolytic anemia, neurologic deficit, and renal failure. Capillaries and arterioles in multiple organs show platelet and fibrin thrombi. The pathogenesis of the disease is obscure but there are suggestions of immune origin-immunologic response against endothelial cells as a basis for the widespread microthrombi. Treatment includes administration of corticosteroids, platelet aggregation-inhibiting substances, and exchange transfusion. (**Ref. 1,** p. 619)

714. **(E)** Constituting about 10% of serum immunoglobulins, IgM is a 19S macromolecule with a molecular weight of 900,000. IgM, secreted into the blood in the early stages of primary antibody response, is particularly effective in combating bacterial infections. It is the first antibody to be produced by developing B cells. (**Ref. 8,** p. 118; **Ref. 6,** p. 822)

715. **(D)** IgE has the lowest serum concentration of the immunoglobulins. It binds with high affinity to target cells via a site in the Fc region and to antigens (allergens) through the Fab portion. It is produced mainly in the lining of the respiratory and intestinal tracts. IgE does not cross the placenta, neither do IgE-antigen complexes bind complement by the classical pathway. Antiallergen IgE can be detected by three different methods: skin tests, radioallergosorbent assay (RAST), and release of histamine from leukocytes. (**Ref. 8,** p. 118; **Ref. 6,** p. 822)

716. **(D)** Peutz-Jeghers syndrome (PJS) is characterized by gastrointestinal polyps associated with melanin pigmentation of the buccal mucosa, lips, and digits. Many of the polyps are located in the small intestines but may also be found in the stomach and colon. Despite the morphologic resemblance of the polyps to those seen in familial multiple polyposis, the polyps in PJS rarely give rise to cancer. The reason for this benign behavior is unclear; the polyps are believed to be hamartomatous growths rather than true neoplasms. (**Ref. 2,** p. 666; **Ref. 1,** p. 811)

717. **(C)** Familial adenomatous polyposis of the colon is characterized by the presence of innumerable neoplastic polyps that may cover virtually the entire colonic mucosa and may sometimes extend into the higher levels of the intestinal tract. Usually the polyps do not appear before the second or third decade of life. The polyps are usually small, pedunculated adenomas which when closely packed give a furry appearance to the mucosa. There is a high incidence of malignant transformation and several polyps may become malignant concurrently. The gene responsible for this disease has been located on the long arm of chromosome 5 (5q21). (**Ref. 2,** p. 688; **Ref. 1,** p. 813)

718. (C), 719. (B) This classification of diseases of immunological origin (hypersensitivity diseases) is based on the immunological mechanisms that mediate the disease. In type I, in which the reaction may be local or systemic, the immune reactions produce vasoactive substances from mast cells or basophils which act on blood vessels or smooth muscles. In humans, the reactions are mediated by IgE antibodies. In type II reactions, humoral antibodies, either IgG or IgM, bind to antigens on cell surfaces causing phagocytosis of lysis of the target cell. Two types of antibody-dependent mechanisms are involved in this type of reaction: complement-mediated cytotoxicity and antibody-dependent cell-mediated cytotoxicity. Type III reactions involve the formation of circulating or extravascular immune complexes and the activation of the complement cascade with the production of biologically active fragments. These reactions are induced only by complement-fixing antibodies—IgG and IgM. In type IV, immunological reactions are mediated by sensitized T lymphocytes. (**Ref. 1,** pp. 177–190)

720. (G) Found most commonly in Japan, the Caribbean basin, southwest United States, and West Africa, adult T cell lymphoma/leukemia is an uncommon aggressive disease which is thought to be caused by HTLV-1. Clinically, patients manifest skin lesions, generalized lymphadenopathy, hepatosplenomegaly, and hypercalcemia. The central nervous system, lungs, and pleura may also be involved. The tumor cells are CD4+ and may express IL-2 receptors. The prognosis is very poor, less than 50% surviving after six months in spite of chemotherapy. (**Ref. 2,** p. 1084; **Ref. 1,** p. 642)

721. (D) Burkitt lymphoma occurs as an endemic disease in certain parts of Africa and sporadically in other parts of the world including the United States. Both types are similar histologically. They show certain differences, however, in clinical and virologic findings. Both forms occur in children and young adults. Whereas the African tumors arise most commonly in the mandible or maxilla, patients with the sporadic form present with abdominal masses. The EBV genome is found in the tumors in 95% of African cases in contrast to 15% in non-African cases. Histologically the tumor is composed of sheets of monotonous small non-cleaved cells with conspicuous nuclei, high mitotic rate and amphophilic, and intensely pyroninophilic cytoplasm; the latter also shows lipid globules. Interspersed among the tumor cells are benign histiocytes creating the typical but not pathognomonic "starry sky" pattern. (**Ref. 2,** p. 1083; **Ref. 1,** p. 641)

722. (A), 723. (G) The different morphology of necrosis occurring in tissue probably reflects variation in cell composition, speed of necrosis, and type of injury. The four distinctive types of necrosis are coagulative necrosis, most commonly due to sudden, severe ischemia of the kidneys (acute tubular necrosis), heart, and adrenals, but also may occur after chemical injury eg, the ingestion of mercuric chloride (proximal renal tubular necrosis). Liquefactive necrosis results from the action of powerful hydrolytic enzymes and is characteristic of ischemic destruction of brain tissue and is also commonly encountered in all focal bacterial lesions, particularly those due to pyogenic microorganisms. Enzymatic fat necrosis is a highly specific morphologic pattern of fat cell death resulting from the action of lipase of fat deposits as is observed in acute pancreatic necrosis. Caseous necrosis, so called because of its characteristic gross appearance that resembles clumped, cheesy material, has been attributed to the capsule of the tubercle. (**Ref. 1,** p. 17; **Ref. 3,** pp. 15–19)

724. (C) Historically, lobar pneumonia differs from bronchopneumonia in that the former involves an entire lobe while in the latter, patchy involvement of the lung is the rule. The common use of antibiotics has blurred this distinction. In spite of this, 95% of lobar pneumonias are caused by *Streptococcus pneumoniae* (pneumococcus). Clinically the onset of the disease is sudden and acute with fever, chills, and cough productive of rusty sputum. The four stages of the disease—congestion, red hepatization, gray hepatization, and resolution, are usually short and no more well defined than in the preantibiotic era. The infection may be complicated by pleuritis, pleural effusion, pyothorax, empyema, and very rarely, fibrosis. (**Ref. 2,** pp. 566–569)

725. (**B**)   About 1% of lobar pneumonias may be caused by *Klebsiella pneumoniae*. Typically, however, the bacterium causes bronchopneumonia. In addition to alcoholics, patients with diabetes mellitus, chronic pulmonary disorders, and other debilitating illnesses are at risk for this infection. The thick gelatinous capsule of the bacteria explains the mucoid appearance and feel of the cut surface of the involved lung. The infection is often complicated by abscesses and bronchopleural fistula. (**Ref. 2,** p. 568)

References

1. Cotran RS, Kumar V, Robbins SL: *Robbins Pathologic Basis of Disease.* 5th ed, Philadelphia, WB Saunders Co, 1994.
2. Rubin E, Farber JL: *Pathology.* 2nd ed, Philadelphia, JB Lippincott Co, 1994.
3. Chandrasoma P, Taylor CR: *Concise Pathology.* 1st ed. Norwalk, Appleton & Lange, 1991.
4. Isselbacher KJ, Braunwald E, Wilson JD, Martin JB, Fauci AS, Kasper DL (eds): *Harrison's Principles of Internal Medicine.* 13th ed. New York, McGraw-Hill, 1994.
5. Lily LD (ed): *Pathophysiology of Heart Disease.* Philadelphia, Lea & Febiger, 1993.
6. Henry JV (ed): *Clinical Diagnosis and Management by Laboratory Methods.* 18th ed. Philadelphia, WB Saunders Co, 1991.
7. McClatchey KD (ed): *Clinical Laboratory Medicine.* 1st. ed. Baltimore, Williams & Wilkins, 1994.
8. Stites DP, Terr AI (eds): *Basic and Clinical Immunology.* 7th ed. Norwalk, Appleton & Lange, 1991.
9. Ganong WF: *Review of Medical Physiology.* 16th ed. Norwalk, Appleton & Lange, 1991.

5

Pharmacology

Joseph J. Krzanowski, Jr.

DIRECTIONS (Questions 726 through 731): Each of the questions or incomplete statements below is followed by five suggested answers or completions. Select the ONE that is best in each case.

---

726. All of the following are true statements about morphine EXCEPT
   A. morphine-induced analgesia occurs as a consequence of binding to mu receptors
   B. repeated administration of morphine results in the development of tolerance
   C. administration of morphine to a pain-free person may be perceived as unpleasant
   D. both the perception of pain and the reaction to pain are eliminated by morphine
   E. the effects of morphine are reversed by naloxone

727. Decreased blood pressure following the inhalation of halothane is most likely due to
   A. arterial smooth muscle relaxation
   B. venodilation
   C. depression of the heart
   D. vasomotor center suppression
   E. histamine release

728. Digoxin
  A. inhibits A-V nodal conduction
  B. is metabolized in the liver
  C. antagonizes epinephrine-induced arrhythmias
  D. stimulates beta adrenergic receptors
  E. has a half-life of approximately 6 hours

729. It may be desirable to produce acute bronchodilation for the management of bronchial asthma in a patient who has altered cardiac rhythm. Which of the following agents would be the most effective agent?
  A. phentolamine
  B. albuterol
  C. methoxamine
  D. metoprolol
  E. phenylephrine

730. Thiopental
  A. may cause laryngospasm
  B. produces acceptable levels of analgesia
  C. has a short duration of action due to rapid metabolism
  D. causes acceptable levels of skeletal muscle relaxation
  E. is considered a CNS stimulant

731. Select the compound acting on the loop of Henle to inhibit NaCl reabsorption.
  A. acetazolamide
  B. ethacrynic acid
  C. hydrochlorothiazide
  D. spironolactone
  E. mannitol

DIRECTIONS (Questions 732 through 736): Each group of questions below consists of lettered headings followed by a list of numbered words, phrases, or statements. For each numbered word, phrase, or statement, select the ONE lettered heading that is most closely associated with it. Each lettered heading may be selected once, more than once, or not at all.

    A. estrogen
    B. progesterone
    C. thyroxin
    D. insulin
    E. cortisone

732. Administration of this compound is likely to increase susceptibility to infection

733. Osteoporosis will be prevented or arrested by the administration of this agent

734. Orally administered sulfonylureas cause this compound to be released into the circulation

735. Propylthiouracil will inhibit the synthesis of this compound

736. The use of this agent for prolonged periods may lead to acute adrenal insufficiency

---

DIRECTIONS (Questions 737 through 745): This section consists of situations, each followed by a series of questions. Study each situation, and select the ONE best answer to each question following it.

CASE HISTORY (Questions 737 and 738): A 16-year-old female presents with undiagnosed abdominal pain. She is not pregnant, denies any drug use, but has continuous nausea and episodic vomiting. Her history does not indicate any specific cause for the nausea and vomiting. Diagnostic procedures are instituted and she is sent home with a prescription for prochlorperazine. Twenty-four hours later she appears in the emergency room with severe spasms of the neck and facial muscles.

737. The above case is an example of
  A. phenothiazine-induced tardive dyskinesia
  B. a pseudo-Parkinsonian reaction
  C. a drug-induced dystonic reaction
  D. inappropriate use of phenothiazines
  E. an hysterical reaction

738. The appropriate management of this adverse reaction is
  A. administration of an anticholinergic agent
  B. to let the drug effect wear off
  C. to administer a skeletal muscle blocking agent intravenously
  D. to give an intravenous injection of dantrolene
  E. to treat the patient with a cholinergic agonist

CASE HISTORY (Questions 739 through 741): In discussing medication with a friend you learn that he is taking a variety of pain medications for a sports injury. He informs you that he takes acetaminophen, aspirin, and ibuprofen for a knee he twisted while water skiing. The pain relief is not adequate and he is now considering the latest over-the-counter medication, naproxen. He has a prescription for a combination product (Percocet) but does not take it because of its side effects.

739. Side effects of Percocet may include all of the following EXCEPT
   A. constipation
   B. nausea and vomiting
   C. respiratory depression
   D. urinary urgency
   E. restlessness

740. The use of which of the following agents would NOT be beneficial in injury where inflammation is present?
   A. ibuprofen
   B. aspirin
   C. naproxen
   D. piroxicam
   E. acetaminophen

741. The use of which two agents in combination is an appropriate therapeutic approach to pain management?
   A. ibuprofen/aspirin
   B. acetaminophen/aspirin
   C. acetaminophen/naproxen
   D. ibuprofen/naproxen
   E. aspirin/oxycodone

CASE HISTORY (Questions 742 through 745):   Your grandmother heard ads on television and read ads in the newspaper about the new histamine blocking agents and is confused. She looked up these compounds and found a wide range of agents listed as histamine blockers, things like cimetidine, astemizole, ranitidine, diphenhydramine, and meclizine. Since you are a medical student (and a grandson), she decides to ask you some questions about these agents.

742. Which of these agents would you recommend for her if she wanted a medication for her seasonal allergy but needed to be sure she was alert and able to drive during the day?
   A. chlorpheniramine
   B. astemizole
   C. ranitidine
   D. diphenhydramine
   E. meclizine

743. Your parents are going on a cruise and they heard that histamine blockers are helpful in preventing "sea sickness." What compound should be taken?
   A. chlorpheniramine
   B. astemizole
   C. ranitidine
   D. diphenhydramine
   E. meclizine

744. One of the references referred to an H_2 blocker. Which compound is that?
   A. chlorpheniramine
   B. astemizole
   C. ranitidine
   D. diphenhydramine
   E. meclizine

745. If these can be used as sleep aids, which one would be preferred?
   A. chlorpheniramine
   B. astemizole
   C. ranitidine
   D. diphenhydramine
   E. meclizine

DIRECTIONS (Questions 746 through 750): Each group of questions below consists of lettered headings followed by a list of numbered words, phrases, or statements. For each numbered word, phrase, or statement, select the ONE lettered heading that is most closely associated with it. Each lettered heading may be selected once, more than once, or not at all.

    A. redistribution
    B. phase I reaction
    C. idiosyncratic reaction
    D. first-pass effect
    E. phase II reaction

746. Conjugation

747. Metabolism of a drug by oxidation, reduction, or hydrolysis

748. A phenomenon which explains the short duration of action of thiopental

749. Nitroglycerin is administered sublingually to avoid this

750. A genetically determined abnormal response

DIRECTIONS (Questions 751 through 805): Each of the questions or incomplete statements below is followed by five suggested answers or completions. Select the ONE that is best in each case.

751. Which of the following statements is true of heparin?
    A. it inhibits several steps in the intrinsic pathway of blood clotting
    B. its dosage may be adjusted by estimating the patient's clotting ability via the bleeding time
    C. it should not be administered intravenously because of the instant impairment of blood clotting
    D. it interacts with drugs which inhibit the liver microsomal enzyme system
    E. it should never be combined in therapy with an oral anticoagulant

752. In the following examples of drug interactions, in which case is the effect of A to increase the pharmacological effect of B?
   A. A induces the metabolism of B
   B. A displaces B from plasma protein binding sites
   C. A inhibits the tubular reabsorption of B
   D. A increases the tubular secretion of B
   E. A inhibits the absorption of B

753. Theophylline may cause all of the following effects EXCEPT
   A. tachycardia
   B. competitive antagonism of adenosine receptors
   C. smooth muscle relaxation
   D. CNS depression
   E. increased gastric acid secretion

754. Which of the following classes of drugs may induce sleep with the fewest deviations from a physiologic sleep pattern?
   A. phenothiazines
   B. barbiturates
   C. butyrophenones
   D. benzodiazepines
   E. volatile anesthetics

755. Figure 5.1 represents the concentration of a drug in serum samples obtained at various times after the intravenous injection of the drug. The serum half-life of the drug is
   A. 1 hour
   B. 2 hours
   C. 4 hours
   D. 8 hours
   E. 16 hours

756. Which of the following is the drug of choice for the reversal of pancuronium-induced neuromuscular blockade?
   A. neostigmine
   B. physostigmine
   C. diisopropylfluorophosphate
   D. atropine
   E. gallamine

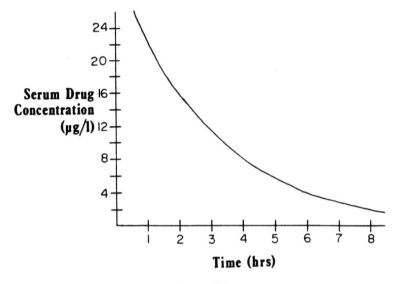

Figure 5.1

757. Drug metabolism usually results in all of the following EXCEPT
   A. rendering the drug more polar
   B. increasing the water solubility of the drug
   C. increasing the duration of action of the drug
   D. increasing the rate of renal excretion of the drug
   E. altering the drug to yield an inactive metabolite

758. Advantages of isoflurane over halothane as a general anesthetic include all of the following EXCEPT
   A. lesser degree of biotransformation
   B. decreased incidence of postoperative chemical hepatitis
   C. fewer catecholamine-induced arrhythmias
   D. more pleasant odor permitting inhalation induction
   E. less depression of cardiac output

759. All the following are effects of the combination oral contraceptive preparations EXCEPT
   A. creating an environment in the vagina inhospitable to sperm
   B. prevention of ovulation

    C. facilitation of regular endometrial sloughing
    D. an increased likelihood of developing ovarian carcinoma
    E. adverse effects similar to those experienced during pregnancy

760. Succinylcholine
    A. causes depolarizing neuromuscular blockade
    B. is dependent upon liver cholinesterase enzymes for its metabolism
    C. action may be reversed by the administration of neostigmine
    D. causes spastic muscle paralysis
    E. has an additive effect with previously administered *d*-tubocurarine

761. A medical student finds himself afflicted with venereal disease caused by *Treponema* (syphilis), *Neisseria* (gonorrhea), and *Chlamydia* (nongonococcal urethritis). Which of the following agents used singularly is likely to cure his three afflictions?
    A. procaine penicillin G
    B. ampicillin
    C. cephalothin
    D. streptomycin
    E. tetracycline

762. Which of the following effects would NOT be seen in a patient who has ingested a toxic dose of aspirin?
    A. respiratory alkalosis
    B. increased carbon dioxide production
    C. hyperventilation
    D. miosis
    E. uncoupling of oxidative phosphorylation

763. Premature labor may be slowed or arrested via the administration of
    A. a β_2-adrenergic agonist
    B. an ergot derivative
    C. an α-adrenergic agonist
    D. a muscarinic agonist
    E. a ganglionic antagonist

764. Induction of general anesthesia is determined by all of the following EXCEPT
   A. affinity of anesthetic molecules for specific CNS receptors
   B. rate of pulmonary ventilation
   C. solubility of the anesthetic agent in blood
   D. solubility of the anesthetic agent in fatty tissues
   E. rate of blood flow in the brain

765. Which of the following is NOT a property of barbiturate hypnotic agents?
   A. development of tolerance
   B. induction of liver microsomal enzymes
   C. respiratory depression
   D. analgesia
   E. suppression of REM sleep

766. The major drawback to antianginal use of propranolol is
   A. exacerbation of congestive heart failure
   B. increased blood pressure
   C. urine retention
   D. blurred vision
   E. diabetes-like hyperglycemia

767. During the generation of arrhythmias, an important determination of conduction velocity in the heart is
   A. action potential duration (APD)
   B. effective refractory period (ERP)
   C. ERP/APD ratio
   D. maximum rate of repolarization
   E. maximum rate of rise of action potential upstroke

768. A patient is being treated with warfarin subsequent to suffering a pulmonary embolus. Phenobarbital is later prescribed for night-time sedation. Which alteration in warfarin dosage is indicated?
   A. a decrease because its metabolism has been inhibited
   B. a decrease because its excretion has been reduced
   C. an increase because its gastrointestinal absorption has been impaired
   D. an increase because its metabolism has been stimulated
   E. an increase because its binding to plasma proteins has been blocked

769. The local anesthetic lidocaine
   A. is metabolized primarily by circulating butyrylcholinesterase
   B. may also be used as an anticonvulsant
   C. blocks nerve conduction by interfering with sodium conductance
   D. greatly decreases the resting potential of peripheral nerves
   E. acts on the extracellular surface of the nerve membrane

770. Clear evidence of physical dependence characterized by a withdrawal phenomenon is most difficult to demonstrate with
   A. phenobarbital
   B. morphine
   C. marijuana
   D. ethyl alcohol
   E. meprobamate

771. Which of the following agents is contraindicated in a person with a history of narrow-angle glaucoma?
   A. pilocarpine
   B. atropine
   C. acetazolamide
   D. neostigmine
   E. succinylcholine

772. Which of the following synthetic corticosteroids has mineralocorticoid (sodium-retaining) activity?
   A. prednisone
   B. triamcinolone
   C. dexamethasone
   D. paramethasone
   E. betamethasone

773. An agent NOT indicated for the treatment of tuberculosis is
   A. isoniazid
   B. dapsone
   C. streptomycin
   D. rifampin
   E. ethambutol

774. Which of the following drugs is NOT usually considered to be ototoxic?
    A. vancomycin
    B. streptomycin
    C. ethacrynic acid
    D. aspirin
    E. chloramphenicol

775. Amyl nitrite is used in the emergency treatment of cyanide poisoning because it
    A. oxidizes hemoglobin
    B. irreversibly binds cyanide
    C. competes with cyanide for binding to cytochromes
    D. prevents shock
    E. inhibits tubular reabsorption of cyanide

776. Poisoning with an organophosphate cholinesterase inhibitor can be treated with
    A. edrophonium
    B. carbachol
    C. pralidoxime
    D. nicotine
    E. ephedrine

777. The positive inotropic effect of digoxin
    A. is associated with an increase in the rate of force development
    B. is dependent upon a normal cardiac rhythm
    C. is antagonized by β-adrenergic blockers
    D. is due to a prolongation of the contractile process
    E. results because all phases of systole are prolonged

778. Which of the following diuretic combinations will produce the most effective diuresis with minimum potassium depletion?
    A. acetazolamide plus furosemide
    B. ethacrynic acid plus furosemide
    C. spironolactone plus potassium chloride
    D. spironolactone plus furosemide
    E. hydrochlorothiazide plus bumetanide

779. In the presence of a noncompetitive antagonist, the agonist's
  A. apparent potency is decreased
  B. maximum efficacy is decreased
  C. ED_{50} is increased
  D. ED_{50} is decreased
  E. log dose-response curve is shifted to the right

780. Which of the following agents is most useful in the treatment of absence seizures (petit mal epilepsy)?
  A. phenobarbital
  B. diazepam
  C. ethosuximide
  D. phenytoin
  E. primidone

781. Which of the following methods of drug administration results in the most rapid distribution of the drug in peripheral tissues?
  A. intramuscular injection
  B. subcutaneous injection
  C. intrathecal injection
  D. transdermal administration
  E. oral ingestion

782. A drug is administered repeatedly at an interval of every two half-lives of the drug. Plateau concentrations in the circulation will be attained essentially after the
  A. first dose
  B. second dose
  C. fourth dose
  D. sixth dose
  E. eighth dose

783. Which of the following constituents of plasma is likely to be increased instead of decreased by thiazide diuretics?
  A. sodium
  B. potassium
  C. chloride
  D. magnesium
  E. uric acid

784. A sympathetically innervated tissue or organ most likely to be stimulated upon the administration of methacholine is the
    A. heart
    B. urinary bladder
    C. sweat gland
    D. radial muscle of the iris
    E. pilomotor muscle

785. Megaloblastic anemia during pregnancy is treated with
    A. ferrous sulfate
    B. pyridoxine (vitamin B_6)
    C. folic acid
    D. riboflavin
    E. cyanocobalamin (vitamin B_{12})

786. Lithium carbonate is considered to be specific therapy for
    A. prevention of delirium tremens (DTs)
    B. schizophrenia
    C. reactive depression
    D. manic-depressive psychosis
    E. hallucinogen overdosage

787. In humans an intravenous injection of histamine results in all of the following EXCEPT
    A. a fall in systemic blood pressure
    B. an increase in gastric acid secretion
    C. constriction of CNS blood vessels
    D. bronchoconstriction
    E. dilation of terminal arterioles

788. The combination-type oral contraceptive pill contains
    A. an androgen and a progestin
    B. an androgen and an estrogen
    C. an estrogen and a progestin
    D. estrogen from pregnant mares' urine
    E. FSH and LH

789. Tinea (ringworm) infections may be treated with topical application of

A. griseofulvin

B. tolnaftate

C. bacitracin

D. neomycin

E. nitrofurazone

790. The liver microsomal drug metabolizing system carries out all of the following reactions EXCEPT

A. acetylation

B. aromatic hydroxylation

C. glucuronide conjugation

D. N-demethylation

E. sulfoxidation

791. Aspirin and acetaminophen both

A. inhibit prostaglandin biosynthesis equieffectively

B. are effective antipyretic agents

C. have a high incidence of causing epigastric distress

D. have uricosuric effects

E. have equal anti-inflammatory action

792. Dimercaprol is indicated in poisoning from which of the following heavy metals?

A. iron

B. cadmium

C. mercury

D. zinc

E. lead

793. Which of the following effects of chlorpromazine CANNOT be explained on the basis of its blockade of dopamine receptors?

A. antiemesis (decrease in vomiting)

B. orthostatic hypotension

C. tardive dyskinesia

D. galactorrhea

E. Parkinsonian syndrome

794. Regarding triiodothyronine (T_3)
   A. it is less potent than thyroxine (T_4)
   B. it is converted to thyroxine in peripheral tissues
   C. it is effective orally
   D. release from the thyroid gland is inhibited by propylthiouracil
   E. it is bound more tightly to thyroid-binding globulin than thyroxine

795. Carbidopa is used in conjunction with levodopa in Parkinson disease
   A. to decrease peripheral metabolism of levodopa
   B. because it facilitates levodopa transport across the blood–brain barrier
   C. because of its central anticholinergic effects
   D. to block dopamine receptors in the basal ganglia
   E. because it inhibits the involuntary movements that frequently accompany levodopa therapy

796. Of the following antineoplastic agents, the one with the highest specificity for malignant tissue is
   A. cyclophosphamide
   B. *l*-asparaginase
   C. vincristine
   D. methotrexate
   E. busulfan

797. Humans are insensitive to the metabolic effects of the sulfonamides because
   A. the sulfonamides cannot gain access to eukaryotic cells
   B. they require preformed folic acid
   C. sulfonamides have no effect on mammalian dihydrofolate reductase
   D. human cells cannot bioactivate sulfonamides to the active compound
   E. they synthesize large quantities of p-aminobenzoic acid

798. An agent that is effective orally against dermatomycoses is
   A. griseofulvin
   B. amphotericin B
   C. nystatin

D. flucytosine
E. tetracycline

799. Aspirin is a weak acid with a pK of 3.5. At physiologic pH (7.4), approximately what percent of aspirin molecules are in the associated (protonated) form?
   A. 0.001%
   B. 0.01%
   C. 0.1%
   D. 1%
   E. 10%

800. Of the following penicillin congeners, the one with the broadest spectrum of action is
   A. penicillin V
   B. methicillin
   C. nafcillin
   D. carbenicillin
   E. oxacillin

801. Assuming a single compartment of digoxin distribution with an apparent volume of distribution of 8 L/kg, intravenous injection of 0.5 mg digoxin in a 62-kg patient would be expected to give an initial plasma digoxin level of
   A. 1.0 ng/mL
   B. 1.0 mcg/mL
   C. 100 ng/mL
   D. 100 mcg/L
   E. 100 mg/L

802. If the dose in Question 801 were insufficient, how much more digoxin could be administered 15 min later without experiencing likely toxicity? (Assume that during the 15 min no digoxin has been metabolized or excreted.)
   A. 0.25 mg
   B. 1.0 mg
   C. 1.5 mg
   D. 2.5 mg
   E. no more can be administered because the plasma levels are already borderline toxic

803. Since a 62-kg person cannot have 496 L of body water, what is the explanation for the apparent volume of distribution for digoxin in Question 801?

    A. digoxin is fat soluble and much is distributed to muscle, adipose tissue, and brain

    B. digoxin is bound extensively to plasma and tissue proteins

    C. digoxin is metabolized extensively by the liver

    D. digoxin is freely filtered by the renal glomerulus and achieves high concentrations in the urine

    E. digoxin does not distribute efficiently to peripheral tissues

804. An injection of which of the following agents is used to help make the diagnosis of myasthenia gravis?

    A. hemicholinium

    B. atropine

    C. nicotine

    D. decamethonium

    E. edrophonium

805. Nitrofurantoin is used only in the treatment of urinary tract infections because

    A. it is only active against urinary tract pathogens

    B. it is too toxic to be administered systemically

    C. it is highly effective in the presence of renal failure

    D. therapy cannot be continued for more than a few days at a time

    E. its half-life is so short that it only achieves bacteriostatic concentrations in urine

DIRECTIONS (Questions 806 through 867): Each group of questions below consists of lettered headings followed by a list of numbered words, phrases, or statements. For each numbered word, phrase, or statement, select the ONE lettered heading that is most closely associated with it. Each lettered heading may be selected once, more than once, or not at all.

Questions 806 through 809

    A. diethylcarbamazine
    B. thiabendazole
    C. praziquantel
    D. pyrantel pamoate
    E. niclosamide

806. The drug of choice in all types of tapeworm infections

807. Drug with a bitter taste which is effective in all types of schistomiasis

808. A depolarizing neuromuscular junction blocker in the hookworm, pinworm, and roundworm

809. Has both amebicidal and schistosomicidal activities

Questions 810 through 813

    A. methotrexate
    B. cyclophosphamide
    C. doxorubicin
    D. fluorouracil
    E. azathioprine

810. May cause congestive heart failure in patients receiving large cumulative doses

811. Must be activated by liver cytochrome P450 for cytotoxic activity

812. A purine analogue used primarily as an immunosuppressive

813. Its cytotoxic activity is potentiated by concurrent administration of allopurinol

Questions 814 through 816

    A. amphotericin B
    B. vidarabine
    C. amantadine
    D. flucytosine
    E. griseofulvin

814. Herpes simplex encephalitis

815. Influenza A_2 prophylaxis

816. Ringworm

Questions 817 through 820

    A. antiarrhythmic action is via α-adrenergic blockade
    B. ventricular premature depolarizations
    C. angina pectoris prophylaxis
    D. conversion of atrial fibrillation to sinus rhythm
    E. treatment of ventricular fibrillation

817. Isosorbide dinitrate

818. Disopyramide

819. Propranolol

820. Nifedipine

Questions 821 through 824

    A. anaphylaxis
    B. tachyphylaxis
    C. induction
    D. supersensitivity
    E. teratogenesis

821. Acute or rapidly developing tolerance to a drug

822. Drug-induced alteration in fetal development

823. Life-threatening acute hypersensitivity reaction

824. Drug-induced increase in enzyme activity

Questions 825 through 830

    A. cyanocobalamin (vitamin B_{12})
    B. thiamine (vitamin B_1)
    C. ascorbic acid (vitamin C)
    D. cholecalciferol (vitamin D)
    E. nicotinic acid (niacin)

825. Beriberi

826. Pellagra

827. Scurvy

828. Wernicke syndrome

829. Rickets

830. Pernicious anemia

Questions 831 through 835

    A. β-lactamase
    B. xanthine oxidase
    C. monoamine oxidase
    D. carbonic anhydrase
    E. aldehyde dehydrogenase

831. Allopurinol

832. Disulfuram

833. Clavulanic acid

834. Tranylcypromine

835. Acetazolamide

Questions 836 through 838

    A. triazolam
    B. tranylcypromine
    C. methylphenidate
    D. lithium carbonate
    E. carbamazepine

836. Manic-depressive illness

837. Insomnia

838. Attention deficit hyperkinetic syndrome

Questions 839 through 843

    A. phenylephrine
    B. epinephrine
    C. physostigmine
    D. isoproterenol
    E. atropine

839. A relatively selective α_1-adrenergic agonist which produces mydriasis

840. Produces both mydriasis and cycloplegia

841. Relatively selective α_1-adrenergic agonist

842. Nonselective β-adrenergic agonist

843. Miosis

Questions 844 through 848

    A. a Class I_B agent that decreases automaticity of ectopic pacemakers
    B. thrombocytopenia is an extra cardiac toxicity
    C. inhibits norepinephrine release from adrenergic nerve endings
    D. potent sodium channel blocker
    E. both activated and inactivated calcium ion channels are blocked

844. Bretylium

845. Quinidine

846. Flecainide

847. Verapamil

848. Lidocaine

Questions 849 through 852

    A. penicillin G
    B. amphotericin B
    C. tetracycline
    D. gentamicin
    E. polymyxin B

849. Antifungal agent

850. Aminoglycoside

851. Used in the treatment of *chlamydiae* and *rickettsiae*

852. Restricted to topical use

Questions 853 through 856

    A. acetazolamide
    B. chlorothiazide
    C. mannitol
    D. spironolactone
    E. ethacrynic acid

853. Osmotic diuretic

854. Inhibits the NaCl transport system

855. Loop diuretic

856. Potassium sparring diuretic

Questions 857 through 859

    A. decreases lipolysis
    B. decreases glycogenolysis
    C. inhibition of insulin secretion
    D. stimulation of insulin secretion
    E. increased serum potassium levels

857. α_2-adrenergic receptor stimulation

858. β_2-adrenergic receptor stimulation

859. Elevated plasma glucose levels

Questions 860 through 864

    A. treatment of infertility
    B. amenorrheic therapy caused by excess prolactin
    C. palliation of prostate cancer
    D. palliation of breast cancer
    E. used in benign prostatic hypertrophy

860. Tamoxifen

861. Clomiphene

862. Flutamide

863. Bromocriptine

864. Finasteride

Questions 865 through 867

    A. labetalol
    B. prazosin
    C. timolol
    D. atenolol
    E. pindolol

865. Selective α_1-adrenergic blocking agent

866. Nonselective β-adrenergic antagonist with no agonist activity

867. Blocks α- and β-adrenergic receptors

DIRECTIONS (Questions 868 through 915): Each of the questions or incomplete statements below is followed by five suggested answers or completions. Select the ONE that is best in each case.

---

868. All of the following agents act via classical drug-receptor interactions EXCEPT
    A. atropine
    B. cimetidine
    C. prazosin
    D. halothane
    E. norepinephrine

869. Characteristics of nondepolarizing neuromuscular blockade include
    A. an initial excitatory effect on striated muscle manifested as fasciculations
    B. inability of the muscle fibers to respond to direct electrical stimuli
    C. well-sustained contraction in response to tetanic stimulation
    D. ability to reverse blockade via administration of an anticholinesterase
    E. potentiation of the blockade after administration of edrophonium

870. Which of the following agents usually is implicated in the induction of hemolytic anemia in persons genetically deficient in glucose-6-phosphate dehydrogenase?
  A. acetaminophen
  B. prednisone
  C. α-methyldopa
  D. lithium
  E. sulfonamides

871. A withdrawal syndrome consisting of rebound hypertension can occur after abrupt cessation of therapy with
  A. hydrochlorothiazide
  B. clonidine
  C. hydralazine
  D. nitroprusside
  E. nifedipine

872. Which of the compounds below do NOT have significant competitive antagonistic activity at the muscarinic receptor?
  A. imipramine
  B. chlorpromazine
  C. digoxin
  D. scopolamine
  E. quinidine

873. Which of the following agents is NOT selective for one type of β-adrenergic receptor?
  A. metaproterenol
  B. nadolol
  C. metoprolol
  D. terbutaline
  E. dobutamine

874. All of the following patients are likely to require supplemental iron therapy EXCEPT
  A. pregnant women
  B. menstruating women
  C. women who are breast feeding infants
  D. children during rapid growth periods
  E. premature infants

875. An intravenous injection of acetylcholine causes a transient decrease in both systolic and diastolic blood pressures and an increase in heart rate. The effects of acetylcholine on heart rate, but not on blood pressure, may be antagonized by
  A. atropine
  B. physostigmine
  C. phentolamine
  D. propranolol
  E. carbachol

876. Parkinsonian-like symptoms induced by antipsychotic agents may be treated with
  A. benztropine
  B. tetracycline
  C. levodopa plus carbidopa
  D. carbachol
  E. levodopa

877. Vomiting may be induced by administration of
  A. apomorphine
  B. chlorpromazine
  C. metoclopramide
  D. dimenhydrinate
  E. canabinoids

878. All of the agents below may lower circulating plasma lipids EXCEPT
  A. nicotinic acid
  B. clofibrate
  C. chlorothiazide
  D. cholestyramine
  E. lovastatin

879. An antihistamine effective in the therapy of peptic ulcer disease is
  A. hydroxyzine
  B. ranitidine
  C. chlorpheniramine
  D. diphenhydramine
  E. promethazine

880. When quinidine is administered to a patient with atrial fibrillation
  A. the ventricular rate may increase dangerously
  B. arterial hypertension usually results if the drug is administered intravenously
  C. thrombi attached to fibrillating atria resolve
  D. sinus rhythm is rarely restored
  E. contractile force development is increased

881. Nifedipine and verapamil both
  A. cause vasodilation
  B. depress atrioventricular nodal conduction
  C. inhibit calcium entry into cells
  D. cause reflex tachycardia
  E. are used to treat digitalis toxicity

882. Advantages of cefoxitin over cefazolin include
  A. longer duration of action
  B. lesser incidence of renal toxicity
  C. greater activity against *Staph. aureus*
  D. greater activity against anaerobic bacteria
  E. it crosses the blood–brain barrier

883. Tolbutamide
  A. inhibits the release of insulin from the pancreas
  B. is metabolized to compounds having long half-lives
  C. may cause alcohol intolerance
  D. is an effective hypoglycemic agent in juvenile-onset diabetes mellitus
  E. increases potassium conductance and decreases calcium ion influx

884. All of the following agents are useful in causing immunosuppression and in decreasing the rejection of transplanted organs EXCEPT
  A. cisplatin
  B. prednisone
  C. azathioprine
  D. cyclosporin
  E. methotrexate

885. Characteristics of anesthesia produced by ketamine include all of the following EXCEPT
  A. profound analgesia
  B. decreased heart rate and blood pressure
  C. little effect on respiration
  D. negligible muscle relaxation
  E. increased cerebrospinal fluid pressure

886. Vitamin D
  A. requires metabolic activation by both the liver and kidney for activity
  B. is a precursor to parathyroid hormone
  C. inhibits calcium absorption in the intestine
  D. decreases bone resorption and promotes bone deposition
  E. is required in the diet

887. All of the agents whose structures are shown in Figure 5.2 are natural products EXCEPT
  A. 1
  B. 2
  C. 3
  D. 4
  E. 5

888. Active metabolites of morphine include
  A. morphine-6-glucuronide
  B. apomorphine
  C. acetylmorphine
  D. codeine
  E. normeperidine

889. Which of the following statements is true of nitroglycerin?
  A. the drug causes smooth muscle contraction
  B. the active form of the drug is the nitrite ion which is liberated via plasma nitroreductases
  C. the drug is usually administered sublingually to avoid liver biotransformation
  D. patients must keep their nitroglycerin tablets dry as they become dangerously explosive when wet
  E. nitroglycerin is effective when administered orally

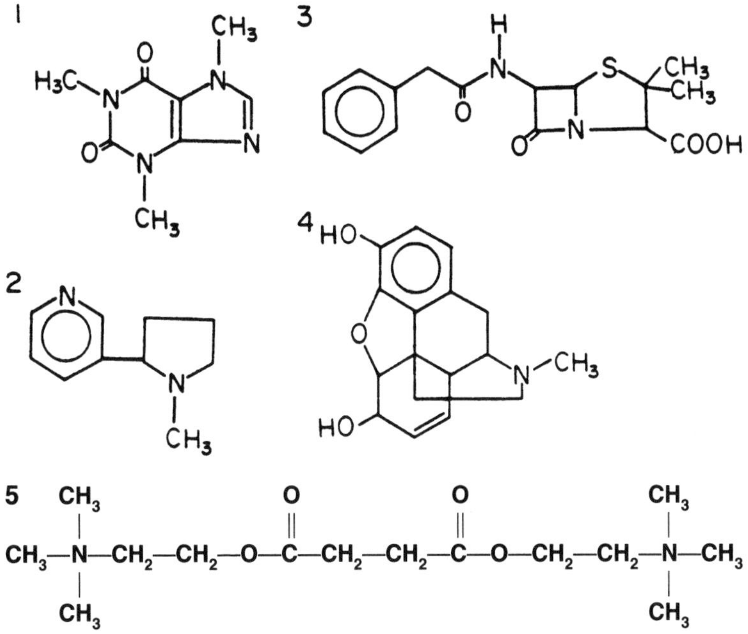

Figure 5.2

890. Which of the following is NOT a long-acting (e.g., 30 min) neuromuscular junction blocking agent?
    A. *d*-tubocurarine
    B. metocurine
    C. pancuronium
    D. succinylcholine
    E. vecuronium

891. Reversal of the neuromuscular blockade caused by the long-acting agents of Question 890 can be achieved by the administration of
    A. neostigmine
    B. isoflurophate
    C. tubocurarine
    D. scopolamine
    E. ipratropium

892. During the reversal of neuromuscular blockade by the agents of Question 891, atropine is administered to counteract which of the following effects?
    A. vomiting
    B. tachycardia
    C. hypertension
    D. increased respiratory secretions
    E. bronchial smooth muscle relaxation

893. Agents which are associated with the production of a syndrome similar to systemic lupus erythematosus include all of the following EXCEPT
    A. streptomycin
    B. procainamide
    C. phenytoin
    D. hydralazine
    E. primidone

894. Antihypertensive agents whose effects on blood pressure are at least partially due to central effects include
    A. minoxidil
    B. reserpine
    C. clonidine
    D. diazoxide
    E. captopril

895. Which of the following agents are routinely used in preventing or treating postpartum hemorrhage?
    A. ergonovine
    B. $PGF_{2\alpha}$
    C. magnesium sulfate
    D. progesterone
    E. ritordrine

896. Considering that the usual skin pathogens are gram-positive cocci, effective topical antimicrobial therapy can be achieved with which of the following used singularly?
    A. neomycin
    B. polymyxin B

   C. nysatin
   D. bacitracin
   E. griseofulvin

897. Epinephrine is effective in treating an acute anaphylactic reaction
     for all of the following reasons EXCEPT it
     A. decreases mucous membrane congestion
     B. antagonizes the effect of histamine on the heart
     C. increases blood pressure
     D. antagonizes the effect of leukotrienes on the bronchi
     E. antagonizes the effect of bradykinin on peripheral vessels

898. Carbon monoxide
     A. is not toxic to humans as long as there is an adequate con-
        centration of oxygen in the atmosphere
     B. has a higher affinity for hemoglobin than oxygen
     C. combines with hemoglobin more rapidly than oxygen
     D. causes oxygen to be released rapidly from hemoglobin in tis-
        sues
     E. toxicity decreases with repeated exposure

899. Chronic ingestion of 100 times the recommended daily allowance
     of which of these vitamins is likely to result in significant toxic-
     ity?
     A. vitamin A
     B. ascorbic acid (vitamin C)
     C. thiamine (vitamin B_1)
     D. cholecalciferol (vitamin D_3)
     E. vitamin B_{12}

900. Which of the following agents is a selective β_2-adrenergic ago-
     nist?
     A. phenylephrine
     B. metaproterenol
     C. isoproterenol
     D. dobutamine
     E. methoxamine

901. Adverse effects due to phenytoin include all of the following EXCEPT
   A. increased seizure frequency
   B. hirsutism
   C. gingival hyperplasia
   D. megaloblastic anemia
   E. increased absorption of calcium

902. Mannitol is
   A. reabsorbed in the proximal tubule
   B. a weak acid
   C. effective in increasing total body water
   D. almost completely reabsorbed from the renal tubule
   E. administered intravenously

903. A hypertensive crisis may be treated with any of the following EXCEPT
   A. trimethaphan
   B. sodium nitroprusside
   C. reserpine
   D. diazoxide
   E. labetalol

904. Transmembrane transport mechanisms without saturability or specificity include
   A. filtration
   B. facilitated diffusion
   C. receptor-mediated endocytosis
   D. active transport
   E. carrier-mediated transport

905. Based on the neurotransmitter aberrations which are thought to be responsible for the symptoms of Parkinson disease, which of the following drug types would you recommend for its treatment?
   A. a serotonin antagonist
   B. a muscarinic agonist
   C. an MAO inhibitor
   D. a dopaminergic agonist
   E. a cholinesterase inhibitor

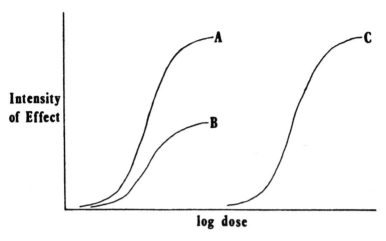

Figure 5.3

906. In Figure 5.3, if curve A represents the log dose-response curve of a full agonist X acting at a particular receptor, which of the following statements is TRUE?
  A. curve C may represent the log dose-response curve of X in the presence of a noncompetitive antagonist
  B. if curve C represents the log dose-response curve of a full agonist Y at the same receptor as X, then Y is a more potent agonist than X
  C. curve B may represent the log dose-response curve of X in the presence of a competitive antagonist
  D. curve B may represent the log dose-response curve of a partial agonist at the same receptor as X
  E. curve A may represent the action of the drug tested and plotted at C in the presence of a competitive antagonist

907. The toxicity of methotrexate can be partially reversed by the administration of
  A. cyanocobalamin (vitamin B_{12})
  B. folic acid
  C. folinic acid
  D. aminopterin
  E. vitamin C

908. Sulfonamides
   A. usually act in a bactericidal manner
   B. act at the 30S ribosomal subunit
   C. are metabolized to little or no extent in vivo
   D. act against both gram-positive and gram-negative bacteria
   E. are antiviral agents

909. Spironolactone is an aldosterone antagonist that
   A. is contraindicated in the presence of hyperkalemia
   B. depresses pituitary ACTH secretion
   C. can produce sodium depletion
   D. interferes with aldosterone biosynthesis
   E. produces edema

910. A carbonic anhydrase inhibitor
   A. is exemplified by acetohexamide
   B. causes alkalinization of the urine
   C. is contraindicated in glaucoma patients
   D. causes a metabolic alkalosis
   E. exacerbates acute mountain sickness

911. Which of the following is NOT true of clonidine?
   A. rebound hypertension can occur if the drug is suddenly discontinued
   B. it produces side effects referable to the CNS
   C. postural hypotension is not a common adverse effect, it is a centrally acting α_2-adrenergic agonist
   D. its primary focus of action is at autonomic ganglia
   E. dry mouth is a common side effect

912. In addition to bacteria, tetracyclines have in vivo activity against
   A. rickettsiae
   B. yeasts
   C. fungi
   D. DNA viruses
   E. gram-positive bacteria

913. The CNS effects of ethyl alcohol are potentiated by concurrent administration of all of the following EXCEPT
   A. diazepam
   B. chlorpheniramine
   C. aspirin
   D. phenytoin
   E. opioids

914. A therapeutic dose of morphine produces all of the following EXCEPT
   A. decreased GI motility
   B. hyperventilation
   C. urinary retention
   D. miosis
   E. nausea

915. Which of the following antineoplastic agents does not act via alkylation of cellular macromolecules?
   A. vincristine
   B. cyclophosphamide
   C. melphalan
   D. mechlorethamine
   E. chlorambucil

DIRECTIONS (Questions 916 through 925): This section consists of situations, each followed by a series of questions. Study each situation, and select the ONE best answer to each question following it.

CASE HISTORY (Questions 916 through 920): A 60-year-old woman has a long history of hypertension and is now in heart failure. For these problems she currently receives digoxin, hydrochlorothiazide, and α-methyldopa. Her cardiac output and blood pressure are now within normal values. Recently she was diagnosed as having temporal arteritis and was placed on high-dose prednisone therapy in an attempt to avert blindness. Shortly after institution of the corticosteroid therapy, she complained of palpitations.

916. Which of the following alterations in plasma constituents is most likely to have occurred in this woman to be responsible for her experiencing palpitations?
   A. hypernatremia
   B. hyponatremia
   C. hypokalemia
   D. hypocalcemia
   E. hypomagnesemia

917. Which of the following ECG changes would help confirm the source of her toxicity as an electrolyte imbalance?
   A. narrowing and increased amplitude of T waves
   B. PR interval shortening
   C. ST segment elevation
   D. clockwise rotation of the electrical axis
   E. T-wave flattening

918. Changing the corticosteroid to which of the following would help diminish the abnormality in Question 966?
   A. prednisolone
   B. cortisone
   C. fludrocortisone
   D. dexamethasone
   E. corticosterone

919. Which of the following other alterations in the therapeutic regimen would tend to reduce the toxic symptoms?
   A. changing the cardiac glycoside from digoxin to digitoxin
   B. changing the diuretic to furosemide
   C. adding reserpine to the antihypertensive regimen
   D. adding triamterene to the diuretic regimen
   E. adding acetazolamide to the diuretic regimen

920. High-dose glucocorticoid therapy for several years is likely to result in all of the following adverse effects EXCEPT
   A. osteoporosis
   B. adrenal atrophy
   C. severe weight loss
   D. cataracts
   E. diminished resistance to infection

CASE HISTORY (Questions 921 through 923): A 30-year-old woman has a 2-day history of burning on urination and urinary frequency. Within the previous 12 hours, she developed a dull pain in the lower back, a fever, and shaking chills. On three occasions during the previous 6 years, she was given an antibiotic by her physician for burning on urination and urinary frequency. Otherwise, she has been in excellent health and has not been hospitalized except for the birth of her son 2 years previously. On physical examination, her vital signs were within normal limits except for her temperature, which was 38.5°C. A complete blood count showed a white count of 20,000/mm^3, 85% of which were polymorphonuclear neutrophils. Other blood values were normal. Urinalysis demonstrated about 25 white cells and 10 gram-negative rods per high-powered field. A clean-catch midstream urine sample was sent for culture, as were several blood samples.

921. Pending the results of the urine and blood cultures, which of the following antimicrobial agents would be the initial drug of choice in this infection?
   A. chloramphenicol
   B. ampicillin
   C. penicillin G
   D. penicillin V
   E. tetracycline

922. Two days after the initiation of the antimicrobial therapy, the patient's condition had not improved. The laboratory reported the blood cultures were negative and the urine culture demonstrated a large number of *Klebsiella pneumoniae* colonies. Thus, the therapy should be changed to the administration of

  A. carbenicillin
  B. methicillin
  C. nafcillin
  D. cephalothin
  E. erythromycin

923. After the patient's bacteriuria subsided, her physician decided to put her on a course of prophylactic chemotherapy to prevent against reinfection. He obtained her previous medical records and found that of her three previous infections, one was due to *Proteus mirabilis* and two were due to *Escherichia coli*. Thus, for prophylaxis, he prescribed

  A. ampicillin
  B. gentamicin
  C. tetracycline
  D. nitrofurantoin
  E. carbenicillin

CASE HISTORY (Questions 924 and 925): A 14-year-old boy has a 2-year history of asthma. His episodes are of moderate frequency and occur on the average of 2 to 4 times per month. The attacks appear to be brought on by emotional stress or physical exertion and almost always occur during waking hours. During the attacks, he becomes severely dyspneic and cyanotic and requires pharmacologic intervention. Immunologic testing has failed to demonstrate hypersensitivity to any antigens.

924. Of the following agents, which would be both effective and LEAST toxic in reversing the acute asthmatic episode?

  A. cromolyn sodium
  B. atropine
  C. epinephrine
  D. ephedrine
  E. terbutaline

925. If it is decided to treat the patient prophylactically, which of the following agents would be most effective in preventing his asthmatic episodes?
   A. ephedrine, inhaled
   B. isoproterenol, orally
   C. chlorpheniramine, orally
   D. theophylline, orally
   E. cromolyn sodium, inhaled

Pharmacology

Answers and Comments

726. (D) Morphine raises the threshold for chronic, dull pain. It is not as effective for sharp, acute pain. Patients may still perceive pain but their reaction may be modified. Morphine stimulates mu, kappa, sigma, and delta receptors; mu receptors are related to supraspinal pain. Tolerance readily develops to opioids. Naloxone is considered a pure antagonist which only acts to reverse the effects of opioids, however it can precipitate a withdrawal phenomenon. (**Ref. 1,** pp. 490, 491, 516; **Ref. 2,** pp. 424, 425, 434)

727. (C) All of the effects listed will lead to a reduction of mean arterial pressure. Halothane and enflurane cause a reduction in cardiac output. Isoflurane reduces blood pressure through arteriolar vasodilation. Other inhalational general anesthetic agents (nitrous oxide) do not cause a decrease in blood pressure at levels used for surgery. (**Ref. 1,** pp. 287, 292, 295; **Ref. 2,** pp. 356–357)

728. (A) A major use of digoxin is to "protect" the ventricles from aberrant electrical activity initiated in atrial muscle. This occurs as a result of inhibiting A-V conduction through an increase in vagal tone. Digoxin is eliminated by renal mechanisms, it has a half-life of 40 hours and it does not act through beta-adrenergic receptors. It inhibits Na^+, K^+ATPase. Epinephrine and digoxin both cause arrhythmias. (**Ref. 1,** pp. 817, 827, 831, 836; **Ref. 2,** pp. 178–179, 184)

729. (B) Albuterol is a beta-adrenergic agonist with selectivity for beta$_2$-adrenergic receptors in pulmonary smooth muscle. Metoprolol, a beta-adrenergic blocking agent, has beta$_1$ selectivity. Phenylephrine and methoxamine are alpha$_1$ agonists with minimal effect on the heart. Metanephrine directly stimulates the heart (beta$_1$ agonist) and phentolamine causes reflex tachycardia due to peripheral vasodilation. Phentolamine also blocks alpha$_2$ receptors resulting in increased norepinephrine combining with cardiac beta receptors. (**Ref. 1,** pp. 204, 205, 226, 234; **Ref. 2,** pp. 118, 125, 132, 286)

730. (A) The CNS depressant thiobarbiturate, thiopental, has a short duration of action due to redistribution of the drug. It only produces transient skeletal muscle relaxation and may have an antianalgesic effect. Bronchospasm and laryngospasm are not uncommon and equipment to assist respiration should be available when thiopental is used. (**Ref. 1,** pp. 301–303)

731. (B) Ethacrynic acid and furosemide are referred to as loop diuretics because of their site of action. They cause short-lived intense diuresis and are sometimes called "high ceiling" agents. Mannitol is an osmotic diuretic. Acetazolamide is a carbonic anhydrase inhibitor acting in the proximal tubule. Spironolactone alters potassium which is coupled to sodium reabsorption. Thiazides act in the distal tubule. (**Ref. 1,** pp. 714, 716, 718, 719, 722, 726; **Ref. 2,** pp. 216–218, 220, 223, 224)

732. (E) The glucocorticoids produce a dramatic decrease in inflammation. They also suppress the immune response. This inhibition of leukocytes and tissue macrophages has the potential to mask signs and symptoms of disease processes and allow bacteria, which under normal circumstances would be destroyed, to proliferate. (**Ref. 1,** p. 1443; **Ref. 2,** p. 545)

733. (A) Postmenopausal osteoporosis can be arrested by estrogen administration. Estrogens improve the intestinal transport of calcium and restore the calcium balance. Usually considerable bone loss occurs before osteoporosis is detected. There is controversy about giving unopposed estrogens prophylactically to all postmenopausal women. (**Ref. 1,** pp. 1394, 1395; **Ref. 2,** pp. 612, 613)

734. (**D**)   While several mechanisms have been proposed to explain the manner in which sulfonylureas act, the predominant view is that they promote insulin release from pancreatic beta cells in the islets of Langerhans. (**Ref. 1,** p. 1484; **Ref. 2,** pp. 595, 596)

735. (**C**)   The formation of thyroid hormone involves iodide trapping in the gland and subsequent oxidation of the iodide to iodine by thyroid peroxidase. The first process is blocked or inhibited by perchlorates while the peroxidase is inhibited by propylthiouracil. (**Ref. 1,** p. 1374; **Ref. 2,** pp. 529, 534, 535)

736. (**E**)   The chronic use of adrenal corticosteroids leads to toxicity associated with fluid and electrolyte imbalance, increased susceptibility to infection, osteoporosis, Cushing syndrome, and other signs related to prolonged use. The other category to toxic effects relates to acute adrenal insufficiency after withdrawal which is too rapid. The presence of corticoids suppresses the pituitary adrenal axis. (**Ref. 1,** p. 1448; **Ref. 2,** p. 551)

737. (**C**)   Phenothiazines can cause tardive dyskinesia which is irreversible. It usually occurs with prolonged drug use. The pseudo-Parkinsonian reaction most often occurs in patients >50 years of age. One of the approved indications for prochlorperazine is treatment of nausea and vomiting. This is most likely an unpredictable dystonic reaction which occurs in patients up to 19 years of age. (**Ref. 1,** pp. 398–400; **Ref. 2,** p. 402)

738. (**A**)   The acute dystonia can be mistaken for an hysterical reaction but it responds dramatically to an anticholinergic or an antiparkinsonian drug. Dantrolene may be useful for a malignant syndrome. The use of a skeletal muscle blocking agent would be inappropriate and the use of a cholinergic agonist would have widespread action which may exacerbate the condition. (**Ref. 1,** pp. 398–400; **Ref. 2,** pp. 402, 403, 892)

739. (**D**)   The oxycodone in this combination product has the potential to cause all of the effects listed except urinary urgency. The side effect associated with opioid analgesics of this type is urinary retention. (**Ref. 1,** pp. 490–495; **Ref. 2,** pp. 425–428)

740. **(E)**   The agents listed are all cyclooxygenase inhibitors and are generally referred to as nonsteroidal anti-inflammatory agents (NSAIDs). Acetaminophen, although widely believed to be the same as aspirin-type compounds, is a weak prostaglandin biosynthesis inhibitor and does not have any significant anti-inflammatory effects. (**Ref. 1,** pp. 641, 656; **Ref. 2,** pp. 499–500, 506)

741. **(E)**   The use of products which have combinations of NSAIDs, or the combination of individual NSAIDs with each other or with acetaminophen, does not provide a rational basis for pain management since these compounds all suppress the same types of pain. Some patients do respond better to one compound or have fewer side effects with a particular compound making selection on this basis rational. However, the combination of an NSAID or acetaminophen with an opioid-type compound provides pain relief from a centrally acting opioid in addition to the pain relief provided by the NSAID-type compounds. (**Ref. 1,** pp. 490, 641; **Ref. 2,** pp. 432, 500)

742. **(B)**   Astemizole is a highly selective H_1-receptor antagonist that does not penetrate into the CNS and has been widely advertised as an agent that does not cause sedation. However, arrhythmias have been caused by this agent, especially in combination with agents that inhibit hepatic drug metabolism or in combination with various antibiotics. (**Ref. 1,** p. 585; **Ref. 2,** p. 234; **Ref. 3,** p. 1861)

743. **(E)**   The most effective agent in the list given is meclizine. It causes little sedation with high antimotion sickness effectiveness. Promethazine is also effective in treating nausea and vomiting associated with surgery or cancer chemotherapy. (**Ref. 1,** p. 587; **Ref. 2,** pp. 234–235)

744. **(C)**   The treatment of gastric ulcers with H_2-receptor antagonists has made this group of compounds one of the most widely prescribed agents in the USA. These compounds have relatively few side effects but do have several drug interactions. (**Ref. 1,** p. 899; **Ref. 2,** p. 237)

745. (D) Sedation is generally thought of as an undesirable side effect of antihistamines. However, for those who have difficulty sleeping, diphenhydramine along with doxylamine and pyrilamine are used by prescription and in over-the-counter as sleep aids. (**Ref. 1,** pp. 584, 588; **Ref. 2,** p. 235)

746. (E) When a drug is converted to a more polar compound and thus more easily excreted, the process is a conjugation reaction. Compounds, or the metabolites of compounds, are often coupled to glucuronate, sulfate, acetate, or an amino acid (glycine). (**Ref. 1,** pp. 13–15)

747. (B) The phase I reaction is metabolism of a pharmacologic agent by hydrolysis (esters), oxidation (microsomal oxidase system), or reduction (endoplasmic reticulum). (**Ref. 1,** pp. 15–16)

748. (A) The thiobarbiturates are first distributed to the brain, thus producing a short (5 to 10 min) period of anesthesia which is useful for short surgical procedures or for induction prior to administration of a volatile general anesthetic. Subsequent administration of this type of agent during the same surgical procedure leads to a progressively longer duration of action. (**Ref. 1,** pp. 13, 301; **Ref. 2,** p. 309)

749. (D) Some compounds must be administered by a route other than oral since they are rapidly metabolized by the liver. Nitroglycerin is a classic example of this type of agent. (**Ref. 1,** p. 8; **Ref. 2,** pp. 42, 164)

750. (C) Some individuals have an abnormal reactivity. This could manifest itself in a response to an extremely low dose of the agent as in the response to primaquine of patients with glucose-6-phosphate deficiency or a requirement for extremely high dose of warfarin in patients with defective receptors. (**Ref. 1,** p. 53; **Ref. 2,** p. 31)

751. (A) Heparin increases the activity of a plasma protein, antithrombin III, which neutralizes the activated forms of factors II, IX, X, XI, XII, and XIII, and of kallikrein. Its primary action is on thrombin (IIa) and Xa. Heparin is usually administered intravenously, and its effect is assessed by measurement of the activated partial thromboplastin time. (**Ref. 1,** p. 1314; **Ref. 2,** pp. 466–467)

752. **(B)** The pharmacologic effect of B is dependent upon the amount of free (unbound) B in the plasma. Thus, by displacing B from binding sites to plasma proteins, A increases the pharmacological effect of B. All of the other processes cited would result in lower levels of A. (**Ref. 1,** pp. 70–71; **Ref. 2,** p. 931)

753. **(D)** Theophylline, a methylxanthine related to caffeine, is used therapeutically to relax bronchial smooth muscle. It causes CNS stimulation, tachycardia, and stimulation of gastric acid secretion. It has been shown to block adenosine receptors; however, current studies are showing that its primary action may be inhibition of phosphodiesterase isozymes. (**Ref. 1,** pp. 623–626; **Ref. 2,** pp. 283–284)

754. **(D)** Insomnia has been and continues to be difficult to manage effectively. Long-term drug therapy is inappropriate. When nonpharmacologic interventions do not succeed, benzodiazepines are the agent of choice due to lower abuse potential and higher therapeutic index when compared with other currently approved agents. However, specific cautions should be observed even with these agents. Benzodiazepines produce the least suppression of REM sleep of all the CNS depressants. (**Ref. 1,** pp. 369–370; **Ref. 2,** p. 316)

755. **(B)** The serum concentration at T = 2 hours is 16 mg/L. The serum concentration has fallen to 8 mg/L by T = 4 hours; thus the half-life is 2 hours. (**Ref. 1,** p. 24; **Ref. 2,** pp. 8, 40)

756. **(A)** Pancuronium is a competitive antagonist of the acetylcholine receptor of the neuromuscular junction. Neostigmine is an acetylcholinesterase inhibitor that increases the concentration of acetylcholine in the synaptic cleft, thus overcoming the effect of pancuronium. While physostigmine has essentially the same activity as neostigmine, it crosses the blood–brain barrier and may produce toxic CNS effects. Atropine would act at muscarinic sites. Gallamine is a pancuronium-type agent. (**Ref. 1,** pp. 177–176; **Ref. 2,** pp. 93, 378)

757. **(C)** Drug metabolism usually results in a decreased duration of action because the drug is rendered more polar, water soluble, and thus more rapidly excreted. While some agents called prodrugs are converted to active compounds, most metabolic transformation results in an inactive metabolite. (**Ref. 1,** p. 13; **Ref. 2,** pp. 6–7)

758. **(D)** Isoflurane has an unpleasant odor. Anesthesia may be maintained with isoflurane after induction with an intravenous agent. (**Ref. 1,** p. 296)

759. **(D)** The questions about oral contraceptives and cancer are unresolved. It does not appear that there is an increase in breast cancer and ovarian cancer has been reported to decrease. Liver cancer may increase (rarely) and uterine cancer incidence is unresolved. (**Ref. 1,** p. 1407; **Ref. 2,** pp. 570, 573)

760. **(A)** Succinylcholine causes depolarizing neuromuscular blockade resulting in flaccid paralysis. It is metabolized primarily by circulating plasma cholinesterase. d-Tubocurarine administered previously antagonizes the action of succinylcholine. (**Ref. 1,** pp. 171–172, 177; **Ref. 2,** pp. 375–376)

761. **(E)** Tetracycline is effective against all three organisms in vivo. Gonococcal infections have become resistant to penicillins. (**Ref. 1,** pp. 1073, 1123–1124)

762. **(D)** Aspirin in high doses uncouples oxidative phosphorylation leading to increased CO_2 production and hyperventilation. A respiratory alkalosis then ensues. As intoxication continues to develop, a metabolic acidosis is present. Miosis is one of the hallmarks of opioid analgesic overdose. (**Ref. 1,** p. 651; **Ref. 2,** pp. 495–496)

763. **(A)** A β_2-adrenergic agonist will inhibit uterine contractions. The other classes of agents either cause uterine contraction (ergot alkaloids, muscarinic agonists, α-adrenergic agonists), or have little effect on the uterus (ganglionic blocker). (**Ref. 1,** pp. 89, 943, 950, 951; **Ref. 2,** pp. 77, 121, 245)

764. (A) General anesthetic molecules do not bind to specific receptors, but nonspecifically associate with cellular membranes. Induction is correlated with the agent's oil/water partition coefficient and its rate of delivery into the body and distribution to the CNS (**Ref. 1,** pp. 271, 281; **Ref. 2,** pp. 352–354, 387–391, 395)

765. (D) The barbiturates have largely been replaced by the benzodiazepines. They still have use for narcoanalysis, epilepsy, anesthetic induction, and emergency management of convulsions. They actually may cause hyperalgesia, that is, an increased sensitivity to pain. (**Ref. 1,** pp. 358–359, 363–364; **Ref. 2,** pp. 311–312)

766. (A) Patients with angina pectoris frequently are also prone to congestive heart failure which propranolol can worsen by virtue of its blockade of cardiac β_1-adrenergic receptors. It actually decreases blood pressure, and its effects on the other organ systems mentioned are negligible. (**Ref. 1,** pp. 238–239; **Ref. 2,** pp. 131– 132)

767. (E) Conduction velocity is determined primarily by membrane responsiveness, that is, the maximum rate of depolarization during phase 0 of the action potential. (**Ref. 1,** p. 842)

768. (D) Reporting of drug interactions involving the oral anticoagulants is increasing. However, one of the classic interactions is that of phenobarbital increasing the rate of metabolism of warfarin via induction of liver microsomal enzymes. (**Ref. 1,** pp. 1319–1320; **Ref. 2,** pp. 469–470)

769. (C) Increased sodium conductance accompanying depolarization is blocked by lidocaine. It has virtually no effect on the resting potential. It penetrates nerve membranes in the unionized form but it has an intracellular site of action. Lidocaine is an amide-type agent which is metabolized by the liver. Ester-types are hydrolyzed by butyrylcholinesterase (pseudocholinesterase). (**Ref. 1,** pp. 312, 318, 320; **Ref. 2,** pp. 363–365)

770. (C) Phenobarbital, morphine, ethyl alcohol, and meprobamate all produce a withdrawal syndrome when administration is terminated in a dependent individual. However, the withdrawal effect due to marijuana is often mild or unclear. (**Ref. 1,** pp. 526, 552–553; **Ref. 2,** pp. 437–439, 447)

771. **(B)** Narrow-angle glaucoma is worsened by agents that cause mydriasis such as atropine. Pilocarpine and neostigmine cause miosis. Acetazolamide results in decreased aqueous humor production. Succinylcholine only rarely increases intraocular pressure, and then, only transiently. (**Ref. 1,** pp. 143–144, 154, 175; **Ref. 2,** pp. 92, 100, 378)

772. **(A)** Prednisone has both glucocorticoid and mineralocorticoid activity. The other agents are exclusively glucocorticoids. (**Ref. 1,** p. 1447; **Ref. 2,** p. 547)

773. **(B)** The development of resistant strains of microorganisms has resulted in treatment with at least two drugs to which drug sensitivity exists. These agents, with the exception of dapsone, are all used for tuberculosis. Dapsone is used for leprosy. (**Ref. 1,** pp. 1157, 1159; **Ref. 2,** pp. 658–659)

774. **(E)** Chloramphenicol causes hematologic toxicity and it should be reserved for conditions where benefits outweigh risks, but is not ototoxic. Vancomycin, streptomycin, and ethacrynic acid may cause permanent deafness. Aspirin causes reversible hearing loss and tinnitus. (**Ref. 1,** pp. 651–652, 724, 1104–1106, 1127–1129, 1139; **Ref. 2,** pp. 219, 496, 640, 647, 683)

775. **(A)** Cyanide binds to the ferric form of cytochrome oxidase. Amyl nitrate is used to oxidize hemoglobin to methemoglobin which effectively competes with cytochromoxidase for cyanide. This keeps cyanide in the peripheral circulation as cyanmethemoglobin and prevents its access to tissues. (**Ref. 1,** p. 1631; **Ref. 2,** p. 166)

776. **(C)** Pralidoxime is a cholinesterase reactivator. Oxime (=NOH) groups have high affinity for phosphorous and can reverse the phosphorylated enzyme if it has not "aged." (**Ref. 1,** p. 141; **Ref. 2,** p. 103)

777. **(A)** Digoxin increases the rate at which force is developed while concurrently shortening systole. The effect is independent

of a normal sinus rhythm and adrenergic stimulation. (**Ref. 1,** pp. 815–816)

778. **(D)** The least potassium depletion is achieved by combining a potassium-sparing diuretic, such as the aldosterone antagonist spironolactone, with an effective diuretic acting via a different mechanism, such as furosemide. (**Ref. 1,** p. 731)

779. **(B)** A noncompetitive (irreversible, nonequilibrium) antagonist decreases the efficacy of the agonist while having no effect of its potency or ED_{50}. The term potency only refers to the amount of a drug required to produce 50% of that drug's maximal response. (**Ref. 1,** pp. 45–47; **Ref. 2,** pp. 12–13, 29)

780. **(C)** The drug treatment of epilepsy has been generally divided into two groups of agents, those used to treat absence seizures and those effective in generalized tonic–clonic episodes. All of the agents listed except ethosuximide are used for generalized tonic–clonic convulsions. Diazepam is used for status epilepticus. (**Ref. 1,** pp. 439, 459; **Ref. 2,** pp. 346–347)

781. **(A)** An intramuscular injection exposes the drug to the largest surface area of vascular tissue of any of the methods listed, and thus results in the most rapid rate of absorption and distribution. (**Ref. 1,** pp. 7–9; **Ref. 2,** pp. 4–5)

782. **(C)** Plasma levels after the first dose are 75% of the plateau levels; after the second dose, 93.8%; fourth, 99.6%; sixth, 99.98%; and eighth, 99.99%. (**Ref. 1,** p. 27; **Ref. 2,** p. 44)

783. **(E)** Thiazide diuretics promote the excretion of sodium, potassium, chloride, and magnesium; other diuretics cause greater changes in extracellular fluid composition. Plasma levels of uric acid increase due to enhanced reabsorption in the proximal tubule and inhibition of tubular secretion of urate; uric acid secretion is blocked and its plasma level increases. (**Ref. 1,** pp. 718–719; **Ref. 2,** p. 221)

784. **(C)** Sweat glands are innervated by sympathetic, cholinergic neurons. The other tissues and organs are innervated by sympathetic, adrenergic fibers. (**Ref. 1,** pp. 86, 126; **Ref. 2,** pp. 70, 87)

785. (C) The megaloblastic anemia that occurs during pregnancy is the result of folate deficiency due to increased demand coupled with marginal diet. Lactation may also cause a deficiency due to the folate lost during nursing. (**Ref. 1,** p. 1305; **Ref. 2,** p. 460)

786. (D) Lithium has virtually no psychotropic activity in normal persons and acts only to reduce the magnitude of the mood swings in manic-depressive illness. Even though the psychotropic effect is limited, lithium has a low therapeutic index and plasma levels need close attention. (**Ref. 1,** pp. 418, 420; **Ref. 2,** pp. 405– 407)

787. (C) CNS blood vessels are dilated by histamine, causing the so-called histamine headache. The physiologic importance of histamine is unknown, however the discovery of H_1, H_2, and H_3 receptors with specific blocking agents has resulted in active investigation of this biogenic amine. (**Ref. 1,** pp. 578–580; **Ref. 2,** pp. 230–232)

788. (C) Oral contraceptives using a combination of an estrogen and a progestin are widely used and highly (99 to 100%) effective. Progestins alone as oral contraceptives are referred to as the "minipill," while estrogen alone has come to be known as the "morning-after pill." (**Ref. 1,** p. 1403; **Ref. 2,** pp. 568, 573, 574)

789. (B) Tolnaftate is a topical antifungal agent. The antifungal activity of griseofulvin occurs only after oral administration. Griseofulvin has very little effect topically. The other three agents are topical antibacterial drugs. (**Ref. 1,** p. 1173; **Ref. 2,** p. 671)

790. (A) Acetylation, although carried out in the liver, is catalyzed by a nonmicrosomal group of enzymes, n-acetyl transferases. (**Ref. 1,** pp. 14–17; **Ref. 2,** pp. 53–55)

791. (B) Both agents inhibit prostaglandin biosynthesis in the CNS and reduce pathologic fever; only aspirin inhibits prostaglandin synthetase in the peripheral tissues. Acetaminophen does not cause gastric distress and can be used in patients with gastric ulcers. It has no anti-inflammatory effect nor is it uricosuric. (**Ref. 1,** pp. 641, 656–659; **Ref. 2,** p. 506)

792. (C) Mercury poisoning responds somewhat to dimercaprol. It should not be used in iron or cadmium poisoning because the heavy metal toxicity may be potentiated. Lead poisoning is treated with $CaNa_2EDTA$. (**Ref. 1**, p. 1609; **Ref. 2**, p. 832)

793. (B) The efferent arc of baroreceptor reflex is antagonized by chlorpromazine by virtue of its α-adrenergic blocking effect. The other actions of the phenothiazine, chlorpromazine, are hypothesized to involve dopamine. (**Ref. 1**, pp. 393, 399, 926; **Ref. 2**, pp. 399, 400)

794. (C) T_3 is effective orally, more potent than T_4, and bound less tightly to thyroid-binding globulin than T_4. T_4 is converted to T_3 in peripheral tissues. Propylthiouracil inhibits the biosynthesis of thyroid hormones. (**Ref. 1**, pp. 1362, 1365, 1374, 1377; **Ref. 2**, pp. 530, 535)

795. (A) Carbidopa inhibits peripheral dopa decarboxylase, thus inhibiting the metabolism of levodopa to dopamine. The concurrent administration of the aromatic L-amino acid decarboxylase inhibitor, carbidopa, with levodopa permits a much lower dose of levodopa with fewer undesirable side effects. (**Ref. 1**, p. 471; **Ref. 2**, p. 386)

796. (B) Most normal cells can synthesize *l*-asparaginase but the cells of acute lymphocytic leukemia cannot and *l*-asparaginase destroys the leukemic cells' essential nutrient. Cyclophosphamide and busulfan are alkylating agents, while methotrexate is an antimetabolite and vincristine blocks mitosis in metaphase; these latter agents act on all tissues. (**Ref. 1**, pp. 1205–1206, 1248; **Ref. 2**, pp. 770–771, 775, 778, 785)

797. (B) Sulfonamide antimicrobial agents inhibit bacterial incorporation of *p*-aminobenzoic acid into folic acid. Mammalian tissues cannot carry out this reaction and require exogenous folic acid. (**Ref. 1**, p. 1048; **Ref. 2**, p. 661)

798. (A) Griseofulvin is effective orally in the treatment of superficial mycoses. It interferes with fungal mitosis and results in the production of uninfected skin, hair, or nails. Amphotericin B and nystatin are not absorbed from the GI tract, and flucytosine and tetracycline, while absorbed well, are not effective against superficial pathologic fungi. (**Ref. 1,** p. 1173; **Ref. 2,** pp. 670–671)

799. **(B)** According to the Henderson–Hasselbalch equation (pH = pK + log [proton acceptor/proton donor]), the ratio of proton acceptor to proton donor is about 10,000. Thus, only about 0.01% of the aspirin molecules will be in the associated form. (**Ref. 1,** p. 4; **Ref. 2,** pp. 2–3)

800. **(D)** Carbenicillin has the broadest spectrum of activity, especially against gram-negative bacilli. (**Ref. 1,** pp. 1078, 1080–1081; **Ref. 2,** pp. 626, 629, 630)

801. **(A)** The patient has an apparent volume of distribution of (8L/kg) (62 kg) = 496 L. 0.5 mg distributed to 496 L gives 0.00101 mg/L, which corresponds to 1.0 ng/mL. (**Ref. 1,** p. 23; **Ref. 2,** pp. 5–6)

802. **(A)** Plasma levels greater than 2.5 ng/mL of digoxin are considered likely to be toxic. Thus, administration of 1.0 mg will raise the plasma level by 2.0 ng/mL to 3.0 ng/mL. (**Ref. 1,** p. 827; **Ref. 2,** p. 183)

803. **(A)** The distribution of digoxin in the body is uneven; it reaches much higher concentrations in heart and muscle due to its hydrophobicity. This leaves little in the plasma. Digitoxin is highly (> 90%) protein bound and it tends to stay in the plasma compartment. Thus the apparent volume of distribution is much greater than the actual volume of distribution. Protein binding of digoxin is approximately 25%. (**Ref. 1,** pp. 23, 828; **Ref. 2,** p. 178)

804. **(E)** Edrophonium is a short-acting acetylcholinesterase inhibitor. The pathology in myasthenia gravis consists of the production of circulating antibodies to the acetylcholine receptor, thus effectively reducing the number of receptors. Because edrophonium inhibits acetylcholine metabolism, muscle strength will be transiently increased because of the greater effective amount of acetylcholine in the synaptic cleft. In a normal person, edrophonium results in too much acetylcholine acting on the motor end plate, causing a depolarizing block and transient muscle weakness. (**Ref. 1,** p. 145; **Ref. 2,** p. 93)

805. **(E)** The half-life of nitrofurantoin is less than one-half hour, too short to permit adequate antibacterial levels anywhere but in the urine. (**Ref. 1,** p. 1061; **Ref. 2,** p. 687)

806. **(E)** Niclosamide is the drug of choice in tapeworm infections. (**Ref. 1,** p. 965; **Ref. 2,** p. 756)

807. **(C)** Praziquantel has a relatively short half-life; however, it effectively increases calcium permeability causing contraction and paralysis of the worm musculature. It is well tolerated orally and effective against all schistosomes which infect humans. (**Ref. 1,** pp. 968, 969; **Ref. 2,** pp. 749, 759)

808. **(D)** Pyrantel pamoate is a neuromuscular blocking agent in the hookworm, pinworm, and roundworm. It does not kill the worm or eggs. (**Ref. 1,** p. 969; **Ref. 2,** p. 761)

809. **(C)** Diethylcarbamazine is used in filariasis. It immobilizes the microfilariae and alters their surface structure making them more susceptible to host defenses. (**Ref. 1,** p. 960; **Ref. 2,** p. 751)

810. **(C)** Doxorubicin may cause a dose-dependent cardiomyopathy. Anthracycline antibiotics cause both acute and chronic cardiomyopathy. (**Ref. 1,** p. 1243; **Ref. 2,** p. 780)

811. **(B)** Cyclophosphamide must be activated by liver cytochrome P-450 to be cytotoxic. However, the liver itself is protected by additional conversion to a 4-ketocyclophosphamide and a carboxyphosphamide. (**Ref. 2,** pp. 1216–1217)

812. **(E)** Azathioprine is a purine analog used primarily as an immunosuppressive, as in the prevention of transplanted organ rejection. (**Ref. 1,** pp. 1236, 1271; **Ref. 2,** p. 808)

813. **(E)** Azathioprine is metabolized by xanthine oxidase, and the xanthine oxidase inhibitor allopurinol causes an increased exposure of the tissues due to the drug. (**Ref. 1,** pp. 1236, 1271; **Ref. 2,** p. 808)

814. **(B)** Vidarabine is effective against certain DNA viruses such as herpes simplex. (**Ref. 1,** pp. 1187–1188; **Ref. 2,** p. 676)

815. (C) Amantadine can prevent influenza A_2 infections if given before or shortly after exposure. It has usefulness in parkinsonism. **(Ref. 1, pp.** 1191–1192; **Ref. 2,** p. 389)

816. (E) Griseofulvin is active against the dermatomycoses. It must be used until the uninfected tissues (skin, nails) replace the infected tissues. **(Ref. 1, pp.** 1173–1174; **Ref. 2, pp.** 670–671)

817. (C), 818. (B), 819. (C), 820. (C), Isosorbide dinitrate, propranolol, and nifedipine are all used prophylactically to prevent attacks of angina pectoris. Propranolol is also used for supraventricular arrhythmias, an activity related to its β-adrenergic blocking action. Isosorbide dinitrate must be used in large doses to be effective. Nifedipine is a calcium channel blocker. Disopyramide is an antiarrhythmic effective against ventricular ectopy. **(Ref. 1, pp.** 772, 779–780; **Ref. 2, pp.** 167–168, 171–172)

821. (B), 822. (E), 823. (A), 824. (C) Tachyphylaxis is the tolerance to a drug that develops rapidly after administration is begun. Anaphylaxis is the full-blown acute hypersensitivity reaction to a drug that is life-threatening due to airway obstruction and cardiovascular collapse. Teratogenic effects of drugs are those adverse drug effects on the fetus which alter its development. Induction is the process by which a drug increases the activity of a metabolic enzyme. **(Ref. 1,** pp. 52–53, 68, 71, 459; **Ref. 2,** pp. 31, 121, 854– 855)

825. (B), 826. (E), 827. (C), 828. (B), 829. (D), 830. (A) Beriberi and Wernicke syndrome are due to a thiamine deficiency, the latter being a consequence of malnutrition in the alcoholic. Pellagra is caused by the deficiency of nicotinic acid, while scurvy results from the dietary lack of ascorbic acid. Rickets results when one is deficient in cholecalciferol, also known as vitamin D. Pernicious anemia is a disease caused by the genetic inability to absorb dietary cyanocobalamin (vitamin B_{12}). **(Ref. 1,** pp. 1300–1301, 1517, 1533, 1538, 1549)

831. (B), 832. (E), 833. (A), 834. (C), 835. (D) Allopurinol inhibits xanthine oxidase and is used to treat gout. Disulfiram inhibits aldehyde dehydrogenase and is used in the treatment of alcoholism. Calvulanic acid is an inhibitor of bacterial β-lactamase, and increases the antimicrobial activity of various penicillin congeners. Tranylcypromine is a monoamine oxidase inhibitor used to treat depression. Acetazolamide inhibits carbonic anhydrase and is used in the therapy of glaucoma. It also is a diuretic but rarely used for this purpose since tolerance develops. (**Ref. 1**, pp. 378–379, 414, 676, 718, 1093; **Ref. 2**, pp. 216, 326, 412, 509, 635)

836. (D), 837. (A), 838. (C) Lithium carbonate prevents the mood swings characteristic of manic-depressive illness and is used in long-term therapy. Triazolam is a benzodiazepine used as a hypnotic to facilitate sleep in insomnia characterized by difficulty "falling" asleep. Methylphenidate is an amphetamine congener with a paradoxical calming effect in children with attention-deficit hyperactivity disorder. (**Ref. 1**, pp. 217, 370, 418; **Ref. 2**, pp. 121, 310, 316, 404)

839. (A) Adrenergic amines which activate α-adrenergic receptors cause contraction of the radial muscle in the eye and will produce mydriasis without cycloplegia. Epinephrine is a nonselective agonist while isoproterenol, the other adrenergic amine listed, is a β-adrenergic agonist. (**Ref. 1**, pp. 88, 217; **Ref. 2**, p. 115)

840. (E) Blockade of muscarinic receptors results in pupillary dilation (mydriasis) and paralysis of accommodation (cycloplegia). Inhibition of cholinesterase with physostigmine may reverse the effects of atropine. (**Ref. 1**, p. 154; **Ref. 2**, pp. 98, 100)

841. (A) Phenylephrine is an agonist at α_1-adrenergic receptors. Isoproterenol is a nonselective β-adrenergic agonist while epinephrine is a nonselective agonist at α- and β-adrenergic receptors. Atropine and physostigmine exert effects through the cholinergic system. (**Ref. 1**, pp. 114, 192, 207; **Ref. 2**, pp. 86, 91, 110, 115)

842. (D) Isoproterenol is the prototype of β-adrenergic amines. It has potent action on the heart and on all smooth muscles, the most prominent of which is its action on airway smooth muscle. The introduction of selective β_2 agonists has led to a decrease in the use of isoproterenol in reversing bronchoconstriction of asthma. (**Ref. 1**, p. 201; **Ref. 2**, pp. 114–117)

843. **(C)** Local application of anticholinesterases to the eye will result in contraction of the sphincter muscle of the iris resulting in miosis. Even though the pupil is contracted to pinpoint size, it still contracts further when exposed to light. (**Ref. 1**, p. 137; **Ref. 2**, pp. 86, 91)

844. **(C)** Bertylium is a class III antiarrhythmic agent which inhibits the release of adrenergic amines from nerve endings. It may cause arrhythmias due to an initial release of catecholamines. It is blocked by agents which inhibit the uptake of adrenergic amines into the nerve ending. (**Ref. 1**, pp. 866–868; **Ref. 2**, p. 206)

845. **(B)** The two major class I_A antiarrhythmic agents, quinidine and procainamide, produce numerous side effects. Procainamide causes a systemic lupus-like syndrome while quinidine causes thrombocytopenia. (**Ref. 1**, p. 856; **Ref. 2**, p. 198-201)

846. **(D)** Flecainide and encainide were developed as potent agents which were orally effective and highly effective in suppressing premature ventricular contractions. However, they were also found to be proarrhythmic in a large-scale test known as the Cardiac Arrhythmic Suppression Trial (CAST) and use of these compounds is now restricted to life-threatening ventricular arrhythmias. (**Ref. 1**, pp. 861–863; **Ref. 2**, p. 205)

847. **(E)** Class IV antiarrhythmic agents, of which verapamil is the prototype, are effective in treating supraventricular tachycardia. They are effective in tissues that fire frequently and where calcium current is involved (the SA and AV nodes). (**Ref. 1**, p. 869; **Ref. 2**, pp. 206–207)

848. **(A)** Lidocaine, class I_B, is widely used to inhibit ectopic activity. It is administered intravenously and is considered the least toxic of the antiarrhythmic agents. Quinidine inhibits sodium channels in the activated state while lidocaine blocks both activated and inactivated sodium channels. Lidocaine shortens the action potential duration making the time available for recovery of a longer duration. (**Ref. 1**, pp. 857, 860; **Ref. 2**, p. 203)

849. **(B)** Both amphotericin A and B are polyene antibiotics. Amphotericin B binds to ergosterol in the fungal cell membrane. This results in the formation of pores causing the loss of cellular ions and subsequent destruction. Bacteria which do not possess ergosterol in the membrane are resistant to this antifungal agent. (**Ref. 1,** pp. 1098, 1106–1107; **Ref. 2,** p. 667)

850. (D) Gentamicin is used for severe infections caused by resistant gram-negative organisms. Nephrotoxicity requires careful adjustment of dosage. (**Ref. 1,** pp. 1108–1109; **Ref. 2,** pp. 648–649)

851. (C) The tetracyclines are broad spectrum agents which are bacteriostatic for both gram-negative and gram-positive bacteria. They enter the cell by both passive diffusion and active transport. Once in the cell they bind to the 30S subunit of the bacterial ribosome. Tetracycline is considered the drug of choice in the above infections. (**Ref. 1,** pp. 1118, 1123; **Ref. 2,** p. 642)

852. (E) Polymyxins are a group of polypeptide compounds which are active against gram-negative bacteria. They are limited to topical use due to their potential to cause nephrotoxicity and because there are more effective and less toxic agents available. (**Ref. 1,** p. 1138; **Ref. 2,** p. 650)

853. (C) Mannitol exerts its action due to an osmotic effect. It is not metabolized but is eliminated by glomerular filtration following intravenous administration. Reabsorption does not occur. Oral ingestion of mannitol could lead to osmotic diarrhea. (**Ref. 1,** p. 714; **Ref. 2,** p. 224)

854. (B) The thiazides were developed in an attempt to produce a potent carbonic anhydrase inhibitor. While these compounds have varying activity as carbonic anhydrase inhibitors, this is not their mechanism of action. They inhibit a poorly understood NaCl transport system in the distal convoluted tubule. (**Ref. 1,** pp. 718–719; **Ref. 2,** p. 219)

855. (E) Ethacrynic acid and furosemide are prototypes of potent short-acting agents which act in the thick ascending limb of the loop of Henle. These agents inhibit a $Na^+/K^+/2Cl^-$ transport system at the luminal side. (**Ref. 1,** pp. 721–722; **Ref. 2,** pp. 217–218)

856. (D) Spironolactone is an aldosterone antagonist which inhibits the cytoplasmic mineralocorticoid receptors. These agents are effective in mineralocorticoid excess whether primary or secondary. (**Ref. 1**, pp. 725–726; **Ref. 2**, pp. 222–223)

857. (C) Stimulation of α_2-adrenergic receptors inhibits insulin release from the islets of Langerhans. These pancreatic cells are richly innervated by adrenergic and cholinergic fibers. β_2-adrenergic blocking agents would also inhibit the release of insulin. Adrenergic receptor stimulation results in increased lipolysis and increased glycogenolysis. (**Ref. 1**, pp. 196, 1466; **Ref. 2**, p. 117)

858. (D) Stimulation of β_2-adrenergic receptors will stimulate insulin release. α_2-antagonists would be expected to increase insulin release. Vagal stimulation also increases the plasma levels of insulin. Serum potassium levels decrease when insulin is released or administered. (**Ref. 1**, pp. 196, 1466; **Ref. 2**, p. 117)

859. (D) Insulin levels are modulated by the autonomic nervous system (cholinergic and adrenergic) and by various neurotransmitters. However, oral ingestion of glucose is the principal stimulus for insulin release. It induces the release of gastrointestinal hormones. (**Ref. 1**, p. 1466; **Ref. 2**, pp. 117, 594)

860. (D) Tamoxifen is an estrogen inhibitor useful in the palliative treatment of postmenopausal women for breast cancer. Optimal activity is observed when estrogen levels are low since estradiol has a tenfold greater affinity for the estrogen receptor. (**Ref. 1**, p. 1256; **Ref. 2**, pp. 574, 583)

861. (A) The partial agonist estrogen, clomiphene, is used to stimulate ovulation in women with ovulation disorders. It causes palpable enlargement of the ovaries. In some patients ovarian cysts may occur. (**Ref. 1**, p. 1396; **Ref. 2**, p. 576)

862. (C) Antiandrogens which antagonize the residual androgen effects after orchiectomy have shown promising activity in prostatic tumors. (**Ref. 1**, p. 1428; **Ref. 2**, p. 784)

863. (B) Bromocriptine binds to dopamine receptors in the pituitary and inhibits prolactin secretion. It has been used effectively in causing regression of prolactin-secreting tumors. (**Ref. 1,** p. 1346; **Ref. 2,** pp. 246, 576)

864. (E) The essential androgen in the prostate is dihydrotestosterone. Inhibition of the 5α-reductase which converts testosterone to the dihydro-derivative has reduced the size of the prostate in benign prostatic hypertrophy. (**Ref. 1,** pp. 1427–1428; **Ref. 2,** p. 580)

865. (B) Prazosin is effective in lowering peripheral resistance. It accomplishes this by blocking α_1-adrenergic receptors and thus does not cause catecholamine-induced tachycardia as observed with the nonselective antagonists. (**Ref. 1,** p. 226; **Ref. 2,** p. 127)

866. (C) Timolol, pindolol, and atenolol are β-adrenergic blocking agents. Timolol is nonselective while atenolol is β_1-selective. Pindolol is nonselective; however, it is unique since it possesses partial agonist activity (intrinsic sympathomimetic activity). (**Ref. 1,** p. 234; **Ref. 2,** p. 131)

867. (A) Labetalol is a unique agent which blocks β-receptors nonselectively and α_1-receptors selectively. The β-receptor activity is approximately fivefold the α-receptor blocking activity. (**Ref. 1,** p. 236; **Ref. 2,** p. 133)

868. (D) Atropine is an antagonist of the muscarinic receptor, cimetidine is an antagonist of the histamine H_2-receptor. Prazosin is a selective α_1 blocker, norepinephrine is an agonist at β_1 and $\alpha_{1,2}$ receptors. Halothane acts via nonspecific interactions with nervous tissues. (**Ref. 1,** pp. 98, 110, 124, 237, 355; **Ref. 2,** pp. 152, 199, 226, 281–282, 899)

869. (D) Nondepolarizing neuromuscular blockade is characterized by fade in the strength of tetanus-stimulated muscle contraction and the reversibility of the block by an anticholinesterase. The muscle fibers retain their ability to respond to direct electrical stimulation. Fasciculations are characteristic of the blockade caused by depolarizing neuromuscular blocking agents. (**Ref. 1,** pp. 374–377; **Ref. 2,** pp. 170–172)

870. (E) Acetaminophen does not cause red cell hemolysis, and neither does lithium; that caused by α-methyldopa is immune in nature. Prednisone is used in the treatment of hemolytic anemia. Sulfonamides cause hemolytic anemia in G-6-PD-deficient persons. (**Ref. 1**, pp. 145, 407–408, 506, 664, 807; **Ref. 2**, pp. 420, 658, 791, 1052, 1456)

871. (B) Rebound hypertension may occur after the abrupt cessation of antihypertensive therapy with agents which act at α_2-receptors in the CNS or with β-adrenergic receptor blocking agents. Agents which cause vasodilation like nifedipine and nitroprusside, or diuretics like hydrochlorothiazide do not cause rebound hypertension. (**Ref. 1**, pp. 792, 797; **Ref. 2**, pp. 146, 150)

872. (C) Chlorpromazine (antipsychotic), imipramine (tricyclic antidepressant), and quinidine (antiarrhythmic) are all known to have antimuscarinic side effects. Scopolamine is an anticholinergic alkaloid. Digoxin has indirect effects resulting in increased vagal tone. (**Ref. 1**, pp. 152, 392, 409, 820, 848; **Ref. 2**, pp. 97, 180, 198, 403, 417)

873. (B) Metaproterenol and terbutaline are selective β_2-adrenergic agonists, while metoprolol is a selective β_1-adrenergic antagonist. Nadolol is a non-selective β-adrenergic antagonist. Dobutamine is a selective β_1 agonist. (**Ref. 1**, pp. 203–204, 234, 236; **Ref. 2**, pp. 117, 119, 131, 286)

874. (B) Most women do not have sufficient iron stores to handle the expansion of red cell mass during pregnancy. There is insufficient iron in mother's milk to accommodate the rapid growth of the breast-fed neonate. Premature infants and children during rapid growth periods may require iron. Except in cases of excessive blood loss, other persons do not require supplemental iron. (**Ref. 1**, p. 1287; **Ref. 2**, p. 452)

875. (D) The tachycardia is reflexly produced in response to the peripheral vasodilation caused by acetylcholine. It is mediated by cardiac β_1-adrenergic receptors which are blocked by propranolol. (**Ref. 1**, p. 124; **Ref. 2**, p. 86)

876. (A) Drug-induced parkinsonism must be treated with CNS-active anticholinergic agents. The use of agents which increase CNS dopamine levels is ineffective. Amantidine is useful in some patients. (**Ref. 1,** pp. 399, 479; **Ref. 2,** p. 402)

877. (A) Apomorphine or syrup of ipecac can be used to induce vomiting. Chlorpromazine has antiemetic effects. Dimenhydrinate and other H_1 blockers with anticholinergic properties inhibit emesis. Canabinoids have useful antiemetic properties in some patients undergoing cancer chemotherapy. Metoclopramide is an antiemetic widely used in cancer chemotherapy. (**Ref. 1,** pp. 56, 926, 928; **Ref. 2,** pp. 411, 508, 624)

878. (C) The thiazides, especially in high doses, cause an elevation in plasma lipids. All of the other agents have hypolipidemic effects. However, decisions to utilize these agents must be based on the pathology. (**Ref. 1,** pp. 721, 877–879; **Ref. 2,** pp. 221, 483–488)

879. (B) Only ranitidine blocks the histamine H_2-receptor, and is therefore effective in decreasing gastric acid secretion. All of the other agents are H_1 antagonists. They are useful in symptomatic treatment of immediate hypersensitivity reactions and also for motion sickness or to produce sedation as a sleep-aid. (**Ref. 1,** pp. 582–583, 587; **Ref. 2,** pp. 236–237)

880. (A) Quinidine has an atropine-like action on the atrioventricular (AV) node, causing a decrease in the nodal refractory period and reducing the degree of AV block. This allows the node to conduct more impulses from the fibrillating atrium to the ventricle, and may cause dangerous acceleration of the ventricular rate. Fibrillating atria frequently have mural thrombi, and if the conversion to normal sinus rhythm occurs, the thrombi may dislodge. Intravenous administration of quinidine routinely results in hypotension. Quinidine has a negative inotropic effect. (**Ref. 1,** pp. 851, 855; **Ref. 2,** pp. 198–199)

881. (C) Nifedipine and verapamil are both calcium channel antagonists. Only verapamil decreases atrioventricular nodal conduction, and this prevents the reflex tachycardia which may accompany systemic vasodilation. Nifedipine has much greater vasodilator action. Calcium channel blockers are contraindicated in digitalis intoxication. (**Ref. 1,** pp. 778–779; **Ref. 2,** pp. 171–172)

882. (**D**) Cefazolin is a first-generation cephalosporin with an extended duration of action. Cefoxitin is a second-generation cephalosporin, and thus has greater activity against gram-negative bacteria, especially anaerobes, and poorer activity against *S. aureus,* as compared to a first-generation cephalosporin. Both agents are minimally toxic to the kidney. (**Ref. 1,** pp. 1088–1090; **Ref. 2,** pp. 632–634)

883. (**C**) Tolbutamide stimulates pancreatic beta cells to release insulin. Thus, it is ineffective in diabetes mellitus of the juvenile onset type which is characterized by an absolute deficiency in insulin. The drug can cause alcohol intolerance and is metabolized to inactive products. Tolbutamide is thought to increase calcium ion influx as a consequence of binding to the ATP-sensitive K^+ channel. (**Ref. 1,** pp. 1484–1487)

884. (**A**) Prednisone (a synthetic glucocorticoid), azathioprine (an antemetabolite), methotrexate (an antimetabolite), and cyclosporin (an antibiotic), are all effective immunosuppressive agents and are used to prevent rejection of transplanted organs. Cisplatin is an antineoplastic agent, which is not an immunosuppressant. (**Ref. 1,** p. 1265; **Ref. 2,** p. 804)

885. (**B**) Ketamine is an excellent analgesic whose primary action is on the limbic system. Thus, respiration and somatic muscle tone are affected little. It also increases CSF pressure. This agent produces cardiovascular stimulation but is not routinely used because of the high incidence of postoperative psychic phenomena. (**Ref. 1,** p. 307; **Ref. 2,** p. 360)

886. (**A**) Vitamin D is structurally unrelated to parathyroid hormone and requires hydroxylation by both hepatic and renal enzymes for biologic activity. It promotes both bone decalcification and intestinal calcium absorption. Vitamin D is synthesized in the skin. (**Ref. 1,** p. 1510; **Ref. 2,** pp. 1533–1534)

887. (**E**) 1 is caffeine, 2 is nicotine, 3 is penicillin G, and 4 is morphine, all of which are natural products. 5 is succinylcholine, a synthetic neuromuscular blocking agent of the depolarizing type. (**Ref. 1,** pp. 180, 489, 619, 1066; **Ref. 2,** pp. 85, 283, 421, 627)

888. **(A)** Conjugation of morphine with glucuronic acid yields a compound more potent than morphine. Heroin is diacetylmorphine. One or both of the acetyl groups may be removed via hydrolysis to yield acetylmorphine and morphine, respectively. Codeine (methylmorphine) can be demethylated and appear as morphine in the urine. Apomorphine produces vomiting. Normeperidine is a metabolite or meperidine, which may have considerable toxicologic importance. (**Ref. 1,** pp. 497, 506–507; **Ref. 2,** p. 424)

889. **(C)** Nitroglycerin relaxes smooth muscle and is inactivated in the liver. Nitrite ion is the active form of the drug; however, it is liberated via nitroreductases located in the target organs. The resulting nitric oxide activates guanylyl cyclase leading to increased cGMP. There is no danger of explosion with the drug. (**Ref. 1,** pp. 768–769; **Ref. 2,** pp. 164–165)

890. **(D)** Succinylcholine, because it is hydrolyzed by pseudocholinesterases (butyrylcholinesterase), has a fleeting action lasting less than 5 minutes. The other agents have actions lasting several times as long. (**Ref. 1,** pp. 176–177; **Ref. 2,** pp. 372–374)

891. **(A)** Neostigmine and pyridostigmine are reversible acetylcholinesterase inhibitors which effectively increase the amount of acetylcholine in the synaptic cleft after a nerve impulse. This higher level of acetylcholine competes with the neuromuscular junction blocking agent for occupation of the acetylcholine receptor. Isoflurophate irreversibly inhibits acetylcholinesterase and is associated with severe toxicity. Scopolamine and ipratropium have no effect on neuromuscular junction blockade. Cholinesterase inhibitors may accentuate the phase I (depolarizing) block by succinylcholine but alleviate the phase II block. Tubocurarine is additive rather than antagonistic. (**Ref. 1,** p. 175; **Ref. 2,** p. 379)

892. **(D)** The acetylcholinesterase inhibitors have the effect of increasing both ganglionic transmission and parasympathetic effects. Increased respiratory secretions, antagonized by atropine, are a problem with acetylcholinesterase inhibitors. Vomiting is not common with acetylcholinesterase inhibitors administered to reverse neuromuscular junction blockade because their administration is not prolonged. The usual effects of the acetylcholinesterase inhibitors on the cardiovascular system are bradycardia and hypotension. In the airways increased acetylcholine induces contraction. (**Ref. 1,** p. 176; **Ref. 2,** p. 91)

893. (A) Hydralazine (antihypertensive), procainamide (class I_A antiarrhythmic), and phenytoin or primidone (anti-epileptics) are all associated with a lupus-like syndrome. (**Ref. 1,** pp. 442, 446, 800, 856; **Ref. 2,** pp. 153, 200, 335)

894. (C) Clonidine acts on an α_2-adrenergic receptors in the brain stem to reduce sympathetic outflow. Reserpine, although having profound CNS effects, owes its antihypertensive activity to depletion of peripheral nerves of their norepinephrine. Diazoxide and minoxidil act on the peripheral vasculature to reduce blood pressure. Captopril is an angiotensin-converting enzyme inhibitor. (**Ref. 1,** pp. 785, 791; **Ref. 2,** pp. 142, 144)

895. (A) Ergonovine and oxytocin effectively contract the uterus and frequently are administered to control bleeding. While $PGF\alpha_2$ does contract the uterus, its use is primarily in the induction of abortion. Ritordrine is a tocolytic, a β_2-selective adrenergic agonist used to delay labor. Magnesium sulfate may be used for seizure control or for delaying labor. Progesterone usually relaxes the uterus. (**Ref. 1,** pp. 948–950, 1399; **Ref. 2,** pp. 121, 246, 271, 525)

896. (D) Bacitracin is active against gram-positive cocci. While neomycin is active against *S. aureus,* group A streptococci are resistant. Polymyxin B is active only against gram-negative bacteria, while nystatin and griseofulvin are antifungal agents. (**Ref. 1,** pp. 1112, 1138, 1140, 1173, 1180; **Ref. 2,** pp. 670–671, 682, 872–873)

897. (B) Bradykinin dilates blood vessels, and leukotrienes LTC_4, LTD_4, and LTE_4 (collectively referred to as SRS-A) constrict the bronchi. Epinephrine constricts blood vessels and increases blood pressure by this mechanism and by direct inotropic action on the heart. It also relaxes bronchial smooth muscle. Epinephrine is ef-

fective in reducing mucous membrane congestion. The direct effect of histamine on the heart is a positive inotropic effect, but this effect is feeble unless a large dose of histamine is injected. (**Ref. 1,** pp. 217, 610; **Ref. 2,** pp. 121, 267)

898. (B) Carbon monoxide shifts the oxygen-hemoglobin dissociation curve to the left, thus oxygen is bound more tightly and is less readily released in tissues. CO combines with hemoglobin at 1/10 the rate of oxygen, but is dissociated from hemoglobin at 1/2400 the rate of oxygen, thus its affinity for hemoglobin is 240 times that of oxygen. (**Ref. 1,** pp. 1618–1619; **Ref. 2,** pp. 823–824)

899. (A) Water-soluble vitamins, such as B_1, B_{12}, and C, cause little toxicity, even in very high doses, because of very effective excretion. However, there is a widespread unfounded belief that large quantities of these water-soluble vitamins is beneficial. Fat-soluble vitamins, such as A, result in specific severe lesions when ingested in large doses. (**Ref. 1,** pp. 1524, 1558)

900. (B) Metaproterenol is selective for β_2-adrenergic receptors. Isoproterenol stimulates both β_1- and β_2-adrenergic receptors, while phenylephrine and methoxamine are selective α_1-adrenergic agonists. Dobutamine stimulates α and β receptors with some selectivity for β_1 over β_2. (**Ref. 1,** pp. 201–204, 207; **Ref. 2,** pp. 110, 117–118)

901. (E) Phenytoin can produce a wide range of side effects and toxicity including all of those listed with the exception of the last. Osteomalacia due to altered vitamin D metabolism and inhibition of intestinal calcium absorption may occur. (**Ref. 1,** pp. 441–442; **Ref. 2,** p. 335)

902. (E) Mannitol is filtered by the glomerulus and is negligibly reabsorbed. It is a nonelectrolyte that has no pharmacologic effects aside from its osmotic activity after intravenous injection. It must be administered intravenously. Oral administration can be used for elimination of gastrointestinal toxins. Total body water is reduced by osmotic diuretics, an action useful for managing increased intracranial pressure. (**Ref. 1,** pp. 714–715; **Ref. 2,** pp. 224–225)

903. (C) Trimethaphan, sodium nitroprusside, and diazoxide may produce the rapid decrease in blood pressure required in the treatment of a hypertensive emergency. Labetalol has become a first-line agent because it does not cause tachycardia. The fall in blood pressure caused by reserpine is rather slow in onset and may be preceded by an increase in blood pressure due to catecholamine release. (**Ref. 1,** p. 810; **Ref. 2,** p. 158; **Ref. 3,** p. 587)

904. (A) Filtration occurs when drugs diffuse through aqueous pores in membranes. Passive nonionic diffusion is the process by which compounds diffuse through the lipoidal portions of membranes. Facilitated diffusion, receptor-mediated endocytosis (pinocytosis), carrier-mediated transport, and active transport use carrier molecules specific for certain compounds and thus are subject to saturability. (**Ref. 1,** pp. 4–5; **Ref. 2,** pp. 2–4)

905. (D) Parkinson disease is characterized by decreased activity of dopaminergic neurons in the caudate nucleus. In the caudate, dopaminergic neurons are antagonized by muscarinic cholinergic neurons; thus in Parkinson disease, there is a relative excess of cholinergic activity. Muscarinic antagonists or a dopamine precursor (L-dopa) plus carbidopa may be employed. (**Ref. 1,** p. 464; **Ref. 2,** pp. 390–391)

906. (D) Curve B may represent the log dose-response curve of X in the presence of a noncompetitive antagonist or the curve of a partial agonist at the same receptor as X. Curve C may represent the log dose-response curve of X in the presence of a competitive antagonist or the curve of an agonist Y of lesser potency than X. (**Ref. 1,** p. 45; **Ref. 2,** p. 16)

907. (C) Methotrexate inhibits dihydrofolate reductase, the enzyme which catalyzes the conversion of folic acid to dihydrofolic acid. Thus, folic acid would be ineffective in reversing methotrexate toxicity, whereas dihydrofolic acid would be effective. Folinic acid (leucovorin) is a clinically useful derivative of dihydrofolic acid. (**Ref. 1,** p. 1223; **Ref. 2,** p. 776)

908. (D) Sulfonamides are broad spectrum and are effective against gram-positive and gram-negative organisms. They are bacteriostatic, antagonize the utilization of *p*-aminobenzoic acid by bacteria, and are extensively metabolized in vivo. (**Ref. 1,** pp. 1047–1048; **Ref. 2,** pp. 661–664)

909. (**A**) Spironolactone is a competitive antagonist of aldosterone binding to its renal receptor. Adverse effects include exacerbation of preexisting hyperkalemia and the production of androgenic effects as a result of its ability to bind to the testosterone receptor. (**Ref. 1,** pp. 726–727; **Ref. 2,** p. 556)

910. (**B**) Inhibitors of carbonic anhydrase raise the urinary pH and inhibit the excretion of hydrogen ions. Thus, a metabolic acidosis ensues. The effect on the eye is to reduce the formation of aqueous humor which lowers intraocular pressure, an effect useful in glaucoma patients. The prototypic carbonic anhydrase inhibitor is acetazolamide; acetohexamide is an oral hypoglycemic agent. Carbonic anhydrase inhibitors have limited usefulness in epilepsy and prevent mountain sickness. (**Ref. 1,** pp. 716–717; **Ref. 2,** p. 216)

911. (**D**) Clonidine acts in the CNS to lower blood pressure, and the blood pressure may rise above pretreatment values if the drug is abruptly withdrawn. It is recommended in combination with drugs acting via different mechanisms of action for moderate and severe hypertension. Orthostatic hypotension does not usually occur. (**Ref. 1,** pp. 792–793; **Ref. 2,** pp. 145–146)

912. (**A**) Tetracyclines are effective in vivo against the rickettsiae and *Chlamydia*. They have no effect on yeasts, fungi, or viruses. Gram-positive bacteria develop resistance to tetracyclines and thus tetracyclines are not used for this purpose since superior agents are available. (**Ref. 1,** p. 1117; **Ref. 2,** pp. 641–642)

913. (**C**) The depressant effects of ethyl alcohol are potentiated by drugs which also have CNS-depressant effects such as sedatives, narcotic analgesics, antianxiety and antipsychotic agents, and antihistamines. Ethanol will potentiate the gastrointestinal and the antiplatelet effects of aspirin. (**Ref. 1,** p. 376; **Ref. 2,** pp. 324–325)

914. (**B**) Morphine in therapeutic doses decreases GI motility and produces urinary retention, nausea, and miosis. It is a CNS depressant that also depresses respiration. (**Ref. 1,** p. 498; **Ref. 2,** pp. 428, 429)

915. (A) Mechlorethamine, melphalan, chlorambucil, and cyclophosphamide are alkylating agents. Vincristine blocks cell division via an inhibition of the formation of the mitotic spindle. (**Ref. 1,** pp. 1209–1211, 1237; **Ref. 2,** pp. 769, 778)

916. (C) Prednisone, having mineralocorticoid activity, exacerbates the potassium depletion caused by other agents, such as hydrochlorothiazide. Hypokalemia in the digitalized patient often causes arrhythmias, in this case manifested as palpitations. (**Ref. 1,** p. 1439; **Ref. 2,** pp. 550–551)

917. (E) Flattening of T waves is indicative of repolarization abnormalities such as would accompany hypokalemia, especially in the presence of digoxin. (**Ref. 1,** pp. 825, 832; **Ref. 2,** pp. 181, 184)

918. (D) Dexamethasone has no mineralocorticoid activity and thus does not cause potassium depletion. (**Ref. 1,** p. 1447; **Ref. 2,** p. 547)

919. (D) Triamterene is a potassium-sparing diuretic that when combined with a thiazide in therapy produces an effective diuresis without causing hypokalemia. (**Ref. 1,** p. 727; **Ref. 2,** p. 223)

920. (C) Glucocorticoid therapy can mimic Cushing syndrome in which central portions become obese while the limbs become wasted. Weight gain is thus common. (**Ref. 1,** p. 1448; **Ref. 2,** pp. 550–551)

921. (B) Most urinary tract infections acquired outside the hospital are due to *Escherichia coli*. Ampicillin is the initial drug of choice because it is usually effective against *E. coli* and nontoxic. However, sulfonamides would most likely be selected because dosing is twice a day. This improves patient compliance. The penicillins are usually ineffective, while chloramphenicol is too toxic, and both chloramphenicol and tetracycline have too broad a spectrum to warrant use in most urinary tract infections. (**Ref. 1,** pp. 1023, 1025; **Ref. 2,** pp. 621, 642, 646, 695–696, 699)

922. (D) Penicillin congeners and erythromycin are usually ineffective against *K. pneumoniae,* and cephalothin is the drug of choice. (**Ref. 1,** p. 1028; **Ref. 2,** p. 697)

923. (D) Ampicillin and tetracycline have too broad a spectrum and probably would permit the emergence of resistant organisms during long-term prophylactic therapy. Gentamicin and carbenicillin must be administered parenterally, and gentamicin is too toxic to warrant use in long-term prophylaxis. Nitrofurantoin is orally effective against most strains of *E. coli* and *K. pneumoniae* and many strains of *P. mirabilis,* and there is rarely a problem with emerging resistant strains. (**Ref. 1,** p. 1061; **Ref. 2,** pp. 686–687)

924. (E) Terbutaline is an excellent bronchodilator and is less cardiotoxic than either epinephrine or ephedrine because of selective action at β_2-adrenergic receptors. Cromolyn sodium is exclusively a prophylactic drug, and atropine is not used as a bronchodilator. (**Ref. 1,** p. 632; **Ref. 2,** pp. 285–287)

925. (D) Theophylline is orally effective, however its margin of safety is narrow. It is the best choice provided for bronchospasm prophylaxis. Ephedrine is not administered by inhalation, while isoproterenol is ineffective orally. Antihistamines such as chlorpheniramine are ineffective in asthma, while cromolyn sodium is more effective in cases of asthma with an atopic etiology. (**Ref. 1,** p. 633; **Ref. 2,** pp. 283–285)

References

1. Gilman AG, Rall TW, Nies AS & Taylor PT: *Goodman and Gilman's The Pharmacological Basis of Therapeutics,* 8th ed. Pergamon Press, New York, 1990.
2. Katzung BG: *Basic & Clinical Pharmacology,* 5th ed. Appleton & Lange, Norwalk, CT, 1992.
3. Bennett DR: *Drug Evaluations Annual 1994,* American Medical Association, Chicago, 1994.

6

Behavioral Sciences
Steven Steury

DIRECTIONS (Questions 926 through 943): Each of the questions or incomplete statements below is followed by five suggested answers or completions. Select the ONE that is best in each case.

---

926. A 78-year-old female is brought to the emergency room because the family felt "she was going crazy." On examination her temperature is 96°F, her face is somewhat puffy, her skin is dry, and her hair is coarse. Which of the following is the most likely diagnosis?
   A. hyperthyroidism
   B. hypothyroidism
   C. hyperparathyroidism
   D. hypoparathyroidism
   E. Addison disease

927. In Zborowski's classic evaluation of different ethnic reactions to pain, which of the following groups tended to be stoical and "objective"?
   A. Jews
   B. Italians
   C. Greeks
   D. "Old Americans"
   E. Mexican Americans

928. Diagnostic criteria for anorexia nervosa do NOT include
   A. disturbance of body image, eg, a feeling of being obese even when emaciated
   B. no known physical illness can explain the weight loss
   C. refusal to maintain body weight at or above a minimally normal weight for age and height (eg, weight loss leading to maintenance of body weight less than 85% of that expected)
   D. refusal to keep body weight over the minimal normal weight for subject's age and height
   E. irregular menstrual periods

929. Gender identity is firmly established and not easily changed by the end of which year of life?
   A. first
   B. second
   C. third
   D. fourth
   E. fifth

930. A 24-year-old female is reported to the police as a missing person by her parents. Her financé had recently broken their engagement, and she had been extremely despondent. When she was found by the police in another state, she was noted to be suffering from amnesia. Which of the following best characterizes her situation?
   A. extinction
   B. fugue
   C. auto-suggestion
   D. schizoid personality
   E. introversion

931. During rapid eye movement (REM) sleep there is
   A. regular respiration
   B. decreased heart rate and blood pressure
   C. muscle atonia
   D. penile erection
   E. none of the above

932. Each of the statements listed below is true of Alzheimer disease EXCEPT
   A. Down syndrome predisposes to Alzheimer disease
   B. the disorder is equally common in both men and women
   C. in rare cases, primary degenerative dementia of the Alzheimer type is inherited as a dominant trait
   D. the brain is atrophied, with widened cortical sulci and enlarged cerebral ventricles
   E. between 10% and 20% of the population over the age of 65 is estimated to have Alzheimer disease

933. In psychosexual development, the last phase is
   A. oral
   B. phallic
   C. latency
   D. genital
   E. anal

934. All of the following are typical autonomic side effects of antipsychotic drugs EXCEPT
   A. constipation
   B. dry mouth and throat
   C. postural hypertension
   D. urinary retention
   E. blurred vision

935. In a patient with organic personality syndrome, a marked change in behavior or personality involving at least one of the following would be found, with the EXCEPTION of
   A. impairment in impulse control
   B. marked apathy and indifference
   C. clouding of consciousness
   D. suspiciousness or paranoid ideation
   E. emotional lability

936. Which of the following is NOT a characteristic of Down syndrome?
   A. marked mental retardation
   B. increased muscle tone
   C. upward-slanting eyes
   D. small, round head
   E. protruding tongue

937. Manifestations of phenylketonuria include all of the following EXCEPT
   A. mental retardation
   B. fair hair and skin of northern Europeans
   C. eczema
   D. hypoactivity
   E. "musty" body odor

938. About what percentage of men remain sexually active in their 80s?
   A. 10
   B. 20
   C. 33
   D. 60
   E. 75

939. Social attachment in man reaches its peak at
   A. 7 months
   B. 1 year
   C. 18 months
   D. 2 years
   E. 7 years

940. Diagnostic criteria for sleepwalking disorder include each of the following EXCEPT
   A. there must be evidence that the episode occurred during REM sleep and that there is abnormal electrical brain activity during sleep
   B. the individual has a blank, staring face while sleepwalking and is relatively unresponsive to the efforts of those trying to communicate with him; he can be awakened only with great difficulty

C. the individual has amnesia for what happened during the sleepwalking episode when he is awakened

D. there is no impairment of mental activity or behavior (although there may initially be a short period of confusion) within several minutes of awakening from the sleepwalking episode

E. there are repeated episodes of arising from bed during sleep and walking about for several minutes to a half-hour, usually occurring during the first third of the major sleep episode

941. All of the following are true of Gestalt therapy EXCEPT that it

A. is a type of psychotherapy that stresses treatment of the whole person

B. was developed by Frederic S. Perls

C. has as its immediate goal the restoration of full awareness to the patient

D. highlights the sensory awareness of the subject's past remembrances and future expectations rather than the present experiences

E. came into existence in the 1960s

942. A 68-year-old male with a diagnosis of "organic brain disease" is noted to have a positive RPR (rapid plasma reagin) on routine blood screening. A VDRL and FTA-ABS are also positive. Which of the following would be the next logical step in his evaluation?

A. CAT scan

B. lumbar puncture

C. cerebral arteriography

D. pneumoencephalography

E. none of the above

943. According to DSM-IV, which of the following statements concerning conversion disorders is NOT true?
  A. the main disturbance is a loss or change in physical functioning which suggests a physical disorder
  B. psychological factors are felt to be causally involved in the symptom
  C. the symptom is not under voluntary control
  D. the symptom cannot, even after appropriate investigation, be explained by a known physical disorder of pathophysiological mechanism
  E. the symptom is limited to pain

DIRECTIONS (Questions 944 through 972): Each group of questions below consists of lettered headings followed by a list of numbered words, phrases, or statements. For each numbered word, phrase, or statement, select the ONE lettered heading that is most closely associated with it. Each lettered heading may be selected once, more than once, or not at all.

Questions 944 through 947

  A. Bender (visual-motor) Gestalt Test
  B. Sentence Completion Test
  C. Thematic Apperception Test (TAT)
  D. Rorschach technique

944. Most useful for revealing personality dynamics

945. May be used to tap specific conflict areas; generally reveals more conscious, overt attitudes and feelings

946. Useful for detecting psychomotor difficulties correlated with brain damage

947. Especially revealing of personality structure; most widely used projective technique

Questions 948 through 950

    A. Gordon Allport
    B. Erik Erikson
    C. Paul Schilder

948. Ego development and psychosexual development

949. Group psychotherapy combining social and psychoanalytic principles

950. Group relations theory; interrelationship between group therapy and social psychology

Questions 941 through 954

    A. avoidant personality disorder
    B. borderline personality disorder
    C. antisocial personality disorder
    D. passive aggressive personality disorder

951. Resistance expressed indirectly through procrastination, dawdling, "forgetfulness"

952. Desires affection and acceptance; hypersensitive to rejection

953. Vandalism, truancy, running away from home before age 15; more common in males

954. Engages in potentially self-damaging acts ranging from gambling to suicide; more commonly diagnosed in women

Questions 955 through 958

    A. Huntington chorea
    B. PKU (phenylketonuria)
    C. Ganser syndrome
    D. parkinsonism

955. A rare disorder most frequently seen in prisoners, in which the subjects respond to questions with completely incorrect and often ludicrous replies, even though the individual has comprehended the sense of the question

956. Rhythmical muscle tremors, referred to as pill rolling, with spasticity and rigid movements, droopy posture, propulsive gait, and masklike facies; it is normally found in later life because of arteriosclerotic alterations in the basal ganglia

957. A congenital metabolic disorder which, if left untreated in infancy, results in mental retardation

958. A progressive hereditary central nervous system disorder characterized by jerking movements and progressive mental decline

Questions 959 and 960

    A. illusion
    B. hallucination

959. A false sensory perception lacking a concrete external stimulus

960. A false perception or misinterpretation of a true sensory stimulus

Questions 961 through 964   (Ego mechanisms of defense are defined as various automatic, involuntary, unconsciously instituted psychological activities that are activated in response to signals of anxiety or other unpleasurable feelings, such as quiet. [**Ref. 6,** p. 126])

    A. reaction formation
    B. displacement
    C. introjection
    D. projection

961. An unconscious defense mechanism which transfers the affective part of an unacceptable idea or object

962. An unconscious defense mechanism in which one attributes to someone else the ideas, thoughts, feelings, and impulses that are part of one's own inner perceptions

963. A defense mechanism where an unacceptable impulse is transformed into its opposite

964. A defense mechanism in which a psychic representation of an object is integrated into one's own ego system

Questions 965 through 968   (In DSM-IV the essential feature of a specific phobia is marked and persistent fear of clearly discernible circumscribed objects or situations. Exposure to the phobic stimulus almost always provokes an immediate anxiety response. Adults recognize that their fear is excessive or unreasonable. Specific phobias, formerly designated as simple phobias, are in the anxiety disorders in DSM-IV. Five subtypes are identified as animal type, natural environmental type, blood-injection type, situational type, and other type. [DSM-IV, p. 405])

    A. fear of pain
    B. fear of heights
    C. fear of strangers
    D. fear of leaving home

965. Acrophobia

966. Algophobia

967. Agoraphobia

968. Xenophobia

Questions 969 through 972

    A. motor aphasia
    B. receptive aphasia
    C. nominal aphasia
    D. syntactical aphasia

969. One is unable to arrange words in their proper sequences

970. One is unable to speak, but is still able to comprehend

971. One has difficulty in finding an object's proper name

972. One is unable to understand the meaning of words or comprehend their own language

---

DIRECTIONS (Questions 973 through 983): Each set of lettered headings below is followed by a list of numbered words or phrases. For each numbered word or phrase select

    A if the item is associated with **A** only
    B if the item is associated with **B** only
    C if the item is associated with both **A** and **B**
    D if the item is associated with neither **A** nor **B**

Questions 973 through 978 (The term "organic" is replaced—in DSM-IV but not yet on the wards of hospitals—with "cognitive impairment." Delirium and dementia, usually associated with organicity, is now a cognitive impairment. They are the most commonly encountered psychiatric disorders in general hospitals. Delirium is usually acute and fluctuating and is characterized by an altered state of consciousness. It may be accompanied by defects in attention, concentration, thinking, memory, and goal-directed behavior. The most readily obvious delirium is alcohol intoxication. Dementia is usually gradual in onset with multiple cognitive defects. The level of awareness and mental alertness is not disturbed in early or mild dementia. The earliest impairment of dementia is poor memory—both inability to learn new information and to recall.)

    A. delirium
    B. dementia
    C. both
    D. neither

973. Memory impairment

974. Onset is usually insidious

975. Stable symptoms which do not typically fluctuate

976. Perceptual disturbances

977. Most commonly found in persons age 30 to 50

978. Sleep–wake cycle is always disrupted

Questions 979 through 983

    A. opioid withdrawal
    B. cocaine intoxication
    C. both
    D. neither

979. Pupillary dilation

980. Bradycardia

981. Fever

982. Nausea and vomiting

983. Perspiration

DIRECTIONS (Questions 984 through 999): For each of the questions or incomplete statements below, ONE or MORE of the answers or completions given is correct. Select

A   if only 1, 2, and 3 are correct
B   if only 1 and 3 are correct
C   if only 2 and 4 are correct
D   if only 4 is correct
E   if all are correct

984. Which of the following disorders fall under the classification of paraphilias?
   1. exhibitionism
   2. sexual sadism
   3. zoophilia
   4. transvestism

985. Marijuana cause all of the following EXCEPT
   1. muscle relaxation
   2. decreased heart rate
   3. nausea, vomiting, and diarrhea on occasion
   4. euphoria

986. Euphoria may be induced by drugs such as
   1. opiates
   2. amphetamines
   3. alcohol
   4. reserpine

987. Mental status evaluation includes the subject's
   1. general physical health
   2. patterns of speech
   3. physical appearance
   4. general affect

988. Which of the following statements is NOT correct concerning delusional disorder
   1. it always interferes with other components of the subject's psychic function
   2. it rarely develops logically from the distortion of a real occurrence

3. it is usually short term
4. it is typified by complicated, very elaborate systematical delusions

989. A person diagnosed as having a histrionic personality disorder may
 1. crave activity and excitement
 2. self-dramatize through exaggerated expression of emotions
 3. overreact to minor events
 4. incessantly draw attention to him or herself

990. The limbic system is comprised of all EXCEPT the
 1. hippocampus
 2. septum pellucidum
 3. cingulum
 4. thalamus

991. Empathy involves all EXCEPT
 1. an awareness of thoughts and feelings expressed by another person
 2. an intellectual processing of information elicited
 3. a response of some type that conveys an understanding of the other person
 4. the empathizer, in effect, "steps into the other person's shoes" and remains there

992. Which of the following is NOT correct?
 1. lithium is an effective antimanic drug
 2. lithium is safe for use in pregnancy
 3. lithium effects on the kidneys (lithium nephropathy) are reversible
 4. lithium side effects such as nausea or diarrhea may persist even at therapeutic levels

993. In the human infant, inborn reflexes include
 1. sucking
 2. grasping
 3. rooting
 4. Babinski

		Directions Summarized		
A	**B**	**C**	**D**	**E**
1, 2, 3	1, 3	2, 4	4	All are
only	only	only	only	correct

994. Psychoanalysis is
1. a system of psychologic therapy developed by Freud
2. the most extensive, intensive, and costly form of psychotherapy available
3. a form of insight therapy
4. a suitable form of treatment for most patients

995. In some humans, REM-state deprivation leads to
1. heightened anxiety
2. decreased appetite
3. increased hostility and irritability
4. improved memory ability

996. Patients with which of the following genetic disorders may have schizophreniclike manifestations?
1. Niemann–Pick disease
2. homocystinuria
3. acute intermittent porphyria
4. Wilson disease

997. Which of the following statements are true concerning superego?
1. it is associated with the internalization of ethical standards of the society in which the subject lives, and it develops by identification with parental attitudes
2. it is one of the three components of the psychic apparatus
3. Freud developed the concept of the superego to describe psychic functions which are expressed in conscience, moral attitudes, and a sense of guilt
4. it is chiefly conscious

998. During orgasm, all occur EXCEPT
1. carpopedal spasm
2. hyperventilation
3. increased blood pressure
4. voluntary vaginal contractions

999. The Wernicke–Korsakoff syndrome
   1. is due to a lack of vitamin B₁
   2. is most often found in chronic alcoholics
   3. involves short-term memory impairment which is irreversible
   4. is four times more common in males than in females

DIRECTIONS (Questions 1000 through 1012): This section consists of a situation, followed by a series of questions. Study the situation, and select the ONE best answer to each question following it.

CASE HISTORY (Question 1000) Bill, a 27-year-old law student, is so compulsive about neatness it drives his roommates nuts. Bill says he knows it bothers his roommates when he makes them get up at 7:00 am on Saturdays to clean the apartment, but he says, "it is a good habit for all of them."

1000. Bill's compulsiveness is probably evidence of
   A. obsessive–compulsive disorder
   B. obsessive–compulsive traits
   C. obsessive–compulsive personality disorder
   D. disorder of brain serotonin system

CASE HISTORY (Question 1001) A 32-year-old single businessman stated that at age 11 his voice "cracked" during an audition for a school play and people laughed at him. He became very anxious when he had to speak in class. He gradually avoided any situation in which he might be called upon or observed, even to answer a roll call. His avoidance of professional meetings were interfering with his work.

1001. The diagnosis for this businessman is
   A. generalized anxiety disorder
   B. specific phobia
   C. social phobia
   D. panic disorder
   E. depersonalization

CASE HISTORY (Question 1002)   Patrick Patient is a 37-year-old rocket scientist who has had diabetes for three years. You are about to suggest he find another doctor because you are so annoyed with him. He is a complaining whiner who is late for his appointments. He procrastinates and delays making future appointments. You have talked with him and his wife about his behavior and they both agree he chronically has had problems with bosses, doctors, and teachers. Although he seems to be very bright, his projects at work are often turned in late. His wife says "the more Pat's supervisor pressures him to hurry up, the slower he gets."

1002. The most likely personality disorder diagnosis is
   A. schizoid personality disorder
   B. schizotypal personality disorder
   C. obsessive–compulsive disorder
   D. passive–aggressive disorder
   E. borderline disorder

CASE HISTORY (Question 1003)   Susan's lover, Judy, was killed in an automobile accident a month after Susan was gang-raped because her supervisor at the factory thought "It would be good if she had real sex." About a week after the death, Susan's friends first noticed that her affect was inappropriate. She giggled whenever she passed a portrait of Judy. Her friends had trouble following her conversation; a psychiatrist friend thought she had loose associations. She could not work because she couldn't follow instructions and bowed on her knees facing north every 15 minutes. (She had been transferred to another location in the company.) She thought Judy was controlling every move she made. She believed the chief of personnel received a broadcast of her thoughts and knew everything she wanted. After a three-day hospitalization and two weeks of outpatient treatment with a neuroleptic, she was "back to her old self." At a follow-up visit five years later, Susan reported she has been in a good relationship for three years and was doing well at her job. She is now a supervisor at another factory. A careful history revealed that the entire illness was limited to less than a month.

1003. The most likely diagnosis of her illness is
   A. homosexuality
   B. schizophrenia
   C. brief psychotic disorder

D. substance-induced psychotic disorder

E. adjustment disorder with mixed mood

CASE HISTORY (Question 1004) You interview Dave Depressed, a 27-year-old recently married stock broker who says he always feels "on the unhappy side." His developmental history reveals the death of his mother at age 6 followed by an increase in his father's drinking and, as Dave puts it, "some sexual abuse from my uncle from about 10 to 12 years of age." He says he has had trouble sleeping for several years. He is always down and fatigued, and feels he will never get better. Despite his troubles, he makes a good living. He is happy he is married and thinks they will have a "good enough" life together. He has recently seen his physician who says "everything is fine." He is on no medications.

1004. Based on the above information, the most likely diagnosis is

A. adjustment reaction with depressed mood

B. dysthymia

C. major depression

D. psychotic depression

CASE HISTORY (Question 1005) In your case assessment of Fred Farthing, a 38-year-old unemployed physician, you determine that his panic disorder started 12 years ago. He seemed to self-medicate his symptoms of panic with alcohol. This self-medication was followed by dependence and this led to several driving-while-intoxicated arrests and suspension of his medical license. He is now depressed. Your understanding is that the panic disorder is the primary problem and that his alcohol dependence and depression are secondary.

1005. You would, therefore, give Dr. Farthing

A. a single DSM-IV Axis I diagnosis

B. three DSM-IV Axis I diagnoses

C. a single DSM-IV Axis I and two Axis II diagnoses

D. two DSM-IV Axis I and one Axis II diagnoses

CASE HISTORY (Questions 1006 through 1008) Jane Smithgate is a 24-year-old medical student who has enjoyed "social drinking" for about 8 years. She has noticed that it now takes her about 4 to 5 beers to get "a buzz." "Before medical school, I would get a buzz with 1 or 2 beers. I guess I am drinking more now."

1006. Ms. Smithgate describes
    A. dependence
    B. tolerance
    C. withdrawal

1007. Based on the data available, does Jane Smithgate meet the DSM-IV criteria of substance dependence?
    A. yes
    B. no
    C. insufficient data

1008. If Jane Smithgate were to use morphine as her drug of choice, and met the criteria for opioid dependence (DSM-IV, 304.00) what withdrawal symptoms might be expected?
    A. hallucinations, tachycardia, and psychosis
    B. hallucinations, tachycardia, psychosis, and seizures
    C. anxiety, restlessness, and vomiting
    D. increased alertness, attention, and concentration
    E. paranoia, suspiciousness, and psychosis

CASE HISTORY (Questions 1009 and 1010) Cathy and Sam were disappointed in their marriage-night lovemaking. Cathy felt devalued and unloved after she noticed Sam grimacing and scowling just at the time he had his orgasm. Sam felt that Cathy lost her arousal during their lovemaking. He felt Cathy's clitoris enlarge at first but then it seemed to get smaller. He also saw that her nipple erection decreased soon after they began making love.

1009. What can you tell Cathy about Sam's grimacing and scowling?
    A. Sam probably was worried about pleasing her
    B. Sam was nervous

C. Sam was not happy with their lovemaking; she should try to please him

D. facial grimacing or scowling is the result of normal involuntary muscle contractions at the time of orgasm in both men and women

1010. What can you tell Sam about Cathy's apparent loss of signs of sexual excitation?

A. Cathy probably was worried about pleasing him

B. Cathy was nervous

C. Cathy was not happy with their lovemaking; he should try to please her

D. just before orgasm the clitoris retracts under the hood or pupuce and may appear smaller. It did not become smaller from loss of arousal. Likewise the nipple erection may seem to diminish as the areoa enlarges around the nipple. In fact the nipple remains erect until after orgasm.

CASE HISTORY (Questions 1011 and 1012) Seven-month-old Tommy is playing happily with a new toy on the floor in his living room. His uncle hides the toy beneath a blanket.

1011. Most likely Tommy will

A. cry until his uncle retrieves it

B. make no attempt to retrieve the toy

C. reach out to remove the blanket

D. be severely emotionally traumatized

1012. According to Erik Erikson, the main task of the infant is to

A. establish a sense of trust

B. develop appropriate schema

C. differentiate from the mother

D. learn to read the mother's cues

DIRECTIONS (Questions 1013 through 1018): Each of the questions or incomplete statements below is followed by five suggested answers or completions. Select the ONE that is best in each case.

1013. According to Kohlberg, most children under 10 make decisions based on
   A. the consequences of their actions
   B. societal rules and norms
   C. the laws of a culture
   D. an implicit understanding of right and wrong
   E. religious training

1014. When interviewing a depressed adolescent, the physician should
   A. never bring up the topic of suicide
   B. inquire directly about suicidal thoughts
   C. inquire indirectly about suicidal thoughts
   D. simply ask the parents about suicidal ideation
   E. focus on the sexual history

1015. Research has shown that early physical maturation among boys often leads to
   A. decreased social status
   B. decreased athletic abilities
   C. increased leadership among peers
   D. increased social adjustment difficulties
   E. poor academic performance

1016. Menarche roughly begins between
   A. 9 and 11
   B. 11 and 14
   C. 14 and 16
   D. 16 and 18
   E. before 8

1017. The etiology of dissociative identity disorder (multiple personality disorder) is thought to be
   A. frontal lobe damage
   B. childhood autism
   C. trauma during childhood

D. lack of formation of basic trust in infancy
E. serotonin dysfunction

1018. The treatment of choice for dissociative identity disorder (multiple personality disorder) is
A. neuroleptics
B. antidepressants
C. behavior therapy
D. insight-oriented psychotherapy
E. carbamazepine

Behavioral Sciences

Answers and Comments

926. (B) Many endocrinopathies, including hypothyroidism, can result in mental changes, and the possible presence of such disorders should be considered in patients presenting with psychiatric manifestations. Severe cases of hypothyroidism have resulted in what has been referred to as "myxedema madness." The symptoms may include depressed affect and paranoia psychosis. (**Ref. 2,** p. 772)

927. (D) Zborowski's classical evaluation of different ethnic reactions to pain revealed that "Old Americans" tended to be more stoical and objective in their responses; Irish more often denied the existence of pain; and Jewish and Italian patients showed more emotional response to pain. (**Ref. 6,** p. 93)

928. (C) Anorexia nervosa is a misnomer because loss of appetite is rare in this disorder. This disorder is more prevalent in industrialized societies, where food is abundant. More than 90% occur in females. The incidence appears to have increased in the past few decades. The diagnosis requires a *refusal* to maintain weight above 85% of expected for height and age. In post-menarche women at least three consecutive menstrual cycles are skipped, eg, there is amenorrhea. (**Ref. 1,** pp. 539–545)

929. (B) Gender identity is demonstrated by the child's ability to label his or her own sex correctly. Most children have developed a sense of gender identity by age 2. Gender stability, the understanding that you stay the same gender throughout life, develops after age 2. In unusual cases of ambiguous genitalia, sexual reassignment should not be attempted after gender identity is established. (**Ref. 9,** p. 27)

930. (B) Fugue is one of the dissociative disorders in which a person suddenly and unexpectedly travels away from their home or workplace; is unable to recall their past; and assumes a new identity or is confused about their identity. After recovery from the fugue—when patients try to understand what happened—there is no recall of what took place during the episode. Fugues are associated with severe stress; the case described would be very unusual. Fugue is more frequent—but still not common—in combat or during natural disasters. (**Ref. 7,** p. 378)

931. (D) REM sleep is marked by vivid dreams and sexual arousal. Respiration, blood pressure, and heart rate are variable. Electromyogram studies show muscle atonia with fine muscle twitches during REM sleep. When a subject is awakened during non-REM sleep the reported thoughts are more organized and not as complex and vivid as in dreaming. Hartman speculated that dreams allow one to work through personal problems. (**Ref. 9,** pp. 420–421)

932. (E) Only 2 to 4% of the population over the age of 65 is estimated to have Alzheimer disease, although the prevalence increases with increasing age, particularly after age 75. Clinically, Alzheimer disease progresses through 3 stages involving speech, later cognition, and finally body control, eg, loss of sphincter control and control of limbs. (**Ref. 5,** pp. 280–281)

933. (D) Psychosexual development is broadly defined as the maturation and development of the sexuality of a person throughout the life cycle. In psychoanalysis, psychosexual development specifically refers to a series of dynamic and crucial developmental stages that each person goes through and that influence basic personality traits in later life. The stages or phases in order of progression are oral, anal, phallic, latency, and genital. (**Ref. 9,** pp. 4, 20–21, 31, 50)

934. **(C)** Postural (orthostatic) hypotension occurs most often during the first few days of treatment, and most patients readily develop a tolerance to it. Other autonomic side effects may include cutaneous flushing, paralytic ileus, miosis, mental confusion, and mydriasis. (**Ref. 7,** pp. 516–517)

935. **(C)** There would be no clouding of consciousness, as occurs in delirium, in a patient with organic personality syndrome. Major reported organic insults include head trauma, heavy metal poisoning, multiple sclerosis, neoplasm, seizure disorders, and vascular disease. (**Ref. 7,** pp. 108, 110)

936. **(B)** Poor muscle tone is characteristic of Down syndrome. In addition to the features noted, subjects with this syndrome are more prone to develop ocular and cardiac abnormalities. Most cases of Down syndrome are associated with trisomy-21, which is usually an environmental rather than a genetic abnormality. (**Ref. 2,** p. 1027)

937. **(D)** Manifestations of phenylketonuria include mental retardation, fair hair and skin, eczema, hyperactivity, and a musty odor to the body. The recessive disorder is treated with a phenylalanine-free diet which may prevent damage to the brain. The disease is transmitted as a simple recessive autosomal Mendelian trait and occurs in about 1 in every 10,000 to 15,000 live births. Patients with this disorder are known to be hyperactive. (**Ref. 2,** p. 1028)

938. **(B)** An important factor that affects the expression of sexuality in old age includes the availability of a suitable partner. Frequency of sexual relationships declines after age 60, but many men and women in their 80s and 90s are sexually active. About 20% of women in their 60s remain sexually active. Relatively few women in their 80s have available sexual partners and therefore are less active. (**Ref. 9,** p. 91)

939. (A) A peak time for social attachment is at about 7 months. This is easily observed. Most children respond fearfully to strangers—thus the term stranger anxiety. Around the age of 7 months, some children show brief wariness toward strangers. Others show striking withdrawal such as crying or clinging to parents. From age 12 to 24 months, children show some stranger anxiety but usually they are less clingy and show less regression. (**Ref. 9,** p. 28)

940. (A) Sleepwalking is a sequence of complex behaviors that are initiated in the first third of the night in non-REM sleep. Sleepwalking usually begins between the ages of 4 to 8. It is more common in boys than girls and about 15 percent of children have an occasional episode. As in other disturbances, a biopsychosocial model is helpful in understanding sleepwalking: it occurs in families; a minor neurological abnormality probably underlies the condition; episodes are more frequent in times of stress and anxiety. (**Ref. 2,** p. 712)

941. (D) Frederick "Fritz" Perls (1893–1970) applied Gestalt Theory to a type of therapy that emphasizes the current experiences of the patient "in the here and now." This therapy has little concern for past remembrances, future wishes, or expectations. A gestalt, a whole, both includes and goes beyond the sum of smaller independent events. (**Ref. 2,** p. 258)

942. (B) A lumbar puncture for evaluation of the cerebrospinal fluid is indicated in patients with syphilis, and is mandatory in patients with possible neurosyphilis. Elevated white blood cells and protein and positive VDRL are consistent with a diagnosis of neurosyphilis which can result in psychiatric symptoms. Neurosyphilis has become rare. However, cases are now seen in patients with AIDS. The disease affects the frontal lobes resulting in personality changes. Delusions of grandeur develop in 10 to 20% of affected patients. (**Ref. 3,** p. 370)

943. (E) The DSM-IV criteria specifically excludes disorders limited to pain or sexual dysfunction from the diagnosis of conversion disorder. Conversion disorders produce symptoms or deficits affecting voluntary motor or sensory function that suggest a neurological or other medical condition. The symptoms are not intentionally produced or feigned, distinguishing this disorder from factitious disorder and malingering. The disorder is accompanied by loss of functioning in social, occupational, or other important areas of functioning and is often accompanied by marked distress. La Belle indifference, eg, emotional indifference to the symptoms, is no longer thought to be a distinguishing feature of this disorder. (**Ref. 1,** pp. 452–457)

944. **(C)** The TAT was designed by Henry Murray and Christiana Morgan in 1943 and contains a series of pictures which the subject uses to create a story. Because pictures are used—even though they are ambiguous—the test stimuli is more structured than the ink blots of the Rorschach test. The TAT has been helpful as a tool for judging motivational aspects of behavior. It is usually not used as a basis for making a DSM-IV diagnosis. (**Ref. 2,** p. 229)

945. **(B)** The Sentence Completion Test responses have been shown to be useful in creating a level of confidence about predictions of overt behavior and may be used to tap specific conflict areas of interest. Usually 75 to 100 sentence stems—such as "I like . . ." or "My mother is . . ."—are given to a subject who is asked to write or say what first comes to mind. The usefulness of the test depends on the openness and cooperation of the subject. (**Ref. 2,** p. 229)

946. **(A)** The Bender gestalt visual motor test was designed by Lauretta Bender in 1930, at Bellevue Psychiatric Hospital, and is used for testing visual-motor coordination in both children and adults. The Bender Visual-Motor Gestalt is used most frequently with adults as a screening device for signs of organic dysfunction. (**Ref. 2,** p. 232)

947. **(D)** The Rorschach technique was created by a Swiss psychiatrist, Hermann Rorschach, who in the early 1900s experimented with obscure inkblots. Surveys have shown this to be one of the most frequently used individual tests in clinical settings throughout the country. This test is useful as an aid in diagnosis. There is a high reliability among experienced clinicians who adminis-

ter the test. It is extremely useful in eliciting psychodynamic formulations, defense mechanisms, and subtle disorders of thinking. (**Ref. 2,** p. 228)

948. **(B)** Erik Erikson (1902–1994) is responsible for making major contributions to the psychoanalytic concept of ego development and psychosexual development. Erikson built onto Freud's theories by concentrating on the child's development beyond latency. He formulated a theory of development that covers the entire span for the life cycle from infancy and childhood through old age and senescence. (**Ref. 2,** p. 260)

949. **(D)** Paul Schilder is associated with using group psychotherapy which combined social and psychoanalytic principles. This work was conducted in the 1930s at Bellevue Hospital in New York. He used the technique of free association and revealed how thoughts and feelings of one subject can stimulate associated thoughts and feelings in another. (**Ref. 7,** p. 1404)

950. **(A)** Gordon W. Allport (1897–1967) was an academician credited with group relations theory involving the interrelationship between group therapy and social psychology. Allport was first to teach the psychology of personality at an American college and was instrumental in establishing the department of social relations. (**Ref. 7,** p. 462)

951. **(D)** Passive–aggressive personality disorder is not a specific DSM-IV disorder. Its traits, however, are well known. A pattern is reflective of passive and indirect resistance to authority, responsibility, and obligations. Associated symptoms may include irritability, whining, discontent. Anger is usually expressed indirectly through resistance: delays, lack of responsiveness, and procrastination. The passive–aggressive patient may undermine his own best interest in medical treatment by failing to carry out treatment plans or procedures. (**Ref. 7,** p. 191)

952. **(A)** An avoidant personality disorder is associated with a desire for affection and acceptance, hypersensitivity to rejection, humiliation, or shame, and low self-esteem. The schizoid personality disordered patient is indifferent to others, which distinguished the two personalities. After initial fearful interactions, these patients often develop a good alliance with their physicians. (**Ref. 7,** p. 189)

953. **(C)** The antisocial patient typically lacks empathy, social responsibility, guilt, and a sense of moral and interpersonal responsibility. A veneer of charm may mask disregard for the regrets and feelings of others; these patients are interested only in meeting their own needs. Repetitive criminal behavior, fights, and impulsivity are common. Antisocial persons may be quite successful having obtained power and position by ruthless exploitation of others and carefully concealing lying and dishonesty. These patients are among the most difficult to treat psychiatrically. (**Ref. 7,** p. 187)

954. **(B)** Borderline personality disordered patients, more often found in women than in men, demonstrate a behavioral pattern of intense and chaotic relationships with fluctuating and extreme attitudes toward others. They demonstrate the defense mechanism of splitting. They may view themselves or others as "all good," or "all bad." Their lives and relationships are chaotic and unstable. Alcoholism, drug abuse, and suicide attempts are common. Depression and anxiety may be treated by psychopharmacology; the underlying personality disorder requires long-term individual psychotherapy. Therapy is difficult because of the patient's difficulty with a trusting, permanent, close relationship. (**Ref. 7,** pp. 187–188)

955. **(C)** Ganser syndrome is a rare disorder most frequently seen in prisoners in which the subjects respond to questions with incorrect and often ludicrous replies, even though the individual has comprehended the sense of the question. Often the answers are approximate, eg, when asked to multiply 4×10, the patient answers "41." This disorder is classified as a dissociative disorder because it is commonly associated with amnesia, fugue, perceptual disturbances, and conversion symptoms. The syndrome was previously classified as a factitious disorder. (**Ref. 2,** p. 651)

956. **(D)** Parkinsonism manifestations include rhythmical muscle tremors referred to as pill rolling, with spasticity and rigid movements, droopy posture, propulsive gait, and mask-like faces. It is normally found in later life because of arteriosclerotic alterations in

the basal ganglia. Depression and dementia are more common in Parkinson disease patients than is expected by chance or explainable by the psychosocial factors of the disease. (**Ref. 2,** p. 110)

957. **(B)** Patients with PKU (phenylketonuria) are usually normal at birth. High PKU levels are toxic and lead to mental retardation. However, if the disease is not recognized and treated, the infant, during the first year of life, can gradually develop mental retardation. Other abnormalities may include delayed psychomotor maturation, tremors, seizures, eczema, tendency to hypopigmentation, and hyperactivity. The behavior is sometimes difficult to distinguish from autism and childhood schizophrenia. (**Ref. 2,** p. 1028)

958. **(A)** Huntington chorea is a rare disease associated with progressive degeneration of the basal ganglia and the cerebral cortex. It is characterized by jerking movements and progressive mental decline. The onset may present at any age, but is most common in late middle life. Males and females appear to be affected in equal numbers. (**Ref. 2,** p. 1160)

959. **(B)** A hallucination is the experience of perceiving a sensory phenomenon when no source of the sensory event occurred in the external world. Hallucinations may be of any of the 5 senses: auditory, visual, tactile, olfactory, or taste. Hallucinations may occur in schizophrenia, mania, depression, or brain disease. (**Ref. 5,** pp. 191–192)

960. **(A)** Illusions are misinterpretations of a real sensory stimulus, eg, a drapery in a darkened room may be misperceived as a human figure. (**Ref. 5,** p. 191)

961. **(B)** Displacement is the redirection of conflicting feelings toward a relatively less important object than the person or situation arousing the feelings. For example, one may be able to tolerate (cause less anxiety) to displace feelings of anger toward the boss onto his assistant. (**Ref. 6,** p. 127)

962. **(E)** Projection is most obvious in paranoid delusions. Intolerable internal feelings (wishes) are first denied ("I do not want to

hurt you") then projected onto another person ("You want to hurt me!"). (**Ref. 9,** p. 256)

963. (A)   Reaction formation is a higher level of defense often seen in neurotic or healthy individuals. It is characteristic of persons with obsessional traits. The wish to be dirty is reversed to excessive concern of cleanliness. The wish to express hate may be transformed into the expression of concern and kindness. (**Ref. 2,** p. 251)

964. (D)   Introjection is an immature defense that is nevertheless very common. A loved object (person) may be taken in to avoid feelings of separateness. In identification with the aggression a resident physician may be harsh or overly demanding of medical students, a trait the resident admires in her mentor. (**Ref. 2,** p. 250)

965. (B)   Acrophobia is the fear of high places. (**Ref. 2,** p. 306)

966. (A)   The fear of pain is termed algophobia. (**Ref. 2,** p. 306)

967. (D)   Agoraphobia is the fear of leaving the familiar setting of the home. (**Ref. 2,** p. 582)

968. (C)   The fear of strangers is referred to as xenophobia. (**Ref. 2,** p. 306)

969. (D)   Aphasia is an acquired disorder of language—comprehension, word choice, expression, and syntax. It is not due to dysarthria, a disorder of the muscles necessary for speech production. (**Ref. 2,** p. 102)

970. (A)   When one is unable to speak, but is still able to comprehend, it is identified as motor aphasia. This is also known as Broca's aphasia. The speech is telegraphic and agrammatical. (**Ref. 2,** p. 102)

971. (C)   Nominal aphasia refers to one who has difficulty in finding an object's proper name. This is also known as anomic aphasia. Speech is often marked by pauses as the word is sought and frequently by vague words as "it" and "thing." (**Ref. 2,** p. 102)

972. (B) Receptive aphasia, also known as Wernicke's, fluent or posterior aphasia, is marked by lack of comprehension of all speech. The bizarre speech of a person with receptive aphasia is fluent but incoherent; often many neologisms are used. **(Ref. 2,** p. 102)

973. (C) Recent memory impairment is associated with delirium. However, both recent and remote impairment are present with dementia. **(Ref. 7,** pp. 101–107)

974. (B) The onset of delirium is acute. However, with dementia the onset is usually insidious. If the onset is acute it is likely to be preceded by coma or delirium. **(Ref. 7,** pp. 101–107)

975. (B) Delirium is associated with clinical features that develop over a short period of time and tend to fluctuate over the course of a day. **(Ref. 7,** pp. 101–107)

976. (A) With dementia misperceptions often are absent; with delirium they are often present. **(Ref. 7,** pp. 101–107)

977. (D) The onset of dementia before the age of 40 is relatively uncommon, and the frequency of onset increases after the age of 60. An age of 60 years or more is a common predisposing factor in delirium. **(Ref. 7,** pp. 101–107)

978. (A) With dementia the sleep–wake cycle is usually normal for age. However, with delirium it is always disrupted. **(Ref. 7,** pp. 101–107)

979. (C) Pupillary dilation is included in the diagnostic criteria for opioid withdrawal as well as for cocaine intoxication. **(Ref. 2,** pp. 425, 443)

980. (D) Tachycardia is a symptom which can be present in cocaine intoxication and is seen within one hour of using cocaine. Additionally, tachycardia is a symptom which can be present due to recent cessation of or reduction in opioid use. **(Ref. 2,** pp. 425, 443)

981. **(A)** Fever is one of numerous symptoms which can be found in opioid withdrawal but is not included among diagnostic criteria for cocaine intoxication. **(Ref. 2, p. 443)**

982. **(B)** Nausea and vomiting are symptoms which can be seen in cocaine intoxication and present within one hour of using cocaine; these symptoms are not present in opioid withdrawal. **(Ref. 2, p. 443)**

983. **(C)** Perspiration is included in the diagnostic criteria for cocaine intoxication as well as opioid withdrawal. **(Ref. 2, pp. 425, 443)**

984. **(E)** Paraphilias are associated with recurrent, intense, sexually arousing fantasies, sexual urges or behaviors involving non-human objects, suffering or humiliation of one's self or one's partner or children or other non-consenting persons. All four listed may be considered paraphilias, but *only if* the behavior sexual urges or fantasies cause clinically significant distress or impairment in social, occupational, or other important areas of functioning. **(Ref. 1, pp. 522–532)**

985. **(B)** Cannabis intoxication is characterized by tachycardia, muscle relaxation, euphoria, and a sense of well-being. In 1982, nearly 65% of 18- to 25-year-olds had tried marijuana. Although it is illegal, it is used regularly by many to produce a sense of well-being. The active agent, tetrahydrocannabinol is sometimes used as an antiemetic in cancer patients undergoing chemotherapy. It also reduces intraocular pressure and has been used medically for this effect. **(Ref. 7, pp. 324–325)**

986. **(A)** Euphoria, which is an enhanced, inappropriate feeling of well-being, can be elicited by substances such as opiates, amphetamines, and alcohol. Because reserpine can actually result in depression, its use is contraindicated in depressed patients since it could result in worsening of their condition or even suicide. **(Ref. 7, p. 576)**

987. **(E)** The mental status examination is collected throughout the psychiatric interview. Specific questions must be asked to address specific areas of the examination, eg, test of memory and presence of hallucinations. Appearance, level of consciousness, psychomotor activity, behavior, and general mood state are observed before and throughout the interview. Speech, thought content, and form orientation and memory are appraised throughout the interview. Insight and judgment are usually determined at the conclusion of the interview. (**Ref. 7,** p. 25)

988. (A) DSM-IV identifies what formerly was known as paranoia as delusional disorder. The delusions are not restricted to those of persecution, but may include grandiose, erotomanic, jealousies, or somatic types also. The delusions are not bizarre but involve situations from real life. Delusions must be present at least one month. This disorder cannot be diagnosed in patients who have ever met the criteria for schizophrenia. The differential diagnosis includes schizophrenia, which differ from delusional disorder by exhibiting bizarre delusions and have grossly impaired functioning. Patients with paranoid personality disorders are not delusional but highly suspicious, fearful, and guarded. Delusions also occur with many medical and neurological illnesses. (**Ref. 2,** pp. 506–509, 736)

989. (E) In addition to the listed behaviors, others which may be seen in a person with a histrionic personality disorder include irrational, angry outbursts or tantrums, and manipulative suicide threats, gestures, or attempts. There are also characteristic disturbances in interpersonal relationships, such as lack of consideration for others, vanity, helplessness, and shallowness. Fundamental to the understanding of this personality disorder is an appreciation of the patient's fundamental insecurity, particularly regarding their self-worth and sexuality. They are sensitive to rejection by others. Psychoanalytic psychotherapy is the treatment of choice for these patients. (**Ref. 7,** pp. 184–185)

990. (D) The limbic system is part of the forebrain and includes hippocampus, the septum, and the cingulate gyrus. The role of the limbic system is not well denied but apparently is associated with emotional behavior. The hippocampus has been implicated in learning and memory and in spatial orientation. (**Ref. 9,** p. 390)

991. (D) Empathy involves a process that enables clinicians to appreciate conscious and unconscious internal experiences of patients. It is a somewhat intuitive capacity that responds to emotional signals of facial expressions, motor activity, speech patterns, and what the patient is talking about. A physician may alternatively think *with* and then *about* the patient. Empathy is contrasted with sympathy. A sympathetic physician is affected by the same things in a parallel or mutual susceptibility that may interfere with good medical care. (**Ref. 8,** p. 2317; **Ref. 6,** p. 443)

992. (B) Lithium is an effective antimanic drug, although the therapeutic response may take several weeks to obtain. Antipsychotic drugs or electroconvulsive therapy may be required to treat mania before the therapeutic effect of lithium is achieved. Lithium carbonate is a simple salt that is excreted by the kidneys. Lithium nephropathy, characterized by tubular interstitial nephritis has been reported. Although mild decreases in glomerular filtration rate occur in some patients treated with lithium, there have been no published reports of irreversible renal failure as a result of chronic non-toxic lithium therapy. (**Ref. 7,** pp. 533–535)

993. (E) In the human infant, inborn reflexes include sucking, grasping, and rooting. The newborn orients reflexively to the mother's breast. The Babinski reflex causes the infant to spread his toes when the plantar aspect of the foot is stroked. The newborn also orients to the human voice and displays visual tracking in the first weeks of life. (**Ref. 2,** p. 37)

994. (D) Psychoanalysis, a system of psychologic therapy, was developed by Freud. Psychoanalysis is the most extensive, intensive, and costly form of psychotherapy available. As a form of insight therapy, there are great demands on the patient and, therefore, only a small minority of patients are appropriate candidates for this form of treatment. For those patients for whom psychoanalysis is the treatment of choice, especially those with personality trait disorders, it is the most economical and effective psychotherapy. Many more patients are appropriate candidates for less extensive psychoanalytically oriented psychotherapy. (**Ref. 7,** pp. 481–484)

995. **(B)** Heightened anxiety, decreased memory, increased hostility, irritability, and hyperphagia may occur in some people after REM-state deprivation. These subjects may also experience greater likelihood of hallucinating with photic stimulation. This is believed to possibly be due to a breakthrough of the dream state into the waking state. (**Ref. 1,** p. 167)

996. **(E)** Patients with genetic disorders such as Niemann–Pick disease, homocystinuria, acute intermittent porphyria, and Wilson disease may have schizophreniclike manifestations. In addition to these genetic disorders, a wide variety of organic disorders can result in schizophrenic symptoms. Therefore, in any psychotic individual a complete history and physical examination, as well as appropriate laboratory studies are mandatory. (**Ref. 13,** p. 187)

997. **(E)** The superego functions largely in an unconscious manner although many values, goals, and aspirations are conscious. Moral values, standards, and prohibitions also have unconscious components that are internalized in the course of development. It is out of love for the parents that the child identifies and internalizes their standards. The superego guides one not only to avoid guilt but to achieve goals and aspirations that regulate (positive) self-esteem and mood. The ego ideal, a part of the superego, matures at least into adolescence, if not even later in life. (**Ref. 6,** p. 123)

998. **(D)** After orgasmic inevitability is reached, orgasm follows. Orgasm includes 4 to 16 involuntary contractions of the lower third of the vagina. Extragenital responses include carpopedal spasm, hyperventilation, myotonia with involuntary contractions of facial muscles causing frowning. Orgasm lasts 3 to 15 seconds. The resolution phase includes relaxation, disgorgement of the genitalia, and emotional well-being. (**Ref. 5,** p. 388)

999. **(E)** Wernicke–Korsakoff syndrome is easy to misdiagnose in the emergency room. It is most often seen in chronic alcoholics, usually men. It is characterized by ophthalmoplegia, nystagmus, impaired recent memory, peripheral neuritis, and ataxia. Treatment with intramuscular B_1 or thiamin may prevent permanent neurologic signs. Hospitalization is usually required to assure treatment and withdrawal from alcohol. (**Ref. 7,** p. 567)

1000. (B) Bill probably is demonstrating traits, not personality disorder. An individual's personality style is exemplified by typical behavior patterns and characteristic responses to life events and stresses. "Trait" describes typical patterns. Personality disorders are marked by an inflexible and pervasive enduring pattern of behavior that leads to significant distress or impairment in social or occupational functions. In obsessive–compulsive personality disorder, the individual is described as oblivious to the fact that other people tend to become very annoyed at delays and inconveniences that result from this behavior. Individuals with obsessive–compulsive disorder have unwanted and senseless but irresistible thoughts, ideas, or impulses. These are symptoms thought to be related to a dysfunction of the brain serotonin neuronal system, but at this time there is no association of dysfunction of serotonin and behavioral traits. (**Ref. 7,** pp. 173, 256; **Ref. 1,** p. 669)

1001. (C) Fear of public speaking is a common fear found in otherwise healthy individuals. An individual with social phobia fears humiliation or embarrassment to such an extent that it interferes significantly with the person's normal routine, occupational or academic functioning, or social activities. Specific phobias (in DSM-III-R this condition was called simple phobias) is the excessive or unreasonable fear of a specific object such as flying, blood, spiders, or snakes. (**Ref. 7,** pp. 244–250)

1002. (D) Personality disorders are marked by an inflexible and pervasive enduring pattern of behavior that leads to significant distress or impairment in social or occupational functions. In DSM-IV this would be coded as personality disorder—not otherwise specified (DSM-IV, 301.9). Passive–aggressive behaviors are a pattern of passive and indirect resistance to authority, responsibility, and obligations. These behaviors are often associated with complaining, irritability, and discontent. Anger is usually expressed indirectly through resistance, delays, and procrastination. (**Ref. 7,** p. 191; **Ref. 1,** p. 629)

1003. (C) Brief psychotic disorder is in response to a significant stressor and lasts for a few days to a month with a return to premorbid functioning. Substance-induced psychotic disorder may present with an identical clinical picture, however, a substance—not stressor—is judged to be the etiological factor. The diagnosis of adjustment disorders usually involve anxiety or mood disturbance and not psychosis. (**Ref. 1,** pp. 303, 627)

1004. (B) Dysthymia was also known before DSM-IV as depressive neurosis. This is a chronic disorder of mood that occurs for most of the day, more days than not, for at least 2 years. It is associated with appetite, sleep changes, and low energy. Hypomania and mania are not associated with this diagnosis. Major depressive disorder may be difficult to distinguish from dysthymia. Major depressive disorder changes a person's "usual" level of thought and behavior and occurs in episodes. The combination of dysthymia and major depression is often referred to as "double depression." (**Ref. 1,** pp. 345–349; **Ref. 7,** p. 200)

1005. (B) Each of Dr. Farthing's diagnoses is an Axis I diagnosis. Axis I represents a deterioration from a previous level of functioning. Axis II diagnosis includes personality disorders and developmental years. More than one diagnosis may be listed on Axis I, II, or III. (**Ref. 1,** pp. 25–27)

1006. (B) Tolerance indicates that a greater dose of a psychoactive drug, eg, alcohol, is necessary to achieve the same physiologic or behavioral effect. Withdrawal is a drug-specific physiologic state that follows cessation or reduction of the psychoactive drug. Dependence is the state in which withdrawal signs and symptoms follow reduction of use of the psychoactive agent. (**Ref. 7,** p. 310)

1007. (C) Although tolerance for alcohol is present, insufficient data is available to determine if the dependence is present. A clinically significant impairment or distress is necessary to meet the diagnostic criteria. This must be manifested by at least 3 of 7 conditions that include tolerance, withdrawal, greater use than intended, desire to cut down use, and impairment of activities in a 12-month period. (**Ref. 1,** p. 181)

1008. (C) Withdrawal from opioids has been described as flu-like symptoms. Individuals who are in withdrawal describe the symptoms as unpleasant. However, compared to withdrawal from alcohol, the symptoms seem mild and are not life-threatening. (**Ref. 7,** p. 329)

1009. (D) These common misperceptions may cause doubt and worry. A physician who is knowledgeable with sexual knowledge and at ease can help avert potential sexual problems. (**Ref. 2,** pp. 655–657)

1010. (D) These common misperceptions may cause doubt and worry. A physician who is knowledgeable with sexual knowledge and at ease can help avert potential sexual problems. (**Ref. 2,** pp. 655–657)

1011. (B) According to Piaget's observations, an object that is covered (disappears) in full view of a 3-month-old seems to no longer exist in the mind of the infant. By 4 months the infant will stare at the place the object was last seen. It is only at 8 months that the average infant will make an effort to find an object that "disappears" in his presence. Piaget's theory deals primarily with cognitive development. Each stage involves a distinct concept of how things work. He described the first 2 years of life as the sensory motor period. (**Ref. 9,** pp. 4–6)

1012. (A) Erikson described 8 specific developmental tasks to achieve psychological maturation. Satisfactory completion of each earlier task prepares one to face the tasks in the next stages. The main task of the infant is to establish basic trust. This sense of trust arises from the baby's experience of tension relief and pleasure through interaction with caretakers. (**Ref. 9,** p. 4)

1013. (A) Gender identity is usually present by 24 months. Gender stability (the understanding that you stay the same gender throughout life) and gender constancy (a recognition that someone stays the same gender even if appearances change, eg, hair style, clothing, etc. (**Ref. 9,** p. 27)

1014. (B) According to analytic theory first proposed by Freud the major psychological event of latency is the further development of defense mechanisms. Repression and denial are typical mechanisms of defense for children of this age. (**Ref. 9**, p. 33)

1015. (C) Boys who experience puberty early are rated as more attractive and class leaders. Later-maturing boys are seen as less mature, more talkative, more restless, and attention-seeking. Early-maturing girls, however, are more vulnerable and less successful than female age peers. They may become self-conscious and withdrawn. Advanced development leads to increased pressure for earlier sexual relations. Later-maturing females may be less conspicuous. (**Ref. 9**, p. 47)

1016. (A) Menarche has begun earlier and earlier over time. The average in 1900 was 14 1/2; in 1980, 12 1/2. Tanner has described 5 stages of development of secondary sexual characteristics that usually occur between 10 and 13 years of age. Tanner notes that it is not deviate for these changes to occur anywhere between 8 and 17. (**Ref. 9**, p. 43)

1017. (C) Although the incidence of this disorder is controversial, most investigators find extreme childhood abuse—often sexual abuse—and other trauma in the developmental history of those patients. Investigators who actively look for patients with this disorder find a 2 to 5% incidence rate. Others believe it is a rare disorder that may be produced iatrogenically in the clinical setting by suggestion or behavioral shaping in patients who are eager to please the doctor. (**Ref. 7**, p. 381)

1018. (D) The most efficacious treatment of dissociative identity disorder is insight-oriented therapy. The treatment is usually long term with frequent testing of trust and boundaries of the therapist. Understanding the patient's development and how she dealt with overwhelming trauma in childhood is necessary before an integration of dissociative parts of the personality can occur. Medications may often be helpful in treating specific symptoms such as anxiety or depressions during on-going psychotherapy. (**Ref. 2**, p. 646)

References

1. Diagnostic and Statistical Manual of Mental Disorders, 4th ed. Washington, DC, American Psychiatric Association, 1994.
2. Kaplan H, Sadock B: *Synopsis of Psychiatry,* 7th ed. Williams & Wilkins, 1994.
3. Kaplan HI, Sadock FJ: *Comprehensive Textbook of Psychiatry,* 4th ed. Volumes I and II. Williams & Wilkins, Baltimore, 1985.
4. Millon T: *Medical Behavioral Science.* WB Saunders, Philadelphia, 1975.
5. Sierles FS: *Behavioral Science for Medical Students.* Williams & Wilkins, Baltimore, 1993.
6. Stoudemire A: *Human Behavior: An Introduction for Medical Students,* 2nd ed. Lippincott Co, Philadelphia, 1994.
7. Stoudemire A: *Clinical Psychiatry for Medical Students,* 2nd ed. Lippincott Co, Philadelphia, 1994.
8. Webster's 3rd International Dictionary, Merriam-Webster, G & C Merriam Co, St. Louis, 1990.
9. Wedding D: *Behavior and Medicine.* Mosby–Year Book, St. Louis, 1990.
10. Werner A, Campbell RJ, Frazier SH, and Stone EM: *A Psychiatric Glossary,* 5th ed. The American Psychiatric Association Publications Office, Washington, DC, 1980.

7

Physiology
David G. Penney

DIRECTIONS (Questions 1019 through 1138): Each of the questions or incomplete statements is followed by four or five suggested answers or completions. Select the ONE that is best in each case.

1019. Cardiac work is most nearly equal to
- **A.** area of the ventricular pressure–volume diagram
- **B.** tension–time index
- **C.** kinetic energy imparted to movement of blood
- **D.** systolic blood pressure
- **E.** heart rate

1020. An isometric twitch is similar to an isotonic twitch in that
- **A.** both produce the same amount of work
- **B.** in both situations, the muscle shortens the same amount
- **C.** activation of the contractile elements are responsible for the tension developed in both types of twitches
- **D.** in both cases the muscle does not shorten
- **E.** in both cases the muscle length changes

1021. The most important factor of those listed below in improving the ability of the heart to increase blood flow to peripheral tissue in exercise is
  A. increased oxygen extraction from the blood by the heart
  B. increased myocardial efficiency independent of the oxygen needs of the organ
  C. increased coronary blood flow
  D. increased venomotor tone
  E. decreased circulatory catecholamines

1022. Stimulation of sympathetic adrenergic nerves to the heart results in
  A. vasoconstriction in all tissues
  B. increased coronary blood flow
  C. increased muscle blood flow
  D. increased skin blood flow
  E. vasodilation in all tissues

1023. If 100,000 cpm of radio-iodinated albumin and 200,000 cpm of radiolabeled red blood cells were injected intravenously and allowed to completely mix in the vascular system without loss, and if the equilibrium concentrations were determined to be 100 cpm/mL of plasma for the plasma indicator and 400 cpm/mL of red cells for the red cell indicator, the plasma volume would be (in mL)
  A. 1000
  B. 250
  C. 200
  D. 500
  E. 100

1024. Reducing carotid sinus transmural pressure will result in
  A. an increased peripheral resistance
  B. a reduction in cardiac contractility
  C. a reduction in cardiac output
  D. atrial premature beats
  E. a reduction in tidal volume

1025. Because of the nature of the oxygen–hemoglobin dissociation curve, one finds that

    A. total capillary oxygen uptake is only slightly influenced by changes in alveolar PO_2, as long as PO_2 remains above 70 torr

    B. the loss of CO_2 into alveoli from pulmonary capillary blood partially inhibits oxygen uptake

    C. breathing 100% oxygen will add half again as much oxygen to pulmonary capillary blood as it contained while breathing air

    D. all people with cyanotic lips have systemic arterial blood PO_2 less than 60 torr

    E. PO_2 must reach 200 mm Hg before significant oxygenation can occur

1026. In severe exercise the oxygen debt is

    A. surplus oxygen borrowed from the inspiratory reserve during exercise

    B. the average oxygen used less the resting oxygen for a similar period of time

    C. oxygen used above resting levels borrowed to provide increased aerobic oxidation

    D. oxygen used after exercise above the resting level and representing in part the anaerobic contribution to work

    E. decreased

1027. The maximum expiratory airflow rate achievable at the middle of one's vital capacity

    A. will usually be greater than that found at a larger state of inflation

    B. will be determined by dynamic airway collapse

    C. will be the same as the maximum flow rate at a point near maximum expired volume

    D. depends only upon the subject's willingness to try hard

    E. is about the same as that seen during maximum exercise

1028. During the slow ejection phase of the left ventricle, the
   A. left atrial pressure is falling
   B. aortic flow velocity is rapidly decreasing
   C. aortic pressure is falling below left ventricular pressure
   D. left ventricular pressure is constant
   E. tricuspid valves are closed

1029. Rapid adaptation of touch sensation is due to
   A. a decrease in firing rate despite continuous deformation of
      the receptor
   B. a return of the receptor to its original conformation despite
      continuous application of pressure
   C. compensating mechanisms at the basal ganglia level
   D. failure of the cerebrum to detect a continuous sensory input
   E. failure of a continuous sensory input to get through the
      reticular activating system

1030. Strictly speaking, the all-or-none law refers to the
   A. strength of muscle contraction
   B. resting potential
   C. action potential
   D. release of transmitter
   E. excitatory postsynaptic potential

1031. Excitable cells (such as nerve and muscle) differ from other cells
   primarily in that only excitable cells
   A. have an electrical potential across their membranes
   B. have an ionic concentration gradient across their mem-
      branes
   C. can undergo rapid, transient changes in membrane potential
   D. have active transport mechanisms
   E. are affected by electrical currents

1032. Concerning the "sodium pump"
   A. the rate of sodium pumping is independent of the internal
      sodium concentration
   B. high-energy phosphate bonds can support the operation of
      the sodium pump
   C. the operation of the sodium pump is independent of potas-
      sium influx

D. the sodium pump is not affected by changes in temperature

E. the process can be explained in terms of facilitated diffusion

1033. Loss of body heat is

A. accomplished chiefly through radiation and water evaporation

B. accomplished chiefly through warming of inspired air and heat loss through urine and feces

C. controlled by the thermoregulatory center in the medulla oblongata

D. independent of environmental conditions

E. independent of neural control

1034. An increase in the osmolality of the extracellular compartment associated with a reduction in volume will

A. stimulate the volume and osmoreceptors and decrease ADH secretion

B. inhibit the volume and osmoreceptors and increase ADH secretion

C. inhibit the volume and osmoreceptors and decrease ADH secretion

D. inhibit the volume and stimulate the osmoreceptors and increase ADH secretion

E. none of the above

1035. When smooth muscle is stretched within physiologic limits

A. the membrane depolarizes

B. action potentials are not elicited

C. the tension that develops is due to elastic elements only

D. syncytial conduction is blocked

1036. The distribution pattern of body hair is determined by

A. androgens in men, but not in women

B. heredity alone

C. sex alone

D. heredity, sex, and androgens

E. heredity in women, androgens in men

1037. In a normal individual, which of the following blood elements has the LOWEST renal clearance?
  A. PAH
  B. potassium
  C. creatinine
  D. inulin
  E. urea

1038. Under basal conditions, the route of greatest water loss is via the
  A. skin
  B. lung
  C. kidney
  D. gastrointestinal tract
  E. sweat glands

1039. The unequal distribution of sodium inside and outside the cell
  A. cannot be expressed by the Nernst equation
  B. does not rule out the possibility that sodium diffuses into the cell
  C. exists because the cell membrane is impermeable to sodium
  D. is unrelated to a sodium pump
  E. is dependent on the active transport of potassium and sodium

1040. The vomiting center is located in the
  A. cerebral cortex
  B. thalamus
  C. hypothalamus
  D. medulla oblongata
  E. cervical spinal cord

1041. In photopic vision
  A. the eye is most sensitive to blue light
  B. the rods are not stimulated
  C. color balance is perceived mainly by the cones
  D. the eye is accommodated to dim light
  E. visual acuity is lower than in scotopic vision

1042. Under normal physiologic conditions, the capillaries
    A. contain more than 25% of the total blood volume
    B. contain a relatively small amount of the total blood volume (about 5%)
    C. have a very rapid blood flow
    D. have a higher blood flow and pressure than the arterioles
    E. none of the above

1043. The term hematocrit means
    A. the percentage of the blood that is red blood cells
    B. the percentage of blood that is plasma
    C. the ratio of the blood volume to the extracellular space
    D. the percentage of new blood formed every 120 days
    E. the average specific gravity of formed elements

1044. The first heart sound occurs during the period of
    A. isotonic contraction
    B. isovolumetric contraction
    C. isovolumetric relaxation
    D. isotonic relaxation
    E. the ST segment

1045. Venoconstriction is elicited by all of the following EXCEPT
    A. hemorrhage
    B. asphyxia
    C. common carotid artery occlusion
    D. lying down
    E. Valsalva maneuver

1046. The opening of the aortic valves is initiated when the
    A. atria contract
    B. ventricles contract
    C. capillary muscles contract
    D. ventricles relax
    E. ventricular pressure exceeds aortic pressure

1047. Atrial contraction causes the
   A. A wave of the atrial pressure curve
   B. C wave of the atrial pressure curve
   C. V wave of the atrial pressure curve
   D. T wave of the ECG
   E. R wave of the ECG

1048. In response to mild exercise the
   A. heart rate increases and stroke volume is decreased
   B. heart rate increases and stroke volume is constant
   C. heart rate increases and stroke volume is increased
   D. stroke volume increases and heart rate is constant
   E. cardiac output increases and heart rate is constant

1049. The P wave of the ECG occurs before the
   A. beginning of atrial contraction
   B. end of atrial contraction
   C. beginning of ventricular contraction
   D. end of ventricular contraction
   E. onset of ventricular ejection

1050. The P wave of the normal electrocardiogram is associated with
   A. auricular repolarization
   B. auricular contraction
   C. auricular depolarization
   D. ventricular repolarization
   E. ventricular systole

1051. In hemodynamics, peripheral resistance is
   A. the resistance to exercise as an aid to circulation
   B. the resistance to blood flow through the systemic circulatory system
   C. peripheral contraction of skeletal muscle that stops blood flow
   D. the dilation of peripheral vessels that causes pooling of blood
   E. resistance to the flow of blood through the lungs

1052. In the normal individual the quantity of hemoglobin in 100 mL of blood averages
  A. 5 mg
  B. 10 mg
  C. 16 g
  D. 10 g
  E. less than 5 g

1053. By definition, the cardiac index is the ratio of
  A. cardiac output to surface area
  B. cardiac output to body weight
  C. cardiac output to work of the heart
  D. stroke volume to surface area
  E. peripheral resistance to surface area

1054. The most important cardiac and vasomotor control centers are situated in the
  A. heart
  B. medulla and pons
  C. cerebrum
  D. cerebellum
  E. peripheral blood vessels

1055. An important function of the cardiac Purkinje system is its ability to
  A. slow the conduction of impulses
  B. speed the conduction of impulses
  C. amplify impulses
  D. delay impulses
  E. select impulses

1056. The venous pulse is
  A. a damped arterial pulse
  B. a result of pressure changes in the heart and neighboring arteries
  C. necessary for proper cardiac filling
  D. diminished in cardiac failure
  E. none of the above

1057. Normally, the greater portion of circulating blood is located in the
  A. heart
  B. large arteries
  C. capillaries
  D. large veins
  E. pulmonary vessels

1058. The electrocardiogram is of great value in the diagnosis of dysrhythmias. For example, any irregularity of the interval between atrial depolarization (P wave) and the QRS complex would be indicative of
  A. abnormality of rhythm
  B. abnormality of conduction
  C. abnormality of contractility
  D. abnormality of automaticity
  E. abnormal contraction and automaticity

1059. Cutting the carotid sinus nerves and the afferent vagal branches from the aortic arch baroreceptors will result in
  A. a decrease in arterial pressure on head-down tilting
  B. partial or total loss of compensatory ability on head-up tilting
  C. a decrease in heart rate and arterial blood pressure
  D. a decrease in cerebral blood flow and venous pressure
  E. no change in control of blood pressure

1060. An increase in ventricular stroke work is obtained by administering a new pharmacologic drug claimed to be a positive inotrope. If the effective (end-diastolic) volume is not increased, the effect of this drug also might represent
  A. homeometric autoregulation associated with an increase in mean aortic pressure, following peripheral vasoconstriction
  B. increased parasympathetic (vagal) activity
  C. heterometric (Frank–Starling) autoregulation
  D. heterometric autoregulation due to increased vagal activity
  E. decreased sympathetic activity

1061. With constant flow through a tube system
  A. reducing the diameter of the tube will reduce lateral pressure
  B. increasing tube diameter will reduce lateral pressure
  C. reducing the tube diameter will reduce flow velocity
  D. increasing tube diameter will increase flow velocity
  E. flow is not affected by tube size

1062. The oxygen dissociation curve is shifted to the right by
  A. decreased CO_2 tension
  B. increased CO_2 tension
  C. increased pH
  D. increased N_2 tension
  E. decreased N_2 tension

1063. The most potent stimulant of ventilation would be
  A. a twofold increase in the P_{CO_2} of inspired air
  B. a twofold increase in the P_{O_2} of inspired air
  C. a 50% decrease in the P_{CO_2} of inspired air
  D. a 50% decrease in the P_{O_2} of inspired air
  E. A and D are equally potent stimuli

1064. Most of the venous CO_2 is in the form of
  A. carbonate
  B. carbonic acid
  C. bicarbonate
  D. dissolved CO_2
  E. oxyhemoglobin

1065. Hyperpnea resulting from moderate exercise is due to all of the following EXCEPT
  A. increased body temperature
  B. joint movement
  C. lowered serum pH
  D. elevated serum P_{CO_2}
  E. increased serum pH

1066. Destruction of the pneumotaxic center located in the pons can cause
  A. apneustic respiration
  B. forceful expiration
  C. accelerated respiration
  D. apnea
  E. none of the above

1067. If the vagus nerves are severed, the respiratory rate
  A. is increased
  B. is decreased
  C. remains constant
  D. ceases
  E. becomes unresponsive to alterations in blood gas content

1068. Oxygen consumption represents the
  A. difference between arterial and venous blood oxygen tension
  B. product of the arterial–venous oxygen saturation difference and blood flow
  C. ratio of arterial to venous oxygen saturation
  D. arterial–venous oxygen saturation difference divided by the arterial flow rate
  E. total oxygen in the lungs

1069. All theories of active transport postulate the
  A. use of energy to accomplish the movement of molecules
  B. presence of a carrier molecule that facilitates the movement of molecules down their concentration gradient
  C. influence of hormones
  D. directional sites in membrane pores
  E. influence of the cortex

1070. In humans, urea is
  A. transported almost exclusively by passive diffusion
  B. concentrated by secretion into the renal tubule
  C. poorly reabsorbed by the renal tubule
  D. actively reabsorbed in significant amounts
  E. none of the above

1071. Active reabsorption of glucose in the kidney occurs in the
    A. proximal tubule
    B. loop of Henle
    C. distal ducts
    D. collecting ducts
    E. Malpighian corpuscle

1072. Under normal conditions, the glomerular filtration rate is most likely to be altered by a change in
    A. glomerular capillary blood flow
    B. glomerular capillary pressure
    C. intracapsular hydrostatic pressure
    D. plasma colloid osmotic pressure
    E. arterial aldosterone levels

1073. Active secretion by the renal tubules is necessary to maintain normal homeostasis of
    A. sodium
    B. potassium
    C. bicarbonate
    D. chloride
    E. glucose

1074. As urine enters the collecting duct it may be
    A. hypotonic
    B. isotonic
    C. hypertonic
    D. A or B, but not C
    E. B or C, but not A

1075. Most of the glomerular filtrate is reabsorbed in the
    A. proximal convoluted tubule
    B. thin loop of Henle
    C. thick loop of Henle
    D. distal convoluted tubule
    E. collecting tubule

1076. Which of the following substances is filtered but NOT reabsorbed by the tubules?
A. xylose
B. plasma proteins
C. inulin
D. NaCl
E. para-aminohippurate

1077. The loops of Henle of the outer cortical nephrons do NOT descend into the inner medulla. Therefore, these nephrons
A. do not participate in the urinary diluting mechanism
B. are functionally unimportant in the renal conservation of sodium and water
C. do not contribute to the medullary osmotic gradient
D. do not play any important role in overall renal function and are simply unimportant vestiges of evolutionary development
E. are necessary for the medullary osmotic gradient

1078. Which of the following combinations of data would lead one to suspect that a patient had the "syndrome of inappropriate antidiuretic hormone secretion" (SIADH)?

	Plasma Osmolality (mOsm/kg)	Plasma Sodium (mEq/L)	Urine Osmolality (mOsm/kg)
A.	286	138	627
B.	263	126	52
C.	286	138	177
D.	263	126	426
E.	300	144	100

1079. Which of the following changes in body fluid volume and/or osmolality would occur to restore osmotic equilibrium after infusion of 500 mL of 5.0% NaCl solution?
A. increased ICF and ECF osmolality only
B. increased ECF volume and decreased ICF volume
C. increased volume and osmolality of both ECF and ICF
D. decreased volume and osmolality of both ECF and ICF
E. decreased HCO_3^- and Na^+ in plasma

1080. Which of the following set of values is indicative of compensated metabolic alkalosis?
   A. $HCO_3^- = 20$ mEq/L, $PCO_2 = 25$ mm Hg, pH = 7.5
   B. $HCO_3^- = 34$ mEq/L, $PCO_2 = 45$ mm Hg, pH = 7.4
   C. $HCO_3^- = 17$ mEq/L, $PCO_2 = 30$ mm Hg, pH = 7.3
   D. $HCO_3^- = 34$ mEq/L, $PCO_2 = 10$ mm Hg, pH = 7.7
   E. $HCO_3^- = 10$ mEq/L, $PCO_2 = 15$ mm Hg, pH = 7.3

1081. The juxtaglomerular apparatus is associated with all of the following EXCEPT
   A. maintaining a normal balance of sodium in the body
   B. nephrons with a long loop of Henle that dip into the renal medulla
   C. participation in the control of aldosterone secretion through the renin–angiotensin system
   D. function as a sphincter around the distal tubules
   E. maintaining normal balance of osmolality

1082. It can be concluded generally that a substance undergoes net secretion into the tubular lumen of the kidney if
   A. the concentration of the substance in the urine is greater than in glomerular filtrate
   B. the concentration of substance in tubular fluid rises as it passes along through the tubule
   C. its clearance exceeds inulin clearance
   D. A and C only
   E. none of the above

1083. Diabetes insipidus, a condition in which there is a marked reduction or absence of ADH, is characterized by a marked sensation of thirst and very marked increases in urine output. In a patient with such a condition (and with complete absence of ADH) without treatment, but with free access to water, the urine output would be about
   A. 3 to 5 L/day
   B. 6 to 8 L/day
   C. 9 to 11 L/day
   D. 15 to 20 L/day
   E. 60 to 80 L/day

1084. Estrogen secretion by the ovary and placenta is influenced by all of the following EXCEPT
  A. follicle-stimulating hormone (FSH)
  B. luteotrophic hormone
  C. luteinizing hormone (LH)
  D. sympathetic nerve activity
  E. progesterone

1085. Which of the following hormones is not secreted by the adenohypophysis?
  A. ACTH
  B. ADH
  C. growth hormone
  D. TSH
  E. FSH

1086. During pregnancy, the maximum rate of secretion of which of the following occurs during the first trimester?
  A. chorionic gonadotropin
  B. estrogen
  C. pregnanediol
  D. oxytocin
  E. hydrocortisone

1087. ACTH is most effective in stimulating the secretion of
  A. hydrocortisone
  B. epinephrine
  C. adrenal androgenic hormones
  D. aldosterone
  E. norepinephrine

1088. When thyroxine is injected
  A. there is no detectable effect for the first 72 hours
  B. the heart is sensitized to epinephrine
  C. the metabolic rate of brain tissues increases after 24 hours
  D. the serum cholesterol level rises
  E. oxidative processes are reduced

1089. The secretion of intrinsic factor occurs in the
  A. paric cell surface receptors for transported proteins
  B. the presence of coated pits

C. formation of membrane vesicles
D. transport of molecules too large to move through the cell membrane by other means
E. no requirement for energy from the cell

1090. The sugars normally found in significant amounts in intestinal chyme include
  A. glucose and fructose
  B. galactose and xylose
  C. mannose and ribose
  D. mannose and xylose
  E. ribose and xylose

1091. Pinocytosis is usually associated with all of the following EXCEPT
  A. specific cell surface receptors for transported proteins
  B. the presence of coated pits
  C. formation of membrane vesicles
  D. the transport of molecules too large to move through the cell membrane by other means
  E. no requirement for energy from the cell

1092. Which of the following is NOT true about erythropoietin?
  A. low partial pressures of oxygen in the blood increase the synthesis of this compound
  B. it is primarily formed in the kidney
  C. it is a hormone that causes an immediate increase in the circulating numbers of red cells
  D. it increases the number of pro-erythroblasts formed
  E. it increases the rate at which the pro-erythroblasts mature into erythrocytes

1093. Which of the following will increase the likelihood of the formation of a blood clot?
  A. increased concentration of prothrombin
  B. decreased Ca^{++}
  C. increased concentration of plasmin
  D. increased antithrombin III
  E. increased platelet rupture

1094. Troponin
A. contains four subunits: troponin I, C, T, and S
B. binds to calcium and tropomyosin
C. is necessary for the binding of actin to myosin
D. contains an essential ATPase
E. binds to heavy myosin during muscle contraction

1095. Deglutition (swallowing)
A. is an entirely voluntary act
B. is an entirely automatic function
C. uses only skeletal muscles
D. depends on a number of reflexively controlled skeletal muscle contractions
E. only includes the action of the esophagus

1096. Growth hormone has all of the following effects EXCEPT
A. the potential to develop ketosis
B. decreased protein catabolism
C. increased glycogen deposition
D. gluconeogenesis
E. increased somatomedin production

1097. Which of the following occur during presynaptic inhibition?
A. hyperpolarization of the presynaptic ending
B. increased transmitter release
C. postsynaptic hyperpolarization
D. presynaptic depolarization
E. postsynaptic desensitization without hyperpolarization

1098. The initial adjustment of ventilation when an individual starts to exercise is caused by
A. increased P_{CO_2} in the blood
B. increased output from the motor cortex to the respiratory centers
C. increased P_{CO_2} in the central nervous system
D. decreased P_{O_2} in the blood
E. decreased pH in the central nervous system

1099. The isohydric principle is important in human systems because
A. it determines the rate of respiration
B. it allows one to evaluate all the extracellular buffer systems by measuring only one
C. it causes all tissues to be at the same pH
D. it does not allow extracellular pH to change beyond physiologically tolerable levels
E. it facilitates the excretion of hydrogen ions in the distal convoluted tubule

1100. Negative intrapleural pressure is maintained by the
A. high pressures in the alveoli
B. low pressures in the alveoli
C. balance between pulmonary capillary pressure and colloid osmotic pressure
D. changes in surfactant concentrations in the alveoli during inspiration and expiration
E. lack of lymphatic exudate into the intrapleural space

1101. Which of the following does not contribute to the resistance of tissue to the development of edema?
A. negative interstitial pressure
B. lymphatic flow
C. lymphatic washout of proteins
D. low capillary pressure
E. decreased plasma proteins

1102. All of the following are possible symptoms of low cardiac reserve as measured in an exercise test EXCEPT
A. anginal pain
B. shortness of breath
C. excessive heart rate
D. premature skeletal muscle weakness
E. increased blood pressure

1103. Respiratory alkalosis due to prolonged hyperventilation is normally accompanied by
- **A.** increased bicarbonate reabsorption in the kidney
- **B.** decreased renal excretion of ammonium
- **C.** dissociation of acid buffers
- **D.** lowering of plasma bicarbonate concentration
- **E.** B and D are correct

1104. Cardiac muscle is like skeletal striated muscle in the following characteristics EXCEPT
- **A.** it is cross-striated
- **B.** the contractile elements are formed from myosin and actin
- **C.** the force of contraction is increased by stretching within limits
- **D.** it has inherent rhythmicity
- **E.** Ca^{++} is involved in excitation-contraction coupling

1105. The mean effective pressure involved in filling the heart is significantly influenced by the following EXCEPT
- **A.** cardiac contractility
- **B.** heart rate
- **C.** ventricular systolic distensibility
- **D.** blood volume
- **E.** intrathoracic pressure during inspiration

1106. A patient is experiencing altered renal function which results in fluid and salt retention. In such a situation one should expect to find
- **A.** increased mean circulatory pressure
- **B.** increased central venous pressure
- **C.** increased blood volume
- **D.** increased mean blood pressure
- **E.** all of the above

1107. Following hemorrhage of a patient, the following would be indications that compensatory changes are still operating effectively EXCEPT
- **A.** tachycardia
- **B.** increasing hematocrit
- **C.** increasing muscle vascular resistance

    D. increasing plasma volume
    E. progressive hypotension

1108. The compliance of a lung that changes 1 L in volume when the intrapleural pressure is lowered by 5 cm H_2O
    A. would be calculated by change in P/change in V
    B. would be calculated by change in V/change in P
    C. would be 5.0 cm H_2O/L
    D. would be 0.20 L/cm H_2O
    E. B and D are correct

1109. Perfusion without ventilation
    A. acts like an arteriovenous shunt
    B. acts like an increased partial pressure of oxygen in the alveoli
    C. leads to depletion of oxygen in the alveoli involved
    D. acts like an increase in dead space
    E. A and C are correct

1110. Which of the following is not a factor favoring the release of oxygen from hemoglobin during its passage through metabolizing tissue?
    A. low temperature
    B. low pH
    C. high P_{CO_2}
    D. low P_{O_2}

1111. Increased blood CO_2
    A. will increase blood pH
    B. has little affect on the carotid body chemoreceptors
    C. will activate the carotid sinus mechanoreceptors
    D. is the most potent stimulus for increasing respiration
    E. shifts the oxygen–hemoglobin dissociation curve to the left

1112. Total body blood volume following hemorrhage is returned to normal by

    A. uptake of fluid from the intracellular and interstitial fluid compartments due to the Bainbridge reflex

    B. increased ADH release which stimulates water uptake by the renal tubules

    C. increased renin release and thence production of angiotensin, stimulating thrist

    D. increased aldosterone release from the adrenal medulla which stimulates water uptake by the renal tubules

    E. B and C are correct

1113. The pontine respiratory center has

    A. afferents directly to motor neurons necessary for respiration

    B. an area that will cause prolonged inspiration if stimulated

    C. its effects through a cortical-medullary reflex arc

    D. an area that is primarily active in controlling the rate of respiration

    E. B and D are correct

1114. Airway resistance is decreased by

    A. decreased vagal efferent activity

    B. increase in lung volume

    C. breathing a less viscous gas than air

    D. breathing through the mouth, rather than the nose

    E. all are correct

1115. In second degree heart (AV) block

    A. the PR interval always lengthens progressively until AV conduction fails, causing the loss of a ventricular depolarization

    B. is caused by a wandering atrial pacemaker

    C. usually involves retrograde conduction to atria

    D. always involves a lost ventricular depolarization every so many P waves

    E. most of the QRS complexes are wide and bizzare

1116. Aldosterone is secreted in response to the following EXCEPT

    A. stress

    B. low plasma angiotensin

    C. low extracellular sodium

D. low extracellular volume

E. high extracellular potassium

1117. At birth

    A. pulmonary vascular resistance falls shortly after the first breath because of arteriolar vasodilation

    B. the initial left atrial pressure rise occurs because the ductus arteriosus has closed

    C. the foramen ovale closes because of umbilical cord clamping

    D. right to left shunting of blood through the ductus arteriosus continues right up till the ductus closes

    E. the adult circulation is functional within a few minutes after birth

1118. Excision of the adrenal glands results in

    A. K^+ retention

    B. death, usually in less than 2 weeks

    C. Na^+ excretion

    D. decreased blood volume

    E. B and D are correct

1119. During a normal menstrual cycle

    A. ovulation is triggered by an increased secretion of FSH

    B. a rapid decrease in the secretion of LH triggers ovulation

    C. estrogen may eventually reduce th LH peak

    D. progesterone rises 5 to 6 days before the LH spikes and drops off afterward

    E. A and B are correct

1120. Spermatogenesis requires

    A. ACTH

    B. androgens

    C. TSH

    D. FSH

    E. B and D are correct

1121. Parathyroid hormone
  A. will be released if Ca^{++} is lowered below normal
  B. if absent will result in decreased plasma Ca^{++} and increased PO_4^- concentration
  C. increases the rate of activation of vitamin D
  D. is secreted by chief cells of the parathyroid gland
  E. all are correct

1122. When an obese but otherwise normal person goes on a diet deficient in calories
  A. body fat is lost at a rate proportionate to the caloric deficiency of the diet
  B. initial weight loss is less than initial fat loss
  C. initial weight loss is primarily due to fat loss
  D. the types of food supplying calories can significantly alter the rate at which weight is lost
  E. A and C are correct

1123. The following are true of the gallbladder EXCEPT it
  A. can be caused to contract by cholecystokinin
  B. can have its contraction blocked by activity of certain sympathetic nerves
  C. is located in the pancreas
  D. stores bile that is continuously secreted
  E. can be caused to contract by vagal activity

1124. Pancreozymin
  A. is the same as cholecystokinin
  B. greatly increases the volume of secretion of the pancreas
  C. decreases HCO_3^- secretion of the pancreas
  D. does not affect enzyme secretion by the pancreas

1125. Motility of the small intestine is
  A. stimulated by distention of the small intestine
  B. characterized by peristaltic waves moving intestinal chyme only a short distance
  C. characterized by mixing waves which divide and recombine the contents of the small intestine
  D. stimulated above a bolus of chyme and inhibited below a bolus
  E. all are correct

1126. The swallowing response
- **A.** does not require sensory information from the pharynx for normal initiation and coordination
- **B.** requires an intact cerebral cortex
- **C.** is a stereotyped largely reflex phenomenon
- **D.** is mediated through unilateral forebrain centers
- **E.** A and C are correct

1127. The act of swallowing is associated with the following EXCEPT
- **A.** closure of the glottis
- **B.** concurrent inhibition of respiration
- **C.** upper esophageal sphincter relaxation when food is placed in contact with the anterior pillars of the pharynx
- **D.** movement of food into the nasopharynx
- **E.** A and C

1128. Salivary secretion
- **A.** is only affected by parasympathetic innervation
- **B.** is primarily stimulated by sympathetic innervation
- **C.** contains several enzymes that are stored in zymogen granules before it is secreted
- **D.** contains the enzyme salivary amylase
- **E.** B and D are correct

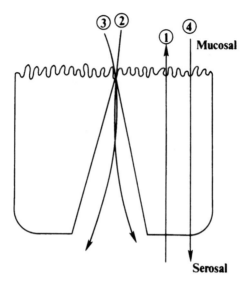

Figure 7.1. (Reproduced, with permission, from Dershwitz M, *National Boards Examination Review for Part 1*, 3rd ed. East Norwalk, Ct: Appleton & Lange; 1987.)

1129. In Figure 7.1, the major pathway(s) for water movement from the mucosal side to the serosal side of the intestinal mucosa are indicated by which arrow(s)?
   A. arrow 1
   B. arrow 2
   C. arrow 3
   D. arrow 4
   E. B and D are correct

1130. Secretin
   A. increases HCl secretion by the stomach
   B. increases pancreatic secretion of HCO_3^-
   C. stimulates pancreatic secretion of lysine
   D. is secreted by the pancreas
   E. all are correct

1131. Complete removal of the stomach will result in
   A. anemia
   B. gross malnutrition

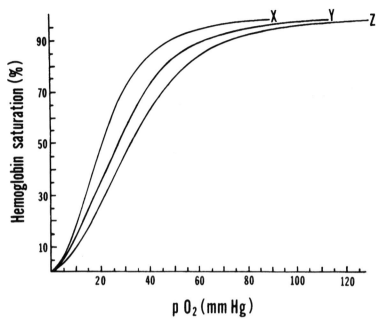

Figure 7.2. (Reproduced, with permission, from Dershwitz M, *National Boards Examination Review for Part 1,* 3rd ed. East Norwalk, Ct: Appleton & Lange; 1987.)

    C. poor protein absorption
    D. metabolic alkalosis
    E. all are correct

1132. In Figure 7.2, a shift from curve Y to curve Z would occur if peripheral tissues developed
    A. a decrease in carbon dioxide
    B. an increase in 2,3-diphosphoglycerate
    C. an increase in myoglobin content
    D. a lower temperature
    E. B and D are correct

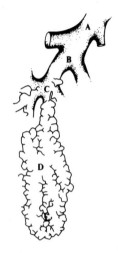

Figure 7.3. (Reproduced, with permission, from Dershwitz M, *National Boards Examination Review for Part 1*, 3rd ed. East Norwalk, Ct: Appleton & Lange; 1987.)

1133. In Figure 7.3, the greatest change in volume during expiration and inspiration would occur at site(s)
  A. A, B, and C
  B. A and B
  C. B and D
  D. C and E
  E. D only

1134. Extremely low arterial oxygen tension (hypoxic hypoxia) may be the result of
  A. hypoventilation
  B. decreased Po_2 in inspired air
  C. low ventilation/perfusion ratio
  D. aveolar–capillary diffusion block
  E. all are correct

1135. In congestive heart failure with complete cardiac decompensation, the patient usually has a
  A. decreased activity of the renin–angiotensin system
  B. heart that can still develop greater force

C. capillary hydrostatic pressure that is greatly elevated
D. decreased retention of Na⁻ and water
E. reduction of extracellular fluid

1136. The following factors alter ventricular function extrinsically EX-
CEPT
   A. CO_2 content of the myocardial blood
   B. oxygen content of myocardial blood
   C. autonomic nervous system
   D. Frank–Starling mechanism
   E. catecholamine content of the myocardial blood

1137. The pulmonary valve opens at a pressure of about
   A. 10 mm Hg
   B. 30 mm Hg
   C. 60 mm Hg
   D. 80 mm Hg
   E. 120 mm Hg

1138. Upon rising to the standing position after remaining recumbent
for many minutes the following are true EXCEPT
   A. venous tone reflexly increases, moving blood toward the
      heart
   B. central blood volume immediately falls as blood drains into
      lower extremities under the influence of gravity
   C. decreased peripheral resistance and bradycardia result
   D. stroke volume, and consequently cardiac output transiently
      decline due to reduced venous return to the heart
   E. arm blood flow transiently decreases as peripheral resis-
      tance reflexly increases

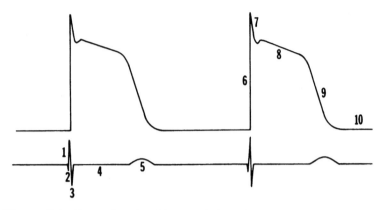

Figure 7.4. (Reproduced, with permission, from Dershwitz M, *National Boards Examination Review for Part 1,* 3rd ed. East Norwalk, Ct: Appleton & Lange; 1987.)

DIRECTIONS (Questions 1139 through 1193): Each group of questions below consists of lettered headings followed by a list of numbered words or statements. For each numbered word or statement, select the ONE lettered heading that is most closely associated with it. Each lettered heading may be selected once, more than once, or not at all.

Questions 1139 through 1143: Refer to Figure 7.4 showing recordings of the intracellular action potentials (top trace) and simultaneous surface electrocardiographic tracings (bottom trace) from ventricular contractile tissue.

    A. T wave
    B. S wave
    C. ST segment
    D. Q wave
    E. R wave
    F. P wave

1139. Deflection #1

1140. Deflection #2

1141. Deflection #3

1142. Deflection #4

1143. Deflection #5

Questions 1144 through 1150

    A. contraction without shortening
    B. shortening under constant tension
    C. synaptic innervation of a number of cells by one fiber
    D. overlapping synaptic innervation of one cell by a number of fibers
    E. spontaneous intermittent discharge of motor units of the nervous system
    F. active contraction of a muscle when pull is exerted upon the tendon
    G. follows stimulation of the contralateral cutaneous nerve

1144. Principle of divergence

1145. Principle of convergence

1146. Stretch reflex

1147. Crossed-extensor reflex

1148. Isometric contraction

1149. Isotonic contraction

1150. Fasciculation

Questions 1151 through 1154

    A. tonic neck reflex
    B. tonic labyrinthine reflex
    C. myotatic reflex
    D. crossed-extensor reflex
    E. optical righting reflex

1151. Accompanies withdrawal reaction

1152. Forelegs extended as neck is dorsiflexed

1153. Right foreleg extends as head turns to the right

1154. Passive extension initiates contraction

Questions 1155 through 1161

    A. apneustic center
    B. pneumotaxic center
    C. medullary respiratory center
    D. apneustic and pneumotaxic centers
    E. chemoreceptor control

1155. Required for rhythmic breathing

1156. Role seems to be similar to that of vagal afferents

1157. Present in the pons

1158. Center for inspiratory drive

1159. Center for expiratory drive

1160. Stimulated by elevated plasma P_{CO_2}

1161. Ablation results in slow, deep breathing

Questions 1162 through 1165

    A. I^{131} albumin
    B. D_2O (heavy water)
    C. thiocyanate
    D. thiocyanate and antipyrine
    E. Fe^{59} tagged erythocytes
    F. Cr^{51} tagged erythrocytes

1162. Total body water

1163. Intracellular fluid volume

1164. Extracellular fluid volume

1165. Plasma volume

Questions 1166 through 1170

    A. myenteric reflex (law of the gut)
    B. gastrocolic reflex
    C. mass movement (peristaltic push)
    D. segmentation
    E. antral systole

1166. Dilation of the intestinal lumen causes contraction above and relaxation below that point

1167. Local contraction and relaxation of the small intestine and colon

1168. Single, vigorous, peristaltic contraction and relaxation of the intestine

1169. Combines mixing and emptying of the stomach

1170. Ingestion of food causes an increase in motility of the large intestine

Questions 1171 through 1175

    A. chemoreceptor affecting blood pressure or respiration
    B. mechanoreceptor affecting blood pressure or respiration
    C. both
    D. neither

1171. Carotid body

1172. Large veins

1173. Lungs

1174. Aortic body

1175. Carotid sinus

Questions 1176 through 1180: Choose from below the area of renal tubule for the major site of

    A. distal tubule
    B. proximal, distal, and collecting duct
    C. Bowman's capsule
    D. ascending limb of Henle loop
    E. collecting duct

1176. Glucose reabsorption

1177. H^+ secretion

1178. K^+ secretion

1179. ADH activity

1180. Tubular filtration

Questions 1181 through 1183: Of the optical defects listed below

    A. astigmatism
    B. myopia
    C. hyperopia

1181. Image falls behind the retina

1182. Image is focused in front of the retina

1183. Images fall at different focal distances as if there were more than one cylindrical lens

Questions 1184 through 1193: Figure 7.5 is a schematic representation of a normal renal tubule. From the figure, indicate the site(s) with which each is most closely associated. Each letter may be used once, more than once, or not at all.

1184. Water permeability

1185. Urea concentration

1186. K⁺ reabsorption

1187. K⁺ secretion

1188. Dilution of solutes

1189. Amino acid reabsorption

1190. Na⁺ reabsorption

1191. Activity of ADH

1192. Concentration of solutes

1193. Active Cl⁻ transport

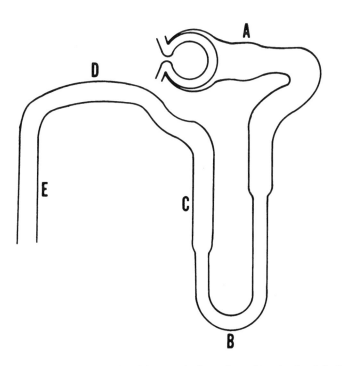

Figure 7.5. (Reproduced, with permission, from Dershwitz M, *National Boards Examination Review for Part 1,* 3rd ed. East Norwalk, Ct: Appleton & Lange; 1987.)

DIRECTIONS (Questions 1194 through 1200): This set of matching questions consists of a list of lettered options followed by several numbered items. For each item, select the one best lettered option that is most closely associated with it. Each lettered heading may be selected once, more than once, or not at all.

A. aorta
B. capillary
C. carotid sinus
D. left atrium
E. left coronary artery
F. left ventricle
G. pre-capillary sphincter
H. pulmonary artery
I. pulmonary vein
J. right atrium
K. right ventricle
L. systemic arterioles
M. systemic artery
N. vein
O. venule

1194. Site where flow occurs mainly during ventricular diastole

1195. Site in the circulation showing the greatest vascular resistance

1196. Artery containing "venous" blood

1197. Class of vessels acting as on–off switch controlling blood flow to vessels whose primary role is exchange

1198. Makes the greatest contribution to the Windkessel effect

1199. Site of primary baroreceptors

1200. Site of heart's primary pacemaker

Physiology

Answers and Comments

1019. (A) The area of the pressure-volume diagram is a very close approximation of cardiac work. (**Ref. 1,** pp. 411–412)

1020. (C) The tension developed by a muscle is always due to the sliding of actin and myosin filaments regardless of whether or not the muscle fiber shortens grossly. (**Ref. 1,** pp. 281–284)

1021. (D) Venoconstriction leads to a redistribution of blood and increased cardiac output during exercise. (**Ref. 1,** p. 485)

1022. (B) Coronary vasodilation is the normal response to cardiac sympathetic stimulation. This response is largely due to local metabolic effects arising from increased oxygen use and a variety of vasodilatory products released. (**Ref. 1,** pp. 514–515)

1023. (A) Total counts albumin injected = plasma volume (mL) counts/mL albumin at equilibrium. (**Ref. 3,** pp. 275–276)

1024. (A) Reducing the pressure presented to the carotid baroreceptors results in an increase in peripheral resistance, returning blood pressure toward normal. (**Ref. 1,** pp. 486–489)

1025. (A) At a P_{O_2} of 70 mm Hg, hemoglobin is approximately 80% saturated with regard to oxygen binding. **(Ref. 1,** pp. 590–593)

1026. (D) After exercise man continues to use oxygen at greater than rest levels. The difference between post-exercise and resting levels of oxygen uptake is known as oxygen debt. **(Ref. 3,** p. 943)

1027. (B) During maximum expiratory effort the pressure exerted on the smaller passages of the lung are sufficient to cause lung collapse. **(Ref. 1,** pp. 570–573)

1028. (B) Aortic flow velocity reaches a maximum during the early rapid phase of ventricular ejection and then decreases. **(Ref. 1,** p. 408)

1029. (A) The capsular structure of the pacinian corpuscle rapidly adapts to the deformation of the tissue because fluid within the capsule redistributes itself so that the pressure becomes essentially equal, reducing the receptor potential. **(Ref. 1,** pp. 122–123)

1030. (C) In a single nerve fiber, a suprathreshold stimulus will always give rise to the same stereotyped response if the resting condition of the fiber is unchanged. **(Ref. 1,** p. 39)

1031. (C) Only living excitable cells respond to a threshold stimulus by a rapid reversible voltage change. This voltage transient is caused by a rapid change in membrane permeabilities to some ionic species (usually Na^+). **(Ref. 1,** pp. 36–40)

1032. (B) The Na^+-K^+ pump exchanges from one extracellular K^+ for one intracellular Na^+ to three Na^+ for two K^+ ions. The actual ratio achieved depends on the relative concentrations of sodium and potassium inside and outside the cell. This pump requires energy, usually in the form of high-energy phosphates and is temperature sensitive as are all chemical reactions. **(Ref. 1,** pp. 19–20)

1033. (A) The major portion of body heat is lost through radiation and water evaporation. (**Ref. 3,** pp. 797–800)

1034. (D) An increase in extracellular fluid osmolality (excess Na^+ and its associated anions) stimulates the osmoreceptors within the supraoptic nuclei of the hypothalamus. Impulses from the nuclei traverse through the pituitary stalk into the posterior pituitary gland, promoting the release of ADH. In addition, the extracellular fluid osmolality increase in physiological situations is the result of extracellular fluid volume being less than normal. The reduction of stretch, which follows, within the kidneys' great veins and the atria thereby reduces nerve signals into the brain to cause an increase in ADH secretion. (**Ref. 3,** pp. 827–829)

1035. (A) Stretch depolarizes smooth muscle and may initiate activity by this mechanism. (**Ref. 1,** pp. 313–314)

1036. (D) The distribution of body hair requires the presence of androgens for the development of the genetic characteristics in both sexes. (**Ref. 3,** pp. 892–893)

1037. (B) Clearance is the quantity of plasma that completely loses its entire content of the substance in question each minute. It is a measure of the effectiveness of the kidney to remove substances from the extracellular fluid. In units of mU/min the clearance of inulin is 125, creatine 140, PAH 585, and urea 70, while potassium is 12. Since inulin clearance is equal to GFR, any clearance value above 125 mL/min is indicative of secretion, while values below 125 indicate reabsorption. (**Ref. 3,** p. 306)

1038. (C) The loss of water in the form of urine represents 60% of the daily water loss. (**Ref. 3,** p. 275)

1039. (E) In most living cells, the Na^+-K^+ is required to maintain the ionic gradients. (**Ref. 3,** pp. 54–55)

1040. (D) The so-called vomiting center is found in the dorsal part of the lateral reticular formation of the medulla oblongata. (**Ref. 3,** pp. 740–741)

1041. (C) The cones are receptors primarily associated with color vision. (**Ref. 1,** pp. 150–152)

1042. (B) The blood content of the capillaries is small, in the range of 300 mL. (**Ref. 1,** p. 363)

1043. (A) The term hematocrit is used to express the percentage of the blood volume, that is, cells. (**Ref. 1,** p. 329)

1044. (B) The first heart sound occurs at the onset of contraction of the ventricles. This is the so-called period of isovolumetric contraction since the volume of blood in the ventricles is not altered during this time period. (**Ref. 1,** pp. 409–410)

1045. (D) Lying down lowers the height of the fluid column that must be supported and tends to decrease venous pressure in the lower part of the body. This facilitates venous return. (**Ref. 1,** pp. 505–507)

1046. (E) The aortic valves open after ventricular pressure exceeds aortic pressure. This is well after the onset of ventricular contraction. (**Ref. 1,** p. 408)

1047. (A) The A wave is caused by atrial contraction. Ordinarily the right atrial pressure rises 4 to 6 mm of Hg during atrial contraction while the left atrial pressure rises about 7 to 8 mm of Hg. (**Ref. 3,** p. 102)

1048. (B) There is increased venous return during exercise due to increased work by skeletal muscle. However, this increased venous return does not appear to increase stroke volume and the cardiac output increase is entirely due to the faster heart rate. In the trained athlete the reverse is true. (**Ref. 1,** p. 534)

1049. (A) The P wave is the electrical recording from the body surface of atrial depolarization and precedes atrial contraction. (**Ref. 1,** p. 408)

1050. (C) The P wave of the normal electrocardiogram is caused by the depolarization of the auricle. (**Ref. 1,** p. 388)

1051. (B) Resistance is the impediment to blood flow in a vessel. Slight changes in the diameter of a vessel cause tremendous changes in its ability to conduct blood. (**Ref. 1,** pp. 443–446)

1052. (C) There is approximately 16 g of hemoglobin per 100 mL of normal blood. (**Ref. 3,** p. 356)

1053. (A) The cardiac output increases approximately in proportion to the surface area of the body. The cardiac output per square meter of body surface area is called the cardiac index. (**Ref. 3,** pp. 221–222)

1054. (B) Located bilaterally in the reticular substance of the lower third of the pons and upper two-thirds of the medulla is an area called the vasomotor center. It is tonically active and maintains vasomotor tone. (**Ref. 3,** pp. 201–202)

1055. (B) Purkinje fibers are larger than the normal ventricular muscle fibers, and they transmit impulses at a velocity of 1.5 to 4.0 m/sec, a velocity about 6 times that in the usual cardiac muscle and 300 times that in the junctional fibers. (**Ref. 3,** pp. 113–114)

1056. (B) The arterial pulse usually disappears in the arterioles. The term venous pulse is used to describe the pressure changes in the large veins near the heart that are due to changes occurring in the heart and adjacent large arteries. (**Ref. 3,** pp. 162–163)

1057. (D) Even after as much as 20 to 25% of the total blood volume has been lost, the circulatory system often functions almost normally because of the variable reservoir system of the veins. (**Ref. 1,** p. 363)

1058. (B) The interval between the P wave and the QRS complex represents the time necessary for conduction of the electrical impulse from the atrium to the ventricle. (**Ref. 1,** pp. 390–391)

1059. (B) The sympathetic discharge responsible for the control of blood pressure during alterations in posture is dependent on the aortic arch and carotid sinus baroreceptors. (**Ref. 1,** pp. 486–488)

1060. (A) Homeometric autoregulation associated with an increase in mean aortic pressure can result in an increase in stroke work. (**Ref. 1**, pp. 431–433)

1061. (A) Bernoulli's principle states that side wall pressure will decrease with increasing velocity. (**Ref. 1**, pp. 438–440)

1062. (B) Increased CO_2 tension causes a decrease in oxygen binding to hemoglobin. (**Ref. 1**, pp. 591–593)

1063. (A) An increase in P_{CO_2} from a normal level of 40 to 73 mm Hg causes a 10-fold increase in alveolar ventilation. An increase in P_{CO_2} stimulates alveolar ventilation not only directly but also indirectly through its effect on hydrogen ion concentration. (**Ref. 3**, pp. 430–431)

1064. (C) Approximately 60% of the CO_2 in venous blood is in the form of bicarbonate. (**Ref. 3**, pp. 440–441)

1065. (E) All of the influences with the exception of a high pH contribute in increased respiration from exercise. In addition to these influences, the higher centers in the central nervous system must have an influence because respiration increases before there is any detectable change in blood chemistry. (**Ref. 3**, pp. 450–452)

1066. (A) Destruction of the pneumotaxic center in the pons often leads to apneustic respiration because the apneustic center is no longer receiving input from the pneumotaxic center. (**Ref. 3**, pp. 452–453)

1067. (B) Vagal input to the respiratory centers is primarily excitatory. As a result, the rate of respiration will decrease following vagal section. The importance of this reflex has been questioned in adults due to data from recent experiments. (**Ref. 3**, pp. 444–445)

1068. (B) The amount of oxygen removed from the blood multiplied by the total blood flow will give the total oxygen consumption. (**Ref. 1**, p. 548)

1069. (A) An active transport system must use some energy for sequestering and transporting particles when these particles reach the cell membrane. (**Ref. 1,** pp. 14–15)

1070. (A) Urea clearance ratios are always less than one and they increase as urine output goes up. These data indicate that urea is transported by diffusion and that water reabsorption concentrates urea in the tubules producing a concentration gradient which encourages the slow movement of urea out of the tubules. (**Ref. 3,** p. 306)

1071. (A) Approximately 80% of the glucose in filtered plasma is reabsorbed in the proximal tubule. (**Ref. 3,** pp. 303–304)

1072. (B) The main driving force for glomerular filtration is the capillary pressure. (**Ref. 3,** pp. 292–294)

1073. (B) Potassium is unusual in that it is both secreted and reabsorbed by the kidney tubules. (**Ref. 3,** pp. 302–305)

1074. (D) Because of the osmotic gradient from top to bottom of the kidney, usine as it enters the collecting tubule can only be hypo- or isotonic but not hypertonic. (**Ref. 3,** pp. 309–310)

1075. (A) Approximately two-thirds of the glomerular filtrate is reabsorbed in the proximal convoluted tubule. (**Ref. 3,** p. 310)

1076. (C) Inulin is neither reabsorbed nor secreted by kidney tubules. (**Ref. 3,** pp. 304–307)

1077. (C) The countercurrent mechanism responsible for the secretion of hyperosmotic urine requires the penetration of the loop of Henle into the renal medulla for the development of a medullary osmotic gradient. (**Ref. 3,** p. 310)

1078. (D) When plasma osmolality and plasma sodium are low, there should be an excretion of water. If, however, the urine osmolality remains high in spite of the low plasma values, inappropriate ADH secretion should be considered. (**Ref. 3,** pp. 314–316)

1079. (B) The infusion of hypertonic saline will result in an expansion of the extracellular volume. The selective permeability and active transport systems will tend to exclude the sodium chloride from the intracellular compartment. The net result will be an expansion of the ECF and a contraction of the ECF due to water loss from osmotic movement across the cell membranes. (**Ref. 3,** pp. 279–280)

1080. (B) During compensated metabolic alkalosis there is a gain of CO_2 in order to return the pH toward normal. The result is increased HCO_3^- and P_{CO_2} and a near-normal pH. (**Ref. 3,** pp. 341–342)

1081. (D) The juxtaglomerular apparatus is important in body sodium and osmolality homeostasis and aldosterone secretion-associated nephrons have a long loop of Henle. (**Ref. 3,** pp. 293–294)

1082. (C) Since inulin is neither secreted nor reabsorbed by the tubules of the kidney, any compound with a clearance greater than inulin probably is secreted into the tubular lumen of the nephron. (**Ref. 3,** p. 300)

1083. (D) In the absence of ADH, urine outputs can reach 10 to 15% of the daily GFR. (**Ref. 3,** p. 865)

1084. (D) Luteotrophic hormone, progesterone, follicle-stimulating hormone, and luteinizing hormone are necessary for the appropriate secretion of estrogen by the ovary and placenta. (**Ref. 3,** pp. 905–910)

1085. (B) Antidiuretic hormone (ADH) is secreted by the posterior pituitary. (**Ref. 1,** p. 897)

1086. (A) Coincident with the development of the trophoblast cells from early fertilized ovum, the hormone chorionic gonadotropin is secreted by the syncytial trophoblastic cells into the fluids of the mother. The rate of secretion rises rapidly to reach a maximum approximately 7 weeks after ovulation and decreases to a relatively low value by 16 weeks after ovulation. (**Ref. 1,** pp. 1015–1018)

1087. (A) ACTH is most effective in stimulating hydrocortisone secretion. ACTH is necessary for aldosterone secretion but increased ACTH will not increase aldosterone secretion. (**Ref. 3,** p. 846)

1088. (B) Thyroxin will sensitize the heart to epinephrine after some delay. The development of this sensitization depends on the up regulation of beta receptors on the myocardium. The result is an increase in heart rate and contractility. (**Ref. 3,** p. 835)

1089. (B) Intrinsic factor for the absorption of vitamin B is secreted by the oxyntic cells of the stomach. (**Ref. 3,** p. 714)

1090. (A) Glucose and fructose are the results of sucrose hydrolysis and are very prominent in intestinal chyme. (**Ref. 3,** p. 718)

1091. (E) Pinoytosis is associated with specific cell surface receptors in the coated pits on most cells. It is an energy-requiring process that may be associated with the use of ATP. (**Ref. 3,** pp. 16–17)

1092. (C) Erythropoietin causes an increase in the formation of red cells in response to low oxygen environments. (**Ref. 3,** pp. 358–359)

1093. (E) Phospholipids released when platelets rupture are a potent stimulator of clot formation. (**Ref. 3,** pp. 394–395)

1094. (A) Troponin is a three subunit protein that controls the access of myosin crossbridges to actin filaments during muscle contraction. (**Ref. 1,** pp. 283–284)

1095. (D) The act of swallowing is a complex combination of voluntary and automatic muscle contractions involving both skeletal and smooth muscle. (**Ref. 3,** pp. 698–700)

1096. (D) Growth hormone promotes protein and glucose sparing, and growth of cartilage through a somatomedin intermediate. (**Ref. 3,** pp. 822–825)

1097. (D) The essential step in presynaptic inhibition is presynaptic depolarization resulting in less transmitter release from the presynaptic ending. The decreased transmitter release gives rise to a smaller excitatory postsynaptic potential and hence inhibition. (**Ref. 3,** p. 489)

1098. (B) The first signal for altered respiration necessary to handle an altered exercise load comes from the central nervous system. (**Ref. 3,** pp. 450–452)

1099. (B) The isohydric principle states that the status of all the buffers in a continuous compartment can be evaluated by measuring the pH and the amount of the constituents of a single buffer system. (**Ref. 3,** p. 334)

1100. (C) The primary force preventing the negative intrapleural pressure from causing the accumulation of fluid in the intrapleural space is the difference between the low pulmonary capillary pressure and the colloid osmotic pressure of plasma. (**Ref. 3,** pp. 418–420)

1101. (E) The development of edema will depend on the capillary hydrostatic pressure exceeding the ability of negative interstitial pressure, lymphatic flow, and lymphatic washout of proteins to maintain normal tissue fluid balance. (**Ref. 3,** pp. 281–283)

1102. (E) Poor cardiac reserve will usually result in a drop in blood pressure during an exercise test. (**Ref. 3,** p. 251)

1103. (E) The alterations associated with respiratory alkalosis are determined by the loss of CO_2 from the lungs. Respiratory alkalosis is a condition in which the primary deficit is in CO_2. Hyperventilation (due to a voluntary effort, hysteria, anoxic anoxia, CNS disease, or to some pharmacologic effect) increases CO_2 elimination leading to a low alveolar and arterial P_{CO_2} and decrease in carbonic acid of the body fluids. Hence, body fluid pH rises and the condition of respiratory alkalosis exists. The kidneys play the major role in compensation by conservation of H^+, reduction of ammonium ion and titratable acid excretion, and by diminishing reabsorption of HCO_3^- from the glomerular filtrate. Hence, urine excretion of the HCO_3^- is increased which results in an increase of the HCO_3^-/CO_2 ratio and a decrease in pH toward normal. Full compensation of this condition is reflected in a lower than normal plasma HCO_3^- level. (**Ref. 3,** pp. 341–342)

1104. (D) Cardiac muscle is similar to striated muscle in that it is cross-striated, the contractile elements are formed from myosin and actin, and the force of contraction is increased by stretching. It is unlike striated muscle in that in certain cells the plasma membranes are considerably more permeable to sodium and calcium which makes the heart muscle membrane potential discharge periodically and confers inherent rhythmicity. (**Ref. 1,** p. 281)

1105. (C) Cardiac contractility, heart rate, blood volume, and intrathoracic pressure all affect the mean filling pressure of the heart. (**Ref. 3,** pp. 221–231)

1106. (E) An increase in salt and water retention would result in increased blood volume which would lead to increased pressure throughout the vascular system. (**Ref. 3,** pp. 316–318)

1107. (E) Following hemorrhage, heart rate increases and vasoconstriction takes place, acting to maintain perfusion pressure. Hematocrit increases as red cells are released from the system, and plasma volume increases as fluid moves out of the tissues and into the vasculature. With any significant blood loss there is an initial decrease in venous return and subsequent decrease in stroke volume and cardiac output which, via the baroreceptors, result in a compensatory increase in sympathetic activity. This causes a tachycardia as well as arterial and venous constriction. Thus, specific increases in vascular resistance in the skin cause those areas to become cool and clammy, resulting in peripheral cyanosis. The initial blood loss and subsequent release of RBCs from the hemopoietic system increases the hematocrit. The vasoconstriction also causes blood shunting to areas of need. Finally, ADH secretin increases water retention while fluid shunting from the GI tract and muscle and from the interstitial spaces (aided by the reduced capillary pressure) move fluids into the vasculature. These aid plasma volume restoration. During this time the Hct will be effected by RBC release from the spleen. (**Ref. 3,** pp. 264–265)

1108. **(E)** The compliance of a lung is the volume change per unit pressure change and is calculated by dividing change in V by change in P. A lung showing a volume change of 1 L with a pressure change of 5 cm H_2O would have a compliance of 0.20. This value represents the comparative stiffness of the lung, with a stiffer lung having less compliance. This occurs with accumulation of fibrous tissue, and/or edema in the alveolar spaces. (**Ref. 1,** pp. 569–570)

1109. **(E)** A low V/P ratio means poor or no ventilation relative to blood perfusion. Hence, the mixed venous blood has a lower O_2 content than normal. So, if alveoli have perfusion without ventilation, the O_2 in the alveoli will be depleted until it is at the level of mixed venous blood. At this point the blood flowing around the alveoli will appear as if it passed through an arteriovenous shunt. (**Ref. 1,** pp. 584–587)

1110. **(A)** The association of oxygen with hemoglobin will be decreased by an increase in temperature, low Po_2, high Pco_2, and low pH. Each of these conditions exist in metabolically active tissue and cause a shift of the oxygen dissociation curve to the right. This enhances the availability of oxygen for the tissue. (**Ref. 3,** p. 438)

1111. **(D)** CO_2 is a potent stimulus for increasing respiration directly and as an agent that increases blood H^+ concentration. Most of this action occurs at the level of the medulla and a smaller portion is due to an influence on the carotid body. (**Ref. 3,** pp. 446–447)

1112. **(E)** Hemorrhage-induced decrease in blood pressure causes a decreased capillary hydrostatic pressure. As predicted by the Starling–Landis equation, this stimulates fluid (mostly water) movement into the vascular compartment. Decreased stimulation of the atrial stretch receptors increases the release of ADH, which increases the reabsorption of water by the kidney tubules. Similarly, plasma renin titer is increased, raising angiotensin concentration, which acts to amplify water conservation and also to stimulate thirst. Aldosterone is released from the adrenal cortex, which further acts to conserve water. (**Ref. 3,** pp. 314–316)

1113. (E) The pontine respiratory center contains the apneustic center, which, if stimulated, will cause apneustic breathing, and the pneumotaxic center which is largely concerned with controlling the rate of respiration. (**Ref. 3,** pp. 444–446)

1114. (E) Airway resistance would be decreased by the changes listed. Airway resistance is a function of the length and diameter of the tubes the atmosphere must pass through and of the viscosity of the gas respired. (**Ref. 1,** pp. 570–572)

1115. (D) Second-degree block can be of two types, the Mobitz I (Wenckebach) and Mobitz II. In Mobitz I, the P-R interval alternates between being of normal length and so long that conduction to the ventricles fails completely, producing the loss of ventricular contraction. In Mobitz II, the P-R intervals are normal, then all of a sudden conduction fails and a beat is dropped. Both result from impaired conduction in the AV junctional tissue. The condition usually involves normal conduction in the atria unless the sinus node is abnormal. The QRS complexes are usually normal. (**Ref. 1,** pp. 390–391)

1116. (B) Aldosterone is secreted as the result of a number of stimuli. The balance of extracellular sodium and potassium is important, as is the control of extracellular volume. In addition, stress and high plasma angiotensin concentration stimulates aldosterone secretion. (**Ref. 1,** pp. 968–970)

1117. (A) The first breath triggers a sharp drop in pulmonary vascular resistance due to arteriolar smooth muscle relaxation, increasing blood flow, and decreasing pulmonary artery pressure. The resulting surge of blood to the left atrium raises left atrial pressure above right atrial pressure and causes the foramen ovale to close functionally. Within a few minutes the umbilical cord is either tied off or closes naturally. The latter process is stimulated by rising Po_2, cold, etc. Next, the ductus venosus closes and the resistance of the systemic circuit rises. With loss of the placental circulation, venous return to the heart decreases, decreasing both atrial pressures. As pulmonary vascular resistance continues to decline, pulmonary artery pressure eventually falls below aortic pressure, at which time, flow through the ductus arteriosus is reversed. This causes pulmonary blood flow and pressure to temporarily increase. Within hours to days after birth the ductus arteriosus closes due to rising arterial O_2 saturation. (**Ref. 2,** pp. 569–570)

1118. (**E**) Aldosterone is necessary for the proper control of Na^+, K^+, and fluid volumes in the body. Hence, a deficiency or a lack of this hormone results in Na^+ loss (no reabsorption), K^+ retention, and massive loss of fluid. (**Ref. 3,** pp. 852–853)

1119. (**C**) Normal ovulation is triggered by a peak in luteinizing hormone secretion which is probably limited by increasing secretions of estrogens. (**Ref. 3,** pp. 902–903)

1120. (**E**) Both testosterone (mediated by LH) and FSH are required for the normal development and maturation of sperm. FSH is required for the establishment of the germinal epithelium while testosterone is necessary for sperm production. (**Ref. 3,** pp. 887–888)

1121. (**E**) Overall the release of parathyroid hormone from the chief cell will result in increased circulating levels of Ca^{++} and decreased plasma phosphate concentration through several mechanisms. One important mechanism is an increased absorption of Ca^{++} from bone, the kidney, and the gut due to activation of vitamin D. The decrease in plasma PO_4^- is a result of its decreased renal tubular reabsorption. (**Ref. 3,** pp. 874–877)

1122. (**A**) During starvation, or at the onset of a calorie-deficient diet, fat is utilized immediately to make up the missing calories. In addition to this fat utilization, there is a loss of body fluid. (**Ref. 3,** p. 782)

1123. (**C**) The gallbladder is the primary storage site of bile, is located in the liver, and can be stimulated to contract by cholecystokinin and vagal activity. Sympathetic activity may, however, be antagonistic. (**Ref. 3,** pp. 721–722)

1124. (**A**) Pancreozymin, also known as cholecystokinin, primarily stimulates the secretion of low volumes of solution containing most of the enzymatic output of the exocrine pancreas. (**Ref. 3,** pp. 702–703)

1125. (E) The motility of the small intestine is characterized by short waves of peristalsis interspersed with mixing waves. In addition, the downward movement of material is facilitated by the fact that a bolus of chyme will stimulate the intestine to contract above the bolus and relax the bolus. (**Ref. 3,** pp. 703–705)

1126. (C) The swallowing response is a stereotyped, largely reflex phenomenon which is mediated through bilateral midbrain centers. (**Ref. 3,** pp. 698–700)

1127. (D) When swallowing occurs, the shift from the more common movement of air in and out of the lungs to the movement of solids or liquids into the stomach requires inhibition of respiration, closure of the glottis, and relaxation of the upper esophageal sphincter. (**Ref. 3,** p. 699)

1128. (D) The only digestive enzyme secreted by the salivary glands is salivary amylase. It is a protein that breaks down starches within the mouth which continues in the stomach for some period of time until the amylase is inactivated by the stomach pH. (**Ref. 3,** pp. 711–712)

1129. (E) Water is absorbed from the lumen of the gut both transcellularly and across the "tight junction" between cells, and may be altered by hormones and prostaglandins either directly or by affecting Na^+ and Cl^- absorption. (**Ref. 3,** p. 731)

1130. (B) The hormone secretin is secreted by the small intestine. It causes increases in fluid and bicarbonate secretion by the pancreas. (**Ref. 3,** p. 719)

1131. (A) The secretion of intrinsic factor by the oxyntic cells is the only essential activity of the stomach. Its absence leads to a fatal anemia due to arrested maturation of RBCs. (**Ref. 3,** p. 737)

1132. (B) Higher temperature, increased concentrations of 2,3-diphosphoglycerate, and P_{CO_2} all shift hemoglobin oxygen saturation curves to the right. (**Ref. 3,** p. 438)

1133. (E) Most of the volume change in the lung occurs in the respiratory bronchioles. They represent the functional unit of the lung for gas exchange. (**Ref. 3,** p. 406)

1134. (E) Hypoxic hypoxia is a problem in normal individuals at high altitudes and may be a complication of pneumonia, asthma, emphysema, and alveolar fibrosis as well as A-V shunting. It occurs when there is any interference with breathing that results in hypoventilation. (**Ref. 3,** pp. 464–466)

1135. (C) Heart failure is a situation in which a number of physiologic mechanisms could be awry. Though the pathophysiology is very complex, one can summarize the situation by considering it a failure of the heart to act as an effective pump. The factors leading to it are numerous including electrical alterations, atherosclerosis of the coronary arteries, valvular deformation, etc. All of these problems can result in a cardiac overload leading to hypertrophy and decompensation. A frequent observation in such patients includes increased renin–angiotensin activation with increased ADH and aldosterone secretion. The overall constant feature in every decompensated individual is an extremely high arteriolar hydrostatic pressure (extremely high resistance) and considerable fluid retention resulting in edema. (**Ref. 3,** pp. 245–246)

1136. (D) Extrinsic control of ventricular function includes the neural and hormonal stimuli to the heart through efferents of the autonomic nervous system, as well as the chemical content of the blood which supplies the heart muscle. The constant sympathetic and parasympathetic impulses ensure that the muscular force of each contraction may be increased or decreased by altering the frequency of impulses in either system. In addition, the level of oxygen, carbon dioxide, and catecholamines in the blood are a second group of controls that are extrinsic in nature. Thus, myocardial hypoxia and/or hypercapnea depress contractility, while contractile force is increased by epinephrine and/or norepinephrine. These controls, along with the intrinsic mechanisms, affect the overall ventricular performance by affecting preload, afterload, and the state of cardiac inotropy. The Frank–Starling mechanism is intrinsic to heart muscle. (**Ref. 1,** pp. 431–434)

1137. **(A)** The pulmonic valve opens at approximately 10 mm Hg, a relatively slight afterload. This is a function of the very low vascular resistance of the pulmonary circuit as compared to that of the systemic circulation. (**Ref. 1,** p. 408)

1138. **(C)** When standing up from a supine position, central blood volume (pool) decreases as the blood (400 mL) flows into the capacitance vessels of the abdomen and legs. This decreases heart preload and results in decreases in central venous pressure, stroke volume, and arterial blood pressure. If the latter change is large enough (orthostatic hypotension), it can produce a "graying out," or a complete "black-out" with syncope. Normally the carotid sinus baroreflex acts within less than 1/2 to 1 second to return blood pressure to, or nearly to, normal, by increasing heart rate, abdominal and limb vascular resistance, and total peripheral resistance. (**Ref. 1,** pp. 506–507)

1139. **(E)**, 1140. **(D)**, 1141. **(B)**, 1142. **(C)**, 1143. **(A)** Transmembrane action potentials of the heart are descriptively labeled as phase 0 for the initial rapid depolarization (spike) including the overshoot. Phase 1 represents the initial rapid repolarization with phase 2 as the slow repolarization phase (plateau). The final repolarization curve is referred to as phase 3, which returns the membrane potential to the resting level (phase 4). Simultaneous recording of the ECG and muscle action potentials indicates that the QRS appears at the beginning of depolarization (phase 0) and the T wave appears during ventricular repolarization (phase 3). During the depolarized state (phase 2) the ECG shows no potential change and represents the ST segment. The QRS complex contains two negative components, the Q and S waves, which represent the initial and final depolarization wave of the septum nearer to the apex of the septum and/or the depolarization of the left side of the septum. (**Ref. 1,** pp. 369, 379)

1144. **(C)** One of the most important principles of organization of the central nervous system is that of divergence. Especially in sensory systems the innervation of many cells by branches from a single fiber distribute one input to a number of different structures. There are two types of divergence in the CNS. One is the "Amplifying" type and the other is divergence into "Multiple

Tracts" type. The former involves an input signal that will spread to a greater number of neurons as the signal moves through successive pools of a nervous pathway. This type is seen in the corticospinal pathway in control of skeletal muscle. In the second type of divergence, the signal is sent in two separate directions from the pool to different paths of the nervous system where it is needed; ie, impulses coursing through the dorsal column of the spinal cord go in two directions as they enter the lower part of the brain: (1)into the cerebellum and (2) into the lower thalamus and cerebral cortex. (**Ref. 3,** p. 502)

1145. **(D)** In the motor portions of the central nervous system, the overlapping synaptic innervation of one cell by a number of fibers, or convergence, is a frequent occurrence for permitting summation, correlation, and sorting of information. Very frequently, it is necessary for signals from multiple incoming nerves to activate the same neuron. This is done by two types of convergence: (1) convergence from a single source and (2) convergence from several different sources. In the former type many terminals from the input side (one incoming fiber tract) end on the same neuron where the action potential summate to bring it up to the threshold potential for discharge. The second type involves input from a number of interneurons that terminate on one neuron to allow summation of information from different sources. (**Ref. 3,** p. 502)

1146. **(F)** The stretch of myotatic reflex consists of an active shortening twitch exerted by a muscle when it is stretched rapidly. The stretch excites the spindles to result in a reflex contraction of the muscle. All skeletal muscles exhibit this reflex and permit recovery of any desired posture or movement from any displacement in any direction. (**Ref. 3,** p. 593)

1147. **(G)** The cross-extensor reflex consists of the stimulation of extensor muscles in the contralateral limb when noxious stimuli are presented to the skin of the bottom of a limb. Hence, flexing of one limb results in an extension of the opposite limb and permits the support of weight of the body when flexion is withdrawing the limb from making its weight-bearing contribution. (**Ref. 3,** pp. 597–598)

1148. (A) Isometric contraction of a muscle occurs when the muscle contracts and does not shorten. The muscle fibers are contracting synchronously and since no movement occurs, no work is being performed. Isometric function is to prevent motion from occurring and thus maintain the position in space. (**Ref. 1,** p. 288)

1149. (B) Isotonic contraction of a muscle is contraction with shortening of that muscle under a constant load. The degree of shortening is directly related to the load upon which it exerts force. Since movement occurs in lifting a load work is performed and its function is one of acceleration. (**Ref. 1,** p. 288)

1150. (E) Fasciculation is the spontaneous contraction of a muscle group integrated by one axon into one motor unit. This finding is indicative of lower motor neuron disease (as in poliomyelitis or axon severance). As the axon atrophies, spontaneous impulses are initiated and the whole motor unit responds in a ripple-like fashion. (**Ref. 1,** p. 306)

1151. (D) The crossed-extensor reflex appears on the contralateral side of the body whenever a withdrawal reaction of sufficient magnitude is elicited. The withdrawal reflexes involve a flexion whenever a cutaneous sensory stimulus on a limb occurs to permit withdrawal. See key to answer 1147. (**Ref. 3,** pp. 597–598)

1152. (A) In the decerebrate preparation, the input from tonic neck receptors has a major effect on tone in the forelimbs. In an organism whose vestibular apparatus has been destroyed, the bending of the neck results in an immediate muscular reflex of a limb or limbs. Thus, bending the head forward causes both forelimbs to relax. This does not occur if the vestibular apparatus is intact and works opposite to the neck reflexes. (**Ref. 3,** pp. 590, 599, 610)

1153. (A) The tonic labyrinthine receptors affect tone in the neck which in turn affects muscle tone in the forelimbs. The labyrinth reflex opposes the neck reflex. Thus, the neck reflex will relax the forelimb when the neck is flexed downward but normally this will be opposed by the labyrinth reflexes which will extend the forelimb when the neck is flexed downward. This occurs because total body equilibrium is necessary and not just of the head alone. Hence, the neck reflex and vestibular reflex must function in an opposite manner. Otherwise the whole body would fall out of balance whenever the neck should bend. (**Ref. 3**, p. 610)

1154. **(C)** The myotatic reflex consists of a muscle contraction when that same muscle is stretched. See key to answer 1146. (**Ref. 3**, p. 593)

1155. **(C)** The medullary respiratory center is responsible for the alternating inspiration that is the essential activity to breathing. The "respiratory" center is composed of several dispersed groups of neurons located bilaterally in the medulla oblongata and pons and divided into 3 major nerve collections: a dorsal respiratory group located in the medulla (dorsal) that can cause inspiration; (2) a ventral respiratory group located in the medulla (ventral) and can cause either expiration or inspiration; and (3) a group called the pneumotaxic center located dorsally in the pons which helps control the rate and patterns of breathing. When the "dorsal" medullary respiratory center is activated it results in inspiration only and never expiration. Expiration at rest results from the passive elastic recoil of the distended chest and lungs and activation of the ventral inspiratory group which is essential for expiration. (**Ref. 3**, pp. 444–445)

1156. **(B)** The role of the pneumotaxic center is to control the rate of respiration and is similar in action to the vagal afferents. The pneumotaxic center switches off the inspiratory ramp signal. Normally, inspiration begins weakly and then steadily increases in a ramp fashion lasting for 2 seconds. Then, it suddenly stops for about 3 seconds. Stopping the ramp earlier will shorten the duration of respiration and this is how the pneumotaxic center controls the rate. It controls the "switch-off" point of the inspiratory ramp and hence, this center's function is to limit inspiration (and in turn control the rate of respiration). This is the exact similar mechanism of vagal activity in the Hering–Breuer inspiratory reflex. The vagi send impulses to the dorsal respiratory group of neurons to "switch off" the inspiratory ramp. The vagi respond to lung inflation via the stretch receptors and will increase the rate of respiration similar to the pneumotaxic center. (**Ref. 3**, p. 445)

1157. (D), 1158.(D), 1159.(C) Both the apneustic and pneumotaxic centers are found in the pons. The apneustic center may supply the drive for inspiration while the medullary respiratory center may be responsible for supplying the drive for expiration. The apneustic center represents an area in the lower portion of the pons whose activity can only be demonstrated when the vagus nerve has been severed and when innervation from the pneumotaxic center has also been eliminated (following midregion pons section). Then the apneustic center sends impulses to the dorsal inspiratory group and prevents the "switch-off" of the inspiratory ramp. Hence, it results in a prolonged inspiration that will overfill the lungs with occasional expiratory gasps. The function of the apneustic center may be to provide an extra stimulus to inspiration but it is normally overridden by signals from the pneumotaxic center and stretch impulses from the vagi to permit normal respiration. Also see answers 1119 through 1125. (**Ref. 3,** pp. 445–446)

1160. (B and C), 1161.(E and B) Ablation of the pneumotaxic center releases the apneustic center from its influence. This results in apneustic or slow, deep breathing. A chemical drive which activates these centers is the level of blood CO_2. Molecular CO_2 readily diffuses across the blood–brain barrier while H^+ and HCO_3^- do not. When blood P_{CO_2} rises, the CSF level will increase and form H^+, which then stimulates the chemoreceptors. So, CO_2 controls respiration by its affect on pH to induce hyperventilation. There is some evidence that the central chemoreceptor area is anatomically separate from the medullary respiratory center. (**Ref. 3,** pp. 444–446)

1162. (B) To measure total body water by a dilution technique, the indicator must be rapidly and evenly distributed through all of the body fluid compartments. Heavy water of D_2O meets these requirements extremely well. (**Ref. 3,** p. 276)

1163. (D) Antipyrine, deuterated water (D_2O) and tritiated water (HTO) are used to measure total body fluids since these distribute uniformly throughout all body fluid. Thiocyanate is used to determine the extracellular fluid. Since the intracellular fluid volume cannot be directly measured, it must be calculated as the difference between total body water and the extracellular fluid volume. About 50 to 60% of the body water is within the cells. (**Ref. 3,** p. 276)

1164. **(C)** The extracellular fluid volume is that volume which is external to the cells and within which there is diffusion equilibrium (excluding proteins). To determine this volume, the indicators utilized are many in number but generally fall into two general groups: the saccharides (as inulin and mannitol) and the radioisotopes of selected ions as Na^+, Cl^-, Br^-, SO_4^-, and thiocyanate. (**Ref. 3,** pp. 276–278)

1165. **(A)** Plasma volume is usually measured as the volume of distribution of a radioactive-tagged plasma albumin and from the dye Evans Blue (T-1824). From the measured plasma volume and a determination of the hematocrit, an estimate of the total blood volume can also be obtained. Plasma volume = (blood volume) (1-Hct). (**Ref. 3,** p. 276)

1166. **(A),** 1167.**(D)** The myenteric reflex assures movement of chyme from top to bottom of the intestine. Segmenting contractions are necessary for the mixing of chyme in the small intestine. Most of the gut mixing and propulsive movements are caused by peristalsis and local constriction of small segments of the gut wall. The propulsive movement is by peristalsis which is an inherent property of smooth muscle. The stimulus is distention which activates the gut wall about 2 to 3 cm above the distention point to cause a contractile ring to appear and initiate peristalsis. The myenteric plexuses is essential for this to appear. It also seems to be "polarized" so that movement is directed toward the anus. In front of this distention point, the gut wall relaxes some few centimeters down and aids in the food being propelled toward the anus. The complex activity of gut contractility and relaxation above and below the distention point is called the "myenteric reflex" or "peristaltic reflex" and referred to as the "Law of the Gut." The segmenting contraction of the small intestine is activated by the entry of the chyme. The resulting stretch initiates local contractions which are spaced at 1-cm interval lengths so that each set of contractions are "segmented." This activity chops the chyme and promotes mixing of food with the small intestinal secretions. (**Ref. 3,** pp. 693–694)

1168. (C) Mass movement accounts for most of the longitudinal movement in the small intestine. The segmenting movement and peristalsis are weak contractions. On occasion, there is a very powerful and rapid peristalsis initiated by irritation of the intestinal mucosa. It is referred to as "peristaltic rush" which is a "mass movement" type (also seen in the colon) forcing the food downward in a large mass into the colon to get rid of the irritating chyme and excess distention. It is inhibited by the extrinsic nervous reflexes to the brain stem and back down to the small intestine. (**Ref. 3,** pp. 703–706)

1169. (E) During antral systole about 10 percent of the antral contents are ejected into the small intestine. The remaining volume is sent forefully back into the fundus of the stomach. These two actions facilitate both gastric emptying and the mixing of chyme in the body of the stomach. (**Ref. 3,** p. 702)

1170. (B) The gastrocolic reflex is a mass colonic movement following gastric distention. Mass movements of the gut following a meal are observed and facilitated by two reflexes: (1) the gastrocolic, and (2) the duodenocolic reflexes. These are activated following the distention of the stomach and/or the duodenum and are dependent upon the extrinsic nerves (the weak reflex still observed following extrinsic nerve section is via the myenteric reflexes). (**Ref. 3,** pp. 702–703)

1171. (A) The carotid body lies in the carotid sinus and it signals changes in the blood gases and flow. This area is a major peripheral chemoreceptor site responding to low P_{O_2}, high P_{CO_2}, reduced flow, and low pH. All of these result in an increase in ventilation, with the goal being to provide an effective and necessary exchange of oxygen into the cell and removal of excess CO_2 and H^+. (**Ref. 3,** pp. 201, 448–449)

1172. (B) The large veins contain stretch receptors that affect blood pressure and respiration. There are stretch receptors which contribute to circulatory control along the pulmonary vessels, other large intrathoracic vessels, kidneys, and in all chambers of the heart. They regulate heart rate, blood pressure, and blood volume by responding to stretch and distortion. In addition they induce venoconstriction. (**Ref. 1,** pp. 420–422)

1173. (C) There are receptors in the lung that are sensitive to both mechanical and chemical stimuli. The lung stretch receptors, via the vagi, affects the frequency of breathing. Early in respiration a large volume change terminates inspiration while late in respiration only a small volume change will terminate respiration. Following vagotomy the stretch effect is abolished. These stretch receptors are responsible for the Hering–Breuer reflex. In addition, there are irritant receptors which are chemically stimulated by increases in any noxious agent (as particulate matter, histamine, bradykinin, sulfur dioxide, ammonia antigens). Such receptor activation leads to augmentation of inspiratory motor neuron activity. This results in airway constriction and rapid, shallow breathing which are attempts to limit the entry of potentially harmful substances into the lung. (**Ref. 1,** p. 604)

1174. (A) The aortic body is largely a chemoreceptor for oxygen and CO_2. It has input to centers active in the control of both respiration and blood pressure. These receptors are particularly sensitive to low Po_2 and to very high Pco_2 as well as a low pH. However, the primary stimuli for these peripheral chemoreceptors is a low Po_2. Hence, any degree of hypoxia will stimulate ventilation. Although both the aortic and the carotid bodies contain these chemoreceptors, it is the carotid body which is the dominant peripheral chemoreceptor area. (**Ref. 3,** pp. 201, 448)

1175. (D) The carotid sinus itself does not contain receptors sensitive to chemical stimuli. (**Ref. 3,** pp. 198–199)

1176. (B) Glucose is actively reabsorbed within the proximal tubule and has a Tm of about 375 mg/min. Since the GRF is about 125 m, theoretical renal threshold for glucose should be about 300 mg to Tm/GFR. The actual glucose threshold, however, is about 200 mg/100 m of arterial plasma, and this represents a glucose venous level of about 180 mg/100 mL. The difference between the actual and theoretical value is a result of renal "splay" owing to the fact that not all of the nephrons have the same Tm and filtration rate for glucose; some glucose may not be reabsorbed when the filtered amount of glucose is below its Tm. (**Ref. 3,** pp. 303–304)

1177. (B), 1178.(A)   The hydrogen ion secretion mechanism is extremely important for acid-base regulation. The ion is secreted both in the proximal and distal tubules as well as in the collecting duct. The H^+ is actively moved across the membrane and for each H^+ ion transported there is one Na^+ that enters the cell. Hence, the Na^+ that is exchanged for H^+ moves down its chemical and electrical gradients. The Na^+ moves via diffusion or by a carrier system. The net result, however, is that a H^+–Na^+ exchange yields one HCO_3 and one Na^+ that can enter the interstitial fluid to be made available as a buffer. K^+ is reabsorbed in the proximal tubule. Secretion is in the distal tubules but in the collecting ducts it is reabsorbed and exchanged for H^+, depending upon the level of Na^+ (a low Na^+ promotes H^+ and K^+ exchange). (**Ref. 3,** pp. 298–300)

1179. (C)   The major site of ADH activity is in the collecting duct (with some activity also in the distal tubule). There it promotes a configurational change in cell pore size to enhance water reabsorption. It is essential for determining the excretion of a hypertonic urine. The stimulus for osmoreceptor activity to enhance ADH secretion appears to be the extracellular Na^+ concentration. (**Ref. 3,** pp. 302–303)

1180. (C)   All substances that will pass through the tubule are filtered at Bowman's capsule, which is richly supplied by the glomeruli. The factors controlling filtration are similar to those in other capillaries (ie, the hydrostatic and osmotic pressure gradients across the capillary vessel walls). Renal filtration is thus mainly controlled by the blood pressure and any alteration in the pressure (as well as the vascular resistance or autoregulations) will affect the degree and extent of renal filtration. (**Ref. 3,** pp. 290–291)

1181. (C)   In the normal eye rays of light which are parallel and reflect from a distant object will fall on the retina. In this situation the relaxed ciliary muscle permits the image to be in sharp focus on the retina and permits the individual to "see" all distant objects clearly. If the object is at a close range, the ciliary muscle will contract to increase refraction of nonparallel light rays in such a fashion that the image of the object at this close range will again focus sharply on the retina. Such an eye, called emmetropic, provides various degrees of accommodation. However, in an eye with a relaxed ciliary muscle in which the parallel rays of light are not bent sufficiently by the lens system, the rays come to a focus after reaching the retina. This situation is referred to as hypermetropia (hyperopia) or "far-sightedness." It results from an eyeball that is either too short or a lens system that cannot refract light sufficiently. Accommodation is attempted by contraction of the ciliary muscle to increase the refractive strength of the lens in order to focus the image on the retina. If this correction is insufficient it requires the placement of a lens in front of the eye which is spherical and convex in shape. This increases the refractive power which is necessary for close vision. The problem of far-sightedness is aggravated with the aging process leading to presbyopia. In this condition the lens becomes less flexible with subsequent loss in accommodation. The decreased capacity of the lens to take a round shape causes difficulty in viewing close objects. The decline in lens flexibility is a continuing process with age and results in a greater difficulty in the ability to read. Since the far point is unchanged while the near point recedes further from the eye, the corrective maneuver is to place a convex spherical lens before the eye. With time and further aging, bifocals or lens with different refractive indices are needed for both reading and work. Presbyopia usually is observed between ages 40 to 50 years and may occur earlier in farsighted individuals. (**Ref. 3**, p. 568)

1182. (B) Myopia is present when a resting eye focuses an image in front of the retina. This condition of "near-sightedness" results from an abnormally long eyeball or by an abnormally great curvature of the cornea or lens. It is not an easy situation to correct since the normal process of accommodation exaggerates the problem. Vision of near objects is not impaired with the near point being very close to normal. However, deficits of far vision seen in myopia can be remedied by the placement of a concave spherical lens before the eye. (**Ref. 3**, p. 568)

1183. (A) The optical defect of astigmatism is mostly the result of an abnormal curvature of the cornea. In the normal eye the cornea is spherical while in astigmatism it becomes egg-shaped (ellipsoid). The defect causes the rays of light that travel in one plane to be bent differently than other rays travelling in another plane. This difference in the bending between two planes may cause one ray to focus on the retina while those in the other planes do not focus on the retina. Hence, in a vertical plane the eye veiws the image as a rectangular object while in a horizontal plane the image is viewed as a curved surface. The light rays which are not bent may be made to do so by the use of a cylindrical lens. This corrective lens must be placed in the same plane as the rays having the abnormal focal point so that its longitudinal axis then is perpendicular to the plane of the astigmatism. (**Ref. 3,** pp. 568–569)

1184. (**A**) Normally, more than 99% of the filtered water is reabsorbed as it passes through the tubules of which 65% (55 mL/min of the cleared 125 mL/min) is reabsorbed in the proximal portion passively by osmotic diffusion. As a substance is reabsorbed (passively, or actively as Na^+), the concentration within the proximal tubule decreases, causing water osmosis out of the tubules. (**Ref. 3,** pp. 289–300)

1185. (**E**) The body normally forms about 25 to 30 g of urea each day and possibly greater amounts in individuals on very high-protein diets. This urea must be excreted in the urine; otherwise uremia will develop. (Normally, the plasma concentration is 26mg/100mL, but in patients with renal insufficiency, it can go up to 200 mg/100 mL.) The rate of urea excretion is dependent upon GFR and plasma concentration. At normal GFR, about 60% of the filtered load is passed through the tubules being higher or lower with changes in GFR. The lower collecting duct has the highest urea concentration, which is passively reabsorbed into the medullary interstitium and causes high concentration. The urea is then reabsorbed into the thin loop of Henle so that it passes upward through the distal tubule and back into the collecting ducts. Hence, urea recirculates through these terminal renal portions several times before it is finally excreted. Despite the recirculation, none of it actually is reabsorbed into the blood, but eventually it is excreted into the urine in a very high concentration even though little water is excreted along with it, thereby demonstrating urea's important role in the execution of highly concentrated urine. (**Ref. 3,** pp. 324–325)

1186. (**A**) K^+ is transported through the tubules in almost identical fashion as sodium. About 65% of filtered K^+ is reabsorbed in the proximal tubules with 25% in the diluting segment of the distal tubules. By the end of the distal tubule, only 10% of filtered K^+ remains. (**Ref. 3,** pp. 300–301)

1187. **(D)** Considerable amounts of K^+ are secreted into the distal tubules. The K^+ is transported in this region of the tubules in a direction opposite to sodium (with the latter entering the cell) but not rigidly coupled with sodium. (**Ref. 3,** pp. 300–301)

1188. **(C)** The diluting segment of the renal tubule is the thick segment of the distal tubule and includes the ascending limb of the loop of Henle. As the name implies, the function of the diluting segment is to dilute the tubular fluid. The cells are specifically adapted for active transport of Na^+ and Cl^- ions from inside the tubular lumen into the peritubular fluid. This transport of negative chloride outward creates about $^+6$ mV charge inside the tubule which causes Na^+ ions to diffuse out from the lumen to peritubular fluid. This segment is also impermeable to water and more impermeable to urea. Hence, the remaining fluid is very dilute (except urea, which is high). (**Ref. 3,** pp. 303–304)

1189. **(A)** Normally, all of the amino acids (as well as proteins, glucose, acetoacetate ions, and vitamins) are completely reabsorbed by active processes in the proximal tubule. (**Ref. 3,** p. 304)

1190. **(A)** See answer 1179, 1186, and 1187. (**Ref. 3,** pp. 298–300)

1191. **(E)** ADH, secreted from the hypothalamic-posterior pituitary system, results in a decrease in urine output. The ADH causes increased water reabsorption from the collecting ducts (and to a slight extent from the late distal tubules as well). The urine that is excreted is thus highly concentrated. (**Ref. 3,** pp. 314–316)

1192. **(B)** The excretion of excess solutes and hence a concentrated urine is dependent upon first creating a hyperosmolality of the medullary interstitial fluid. Normally, body fluid osmolality is 300 mOsm/L while in the medullary tubules it approaches 1200 mOsm/L. In the thick ascending limb this active extrusion of Cl plus passive electrogenic absorption of Na^+ results in an increased medullary osmolality. These, along with K^- and Ca^{++}, are carried downward into the inner medulla by the blood in the vasa recta. Ions are also transported from the collecting duct into the medullary interstitial fluid mainly from active transport of Na^+ and electrogenic passive absorption of Cl^- along with the Na^+. In addition, when ADH concentration is high in the blood, large amounts of urea are also reabsorbed into the medullary fluid from the thin segment of the loop of Henle. The latter passive movement results from the high urea concentration in the medullary interstitium from the collecting ducts and promotes water osmosis out of the descending limb, causing high NaCl concentration to twice normal. Because of the high NaCl concentration the ions move passively out of the thin segment. All these factors cause a marked increase in the medullary interstitial fluid and are referred to as the "countercurrent" fluid flow in the loop. As can be noted, then, there may be occasions when the collecting duct has an equally high fluid concentration as the loop, but it could be lower. The loop is always hyperosmotic. (**Ref. 3,** pp. 308–311)

1193. **(C)** The thick ascending section of the loop of Henle is the diluting segment of the tubule because of its high water impermeability. The cells of this area are also specifically adapted for active transport of Cl ions from inside the tubular lumen into the peritubular fluid. (**Ref. 3,** pp. 308–311)

1194. **(E)** Due to high luminal and tissue pressure in the heart during systole, the bulk of left coronary artery flow occurs during diastole. (**Ref. 2,** p. 562)

1195. **(L)** The arterioles are the greatest single site of vascular resistance in the systemic circulation—about 40% of overall resistance. (**Ref. 2,** pp. 527–528)

1196. **(H)** The pulmonary artery contains venous blood, of the same oxygen saturation (75%) and content (12 to 14 mL/100 mL) as the vena cavae. (**Ref. 2,** p. 512)

1197. **(G)** The pre-capillary sphincters open and close immediately ahead of the capillary beds proper, functioning like on–off switches to control blood flow to one capillary or another. (**Ref. 2,** pp. 529–534)

1198. (A)   The aorta contains much elastin tissue and stores pressure energy during systolic ejection. It gives it back after the aortic valve closes, serving to maintain aortic and arterial blood pressure during ventricular diastole. (**Ref. 2,** p. 512)

1199. (C)   The carotid sinus is the site of the major baroreceptors involved in the second-to-second and minute-to-minute control of arterial blood pressure. (**Ref. 2,** p. 545)

1200. (J)   The wall of the right atrium near its attachment to the superior vena cava is the site of the sinoatrial node, the heart's primary pacemaker. (**Ref. 2,** pp. 494–496)

References

1. Berne RM & Levy MN (eds.): *Physiology,* 3rd ed. Mosby–Year Book, 1993.
2. Ganong WF: *Review of Medical Physiology,* 16th ed. Lange Med. Book, 1993.
3. Guyton AC: *Textbook of Medical Physiology,* 8th ed. WB Saunders, 1991.

Other MEPC titles of interest ...

BASIC SCIENCE

MEPC USMLE Step 1 Review
Fayemi

MEPC: Pathology, 10/e
Fayemi

MEPC: Biochemistry, 11/e
Glick

MEPC: Microbiology, 11/e
Kim

MEPC: Pharmacology, 8/e
Krzanowski

MEPC: Physiology, 9/e
Penney

MEPC: Anatomy, 10/e
Wilson

CLINICAL SCIENCE

MEPC: Medicine, 10/e
Baker

MEPC USMLE Step 2 Review
Chan

MEPC: Psychiatry, 10/e
Chan and Prosen

MEPC: Pediatrics, 9/e
Hansbarger

MEPC: Pediatrics, 8/e
LaCerva

MEPC: Essential Otolaryngology,
  Head and Neck Surgery, 6/e
Lee

MEPC: Surgery, 11/e
Metzler

MEPC: Neurology, 10/e
Slosberg

MEPC: Otolaryngology, Head &
  Neck Surgery
Willett & Lee

STEP 3

MEPC USMLE Step 3 Review
Jacobs

HEALTH RELATED

MEPC: Medical Records, 6/e
Bailey

MEPC: Optometry, 4/e
Casser-Locke

SPECIALTY BOARD REVIEWS

MEPC Specialty Board Review:
  Anesthesiology, 9/e
DeKornfeld

MEPC Specialty Board Review:
  Neurology, 4/e
Giesser

Appleton & Lange Four Stamford Plaza, P.O. Box 120041,
Stamford, Connecticut 06912-0041.